Children's Fractures

MERCER RANG

M.B., B.S., F.R.C.S.(Eng.), F.R.C.S.(C)
Orthopaedic Surgeon, The Hospital for Sick Children and
The Ontario Crippled Children's Centre, Toronto;
Lecturer in Surgery, University of Toronto

With 5 Contributors

J. B. Lippincott Company
Philadelphia · Toronto

ISBN 0-397-50338-5
Library of Congress Catalog Card Number 74-8276
Printed in the United States of America
1   3   4   2

Library of Congress Cataloging in Publication Data

Rang, Mercer.
   Children's fractures.

   Includes bibliographies.
    1. Children—Wounds and injuries.   2. Fractures.
I. Title.   ₍DNLM: 1. Fractures—In infancy and
childhood.   WE180 R196c 1974₎
RD93.5.C4R36   617'.15   74-8276
ISBN 0-397-50338-5

Du sublime au ridicule il n'y a qu'un pas.

From the sublime to the ridiculous is but a single step.

Napoleon

Preface

A parable: The child in the back of the car has a broken arm. The driver stops to ask directions, "Excuse me, can you tell me the way to the Children's Hospital, please"?

A well-meaning pedestrian steps forward to offer advice. "It's really very easy." He begins to describe the *usual* way, rattling through the roads and landmarks to be noted. Before this information has had time to sink in he begins again with another route, "This is the *best* way, I read it in last week's paper." He moves his hands like a deaf mute to indicate turns and so on, before realizing that his instructions have not been comprehended. "Well, perhaps you should take the *easiest* route. It's about 4 miles straight down this road."

Directions about fracture care are a little like this. Advice is varied, requires great attention to detail, and offers every opportunity for the wrong turn to be taken, leaving you in a situation not covered by the instructions. Wise motorists use a map or guide: this book is a Michelin guide to fractures. Information is provided about good places to stop.

Surgeons should plan their routes in advance, so that difficult areas are reconnoitred in the mind's eye before they are encountered. Parents can easily become back seat drivers. They will not like to watch you take a wrong turn and will not be happy to accept your assurances that you can get back on the road again. Soon they will offer continuous advice or seek another driver. If, however, you point out the tricky places in advance, they will not be surprised if you go slowly and will be pleased when a problem is successfully negotiated.

Here, as in most books on fractures, the emphasis is technical. The little that I have included on talking to parents may appear silly to some, but talking is just as important as thinking and doing. The most important quality that the public look for in a doctor is good human relations (according to a recent survey in Ontario). In the survey subjects chose the most important from several qualities: good human relations—46 percent; competence—34 percent, and service—18 percent.

When you treat the next fracture, these figures should be borne in mind. Spend a little time with the parents explaining what will happen. Test the efficiency of your service by phoning up your office or hospital for advice.

In the same survey, some of the public complained about their doctor's competence. Some cited wrong diagnosis and treatment. Others complained that the treatment was too hurried and examination too careless. Few people today are impressed by a perfunctory glance at a radiograph, a badly applied cast, and poorly answered questions. In the present environment where prestige is gained from academic prowess, simple things such as good service and being seen to provide good service are undervalued in our training programs. Everyone has read *Campbell's Operative Orthopaedics,* but how many have read "The Patients' Bill of Rights"?

This book is based on fracture odysseys over the past ten years at The Hospital for Sick Children, Toronto. Each route has been travelled by many children, and I have reviewed as many of these as possible in order to discern the dangers and degrees of danger of each. Many guides to fracture care are romantic accounts, describing classical fractures following an ideal course, but, as anyone knows who has put together a set of teaching radiographs, these are unusual. Children's fractures are usually easy to treat, but they do not always remodel. There are bad results.

The heartening fact emerged that improvements in fracture care are more likely to come from a greater use of the present corpus of knowledge than from advances. Even taking a generous view of the advances in children's fractures during the past 70 years, no technical breakthrough can be recognized. Problems have been better delineated by clinical research, but no new technique has emerged (Fig. 0-1). Internal fixation, aseptic surgery, and radiography are all more than 70 years old. The advances we await are replacement of a crushed growth plate and sustenance of an avascular epiphysis. Instantaneous bone welding would be helpful, but children's fractures heal so speedily that it would have to be a trouble-free method to be acceptable.

I have written this book for the resident in orthopaedics and for everyone else who treats children's fractures. It contains little or nothing about bone healing and I think I left out a picture of a classical supracondylar fracture because most books on fractures include these things. The features of children's fractures that make them different from adult fractures are emphasized. You will find pictures of errors, because these are often more instructive than good results.

A middle section on injuries of the head, trunk, and soft tissues has been included, not because an orthopaedic surgeon should be prepared to elevate a depressed skull fracture, but to heighten awareness of these injuries, and indicate the investigation and treatment so that this may be dovetailed into the orthopaedic management.

MERCER RANG

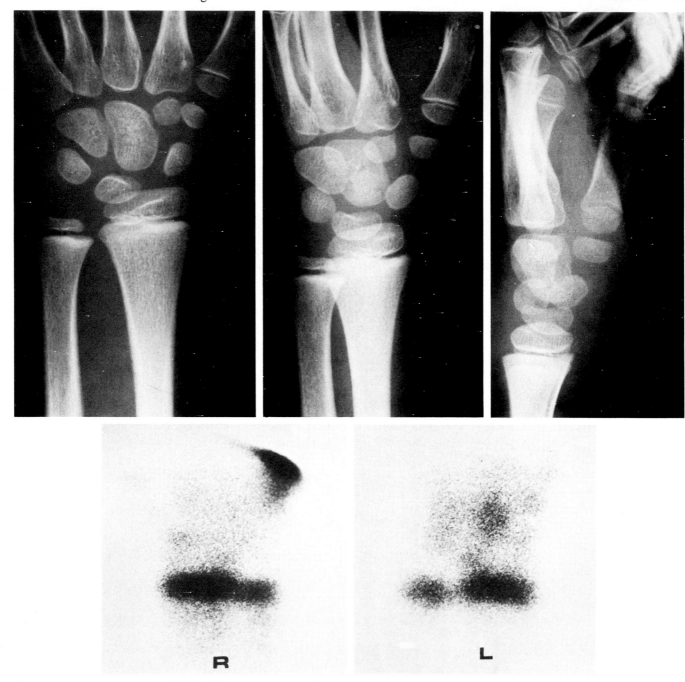

Fig. 0-1. Technetium scanning will demonstrate fractures, including stress fractures, early. Clinical findings suggested a fracture of the left wrist in this child, but the roentgenograph was normal. A scan showed signs of injury to the left capitate bone. Is this a technical breakthrough?

Acknowledgments

I am most grateful to my colleagues Drs. Walter P. Bobechko, Norris Carroll, Donald A. Gibson, Robert Gillespie, and Robert B. Salter of The Hospital for Sick Children, Toronto, for material, for ideas and for reading the manuscript.

Reviews of fractures have been carried out with the assistance of Drs. George Weiss (spine), Alex Finsterbush (radial neck and ankle), Bernard Nolan (pelvis) and Barry Malcolm (trochanteric fractures). Dr. Robert McMurtry kindly summarized his review on meniscectomy in children. Dr. Carl Grant carried out strength testing of bone for Figure 1-3. Dr. Roland Jakob performed experimental work on fractures of the lateral condyle. Illustrations were sent by Drs. Lipmann Kessel, Thomas Barrington, and Charles Zaltz. James Heslin persuaded me that it was a small step to transform an instructional course we presented together into a book. Joyce Parks has edited much of the manuscript, though not as much as she would have liked, and Eva Struthers has prepared the photographs. Also, Dr. Bernard Reilly provided much assistance with radiographs. Dr. E. P. Schwentker read the proofs. Lewis Reines, Editor, and Suzanne Boyd, of J. B. Lippincott Company, were most helpful.

To all these people my grateful thanks.

Contents

1 Children Are Not Just Small Adults 1

    Anatomical Differences 1
    Biomechanical Differences 1
    Physiological Differences 5

2 Injuries of the Epiphysis, Growth Plate, and Perichondrial Ring 7

    Epiphyseal Fractures 7
    Growth Plate Injuries 7
    Injuries of the Perichondrial Ring 17

3 Fracture Care Is a Game of Chess 18

    Traps to Happy Relationships 18
    Traps to Diagnosis 18
    Traps Between You and Correct Treatment 20
    Traps Arising During Treatment 26

4 Fractures with Vascular Damage 28

    Physical Signs 28
    The Three Faces of Arterial Occlusion 28
    Management 30
    Reconstruction of a Damaged Limb 34
    The Severed Limb 35

5 Fractures in Special Circumstances 36

    The Battered Child 36
    Pathological Fractures 39
    Fractures in Special Groups of Patients 41
    Stress Fractures 42
    Lucky Breaks 44
    Second-Hand Cases 44

6 Soft-Tissue Injuries · *Hugh G. Thomson,* M.D., M.S., F.R.C.S.(c), F.A.C.S. ... 47

    Hematoma 47
    Fat Fracture 47
    Foreign Body Penetration 48
    Laceration 48
    Abraded Wounds 53

Wringer Injuries. 54
Avulsed Flaps 58
Degloving Injuries 58
Common Complications 63
Summary. 65

7   Chest and Gastrointestinal Tract · *Sigmund H. Ein,* B.A., M.D.C.M., F.A.A.P., F.A.C.S., F.R.C.S.(C). 66

Initial Care of Severe Injuries. 66
Chest Injuries 68
Abdominal Trauma 69
Initial Management 70
Intraperitoneal Hemorrhage 70

8   Genitourinary Trauma in the Pediatric Orthopaedic Patient · *Martin Barkin,* M.D., B.SC. (MED), M.A., F.R.C.S.(C)
and *J. F. Schillinger,* M.D., F.R.C.S.(C). 74

Initial Management of the Traumatized Child. 74
Presentation and Diagnosis of Genitourinary Injuries. 75
Special Techniques for Urologic Evaluation. 75
Specific Injuries of the Upper Tract 76
Ureteral Injuries 77
Vesical and Urethral Injury 77

9   Craniocerebral Injury · *E. Bruce Hendrick,* M.D., B.SC. (MED), F.R.C.S.(C) 78

Examination 78
Diagnosis 80
Treatment 80
Other Problems 81
Prognosis. 82

10   Clavicle 84

Shaft Fractures 84
Medial End 84
Outer End 86

11   Injuries of the Shoulder and Humeral Shaft 87

Fractures of the Scapula 87
Dislocation of the Shoulder 87
Separation of the Proximal Epiphysis 87
Adolescent Type-II Injury. 87
Fractures of the Upper Metaphysis 90
Fractures of the Humeral Shaft 90
Special Problems 91

12   Elbow 93

Diagnosis 93
Reduction and Complications 93
Supracondylar Fractures. 95
Medial Epicondyle 105
Dislocation of the Elbow 108
Fractures of the Lateral Epicondyle 109
Fractures of the Lateral Condyle 109

Fractures of the Medial Condyle 112
Fractures of the Proximal Radius 112
Fractures of the Olecranon. 118
Dislocations of the Elbow Joint 118
Dislocation of the Radial Head 120
Pulled Elbow. 121

13   Radius and Ulna 124

The Mechanism of Injury. 124
Anatomy and Pathology. 124
Individual Fractures. 128
Fracture Dislocations 136
Follow-up Care 140
Conclusions. 140

14   Hand 141

Problems of Finger Fractures 141
Individual Injuries 141
Miscellaneous Injuries 148

15   Pelvis 150

Associated Injuries in 100 Children with Pelvic Fracture 150
Classification. 150
Initial Management 150
Treatment 154

16   Hip 155

Type I Injuries. 158
Transcervical and Basal Fractures 158
Treatment 161
Trochanteric Fractures 164
Dislocation of the Hip 166
Results 167

17   Femoral Shaft 169

Initial Examination 170
Classification 171
Early Problems 173
Late Problems. 178
Supracondylar Fractures. 179

18   Knee Joint 181

Traumatic Hemarthrosis. 181
Tibial Spine. 181
Dislocation of the Patella 183
Fractures of Patella 184
Intraarticular Fractures of the Femur 185
Fractures of the Tibial Plateau 185
Avulsion of the Tibial Tubercle 186
Ligamentous and Capsular Injuries. 186
The Meniscus in Childhood 186

Locking 188
Subluxation of the Proximal Tibiofibular Joint 188
Puncture Wounds and Foreign Bodies 188

19 Tibia 189

Proximal Growth Plate Injuries 189
Proximal Metaphyseal Fractures 189
Diaphyseal Fractures 194
Common Variations 195
Uncommon Variations 196
Complications and Problems 197
Robert Gillespie's Fracture of the Distal Tibial Diaphysis 197
Metaphyseal Fractures 197

20 Ankle 198

Applied Anatomy 198
Problems of Diagnosis 198
Fracture Patterns 200
Miscellaneous Injuries 206

21 Foot 210

Talar Fractures 210
Os Calcis Fractures 210
Midtarsal Injuries 211
Metatarsal Fractures 212
Phalangeal Fractures 215

22 Spine and Spinal Cord 216

General Features 216
Classification 216
Cord Injury Without Fracture or Open Injury 217
Cord Injury With Vertebral Fracture or Dislocation 217
Pattern of Injury Related to Prognosis 218
Vertebral Fractures and Other Injuries 221
A Brief Guide to the Care of Spinal Injuries in Children 223

Appendix 1 Accident Prevention 225

Appendix 2 Grief and Disaster 226

Appendix 3 Writing a Medicolegal Report 227

Appendix 4 The Role of Muscles in Fracture Patterns 229

Appendix 5 References 230

Index 231

Children's Fractures

1

Children Are Not Just Small Adults

Fractures in children differ from those in adults. Because the anatomy, biomechanics, and physiology of a child's skeleton are very different from those of an adult, in children you will see differences in the patterns of fracture, the problems of diagnosis, and the methods of treatment.

ANATOMICAL DIFFERENCES

The most important part of a child's skeleton is composed of radiolucent growth cartilage. Injury can only be inferred from widening of the growth plate or from displacement of adjacent bones on plain or stress radiographs (Fig. 1-1). The periosteum is thicker and stronger and produces callus more quickly and in greater amount than in adults.

BIOMECHANICAL DIFFERENCES

Biomechanics of Bone

Many years ago it was thought that fractures were not so common in children as in older people because "the proportionate excess of the animal over the earthy constituents" made bending of bone possible. However, the osteoid of a child's bone is not significantly less calcified, but the density of a young bone is certainly less. Young bone is more porous (Fig. 1-2); the cortex is pitted and can be cut easily because the Haversian canals occupy such a great part of the bone. In effect, a child's bone is more like Gruyère cheese than cheddar and can tolerate a greater degree of deformation than an adult's bone can (Fig. 1-3). Pores prevent the extension of a fracture line in the same way that a hole drilled through the end of a crack in a window will prevent the crack from extending. Compact adult bone fails in tension only, whereas the more porous nature of a child's bone allows failure in compression as well.

Classification of Children's Fractures

The porous character of a child's bone accounts for the various fracture types (Fig. 1-4):

Buckle Fracture. Compression failure of bone produces a buckle fracture, also called a torus fracture for the resemblance to the raised band around the base of an architectural column (Fig. 1-5). They occur near the metaphysis, where porosity is greatest, particularly in

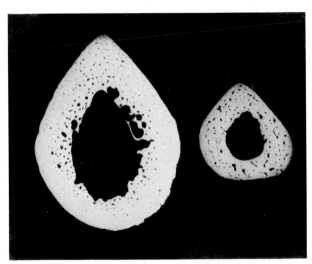

Fig. 1-2. Microradiographs of the distal radial diaphysis of an adult and a child 8 years old. The Haversian canals are larger in the child. Children's bones are more porous than adults'.

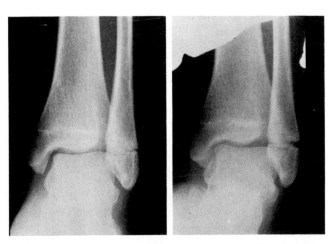

Fig. 1-1. Separation of the fibular epiphysis was only a clinical diagnosis until a stress radiograph was obtained.

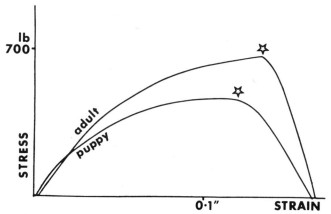

Fig. 1-3. Stress / strain curve for the femurs of a puppy and an adult dog. The curves rise steeply during the elastic phase. The puppy then shows a marked plateau indicating plastic deformation. Fracture occurs at the star. The puppy's bone loses strength more slowly as a greenstick fracture becomes complete. (Courtesy Dr. C. Grant).

younger children. Teen-aged children who do not bear weight for any reason and hence still have porous bones may sustain buckle fractures.

Bend of Bone. Bending of bones, most commonly recognized in the ulna and fibula, can occur without any evidence of acute angular deformity (Fig. 1-6). If you try to break a child's forearm, either post mortem or during osteoclasis, you will find that the bones may be bent 45 degrees or more before the telltale sound of a greenstick fracture is heard. If you stop before the bone fractures you will find that it will slowly, but incom-

pletely, straighten itself out during the course of a few minutes.

Greenstick Fracture. When a bone is angulated beyond the limits of bending, a greenstick fracture occurs. This is a failure of the tension side of the bone; the compression side bends. At the moment of fracture there is considerable displacement—as in most fractures—and then elastic recoil of the soft tissues improves the position (Fig. 1-7). The fracture can hinge open again subsequently owing to muscle pull (Fig. 1-8). Complete closure of the fracture, which is prevented by jamming of spicules, can only be achieved by completing the fracture and momentarily overcorrecting the angulation.

Anyone wishing to study biomechanics further is advised to read J. E. Gordon's *New Science of Strong Materials or Why You Don't Fall Through the Floor.*[2]

The Biomechanics of Growth Cartilage

Ruysch was one of the earliest experimentalists to find (in 1713) that considerable force is required to separate the epiphysis from the metaphysis because they are firmly connected *externally* by the periosteum and *internally* by the mammillary processes existing between the two. In 1820 James Wilson showed that a longitudinal force of 550 pounds was required to detach the epiphysis

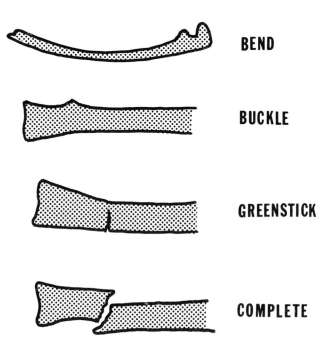

Fig. 1-4. Fracture types in children.

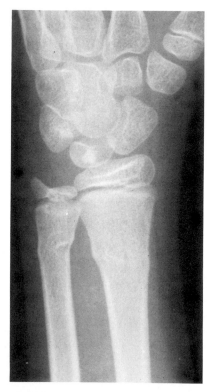

Fig. 1-5. Buckle fracture (child, 10 years). The compressed bone has erupted on the surface in the same way that mountain ranges were pushed up on earth.

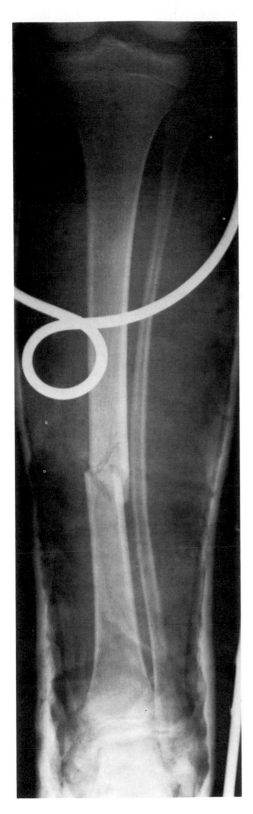

Fig. 1-6. Bending of the fibula (child, aged 12). The position remained unchanged, and no new bone formed around the fibula. Remodelling did not occur, even after 4 years.

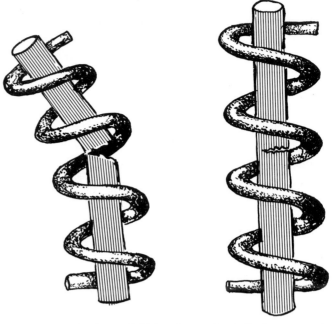

Fig. 1-7. Elastic recoil hides the maximal displacement of a fracture.

from the metaphysis, but that if the periosteum was divided first the force required was only 119 pounds. A few years later, in 1845, Salmon again demonstrated the importance of periosteum. Although he could separate the epiphysis of a newborn's distal femur by hyperextending the knee, he could not produce displacement until he cut the periosteum.

In 1898 John Poland wrote *Traumatic Separation of the Epiphysis,* a book of 900 pages that summarized the state of knowledge to that time. Since then, very little new has been added, and anybody interested in children's fractures must read Poland's book. He was probably the first to show experimentally that it was easy to produce epiphyseal separation but difficult to produce dislocations in children. He wrote, "This is easily understood when the comparatively weak conjugal neighborhood in the young subject is realized. The violence producing the two forms of injury—epiphyseal separation in children and dislocations in adults—is frequently of the same character." (This quotation is more readily understood if you appreciate that the growth plate was once called conjugal cartilage, because it joins two bones intimately together.) Poland concluded that ligaments are stronger than growth cartilage.

At least one attachment of a ligament is to an epiphysis. Hence when a valgus force is applied to the knee of a child, for example, the distal femoral growth plate gives way, whereas in an adult the medial ligament will rupture or detach.

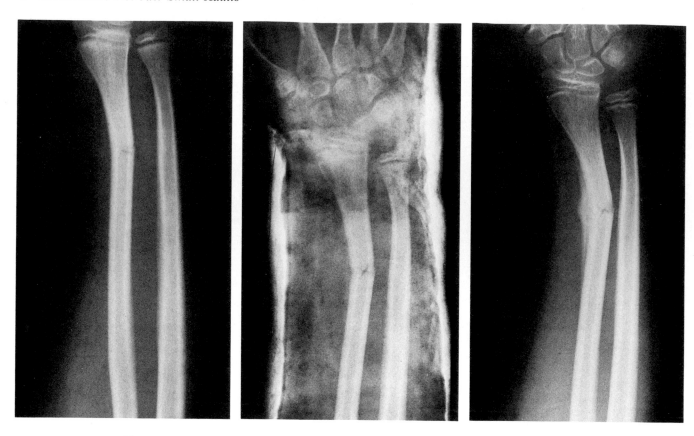

Fig. 1-8. Greenstick fracture of the radius. One cortex has bent; the other is gaping. The initial angulation was acceptable, but it increased and should have been corrected.

Growth cartilage has the consistency of hard rubber. When the plate is thick the epiphysis can be rocked slightly on the metaphysis because of the elasticity of the plate. This property not only protects the bone from injury but also appears to protect the joint surface from the type of crushing injury that is common in adults.

In 1950 Harris revived interest in biomechanical testing of the growth plate.[3] Applying a lateral force to an epiphysis he found that the hormonal environment greatly influences the strength of the bond between epiphysis and metaphysis.

Bright and Elmore in a brief but elegant paper[1] studied the force required to separate the upper tibial epiphysis in a rat (Fig. 1-9). The age of the animal and the direction in which the force is applied are both important factors. The plate is most resistant to traction and least resistant to torsion. Furthermore, the epiphysis can be displaced 0.5 mm. before separation begins.

The Biomechanics of Periosteum

Today it is well recognized that the continuity of the periosteum determines whether or not a fracture is displaced. The periosteum is much thicker, stronger, and less readily torn in a child than in an adult. When

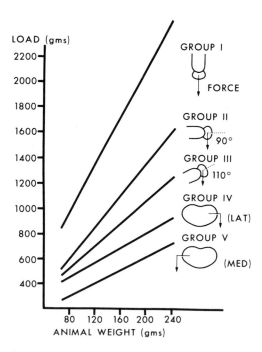

Fig. 1-9. Load required to separate the proximal tibial epiphysis of a rat using forces applied at different angles to the growth plate. (Bright, R. W., and Elmore, S. M.: Physical properties of epiphyseal plate cartilage. Surg. Forum, *19:* 463, 1968)

displacement occurs, the strong hinge of periosteum can help or hinder reduction.

PHYSIOLOGICAL DIFFERENCES

Growth Remodelling

Growth appears to provide the basis for a greater degree of remodelling than is possible in an adult (Fig. 1-10). As a bone increases in length and girth the irregularities produced by a fracture are blurred to some extent, more by rounding the excrescences than by alteration in the alignment of the bone. Valgus and varus and malrotation do not improve (Fig. 1-11).

Overgrowth

A fracture through the shaft of a long bone stimulates longitudinal growth, probably because of the increased nutrition to growth cartilage produced by the hyperemia associated with fracture healing. In practice, an undisplaced fracture of the shaft of the femur will, in the course of a year or two, cause the femur to be about 1 cm. longer than its opposite member.

Progressive Deformity

Permanent damage to the growth plate will produce shortening and often progressive angular deformity. Such complications have been recognized for many years, and in 1888, Lentaigne even diagnosed this condition in an Egyptian mummy.

Complete Fractures

Complete fractures are rarely comminuted in children. This may be because a child's bone is more

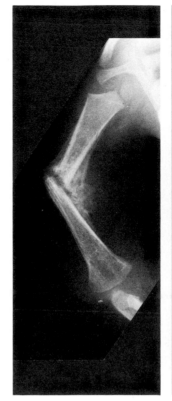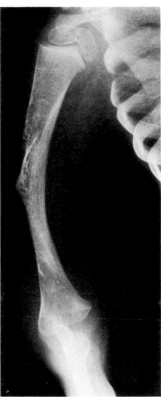

Fig. 1-10. Remodelling in a 15-month-old child. Three years later angulation has diminished from 65 to 30 degrees. The lateral cortex has been eroded. Layers of periosteal new bone are seen medially.

flexible than that of an adult. Some of the force of impact is dissipated in bending the bone, whereas in adults the kinetic energy of impact is entirely used to disrupt the intermolecular bonds in bone.

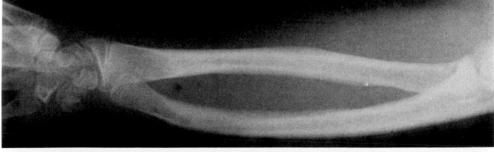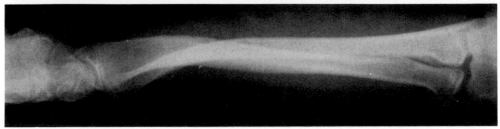

Fig. 1-11. Rounding off the corners in a 16-year-old boy. Two years earlier the radial fracture healed with 30 degrees of dorsal angulation and 90 degrees of malrotation. He now has no range of forearm rotation. Remodelling is not a substitute for reduction.

Nonunion

Nonunion is an adversary almost unknown to the children's orthopaedic surgeon. Displaced intraarticular fractures and the rare shaft fracture with gross interposition may not unite, but otherwise union is easily achieved. The reason for facile union is not known for certain, but the periosteum is actively, not dormantly, osteogenic.

Speed of Healing

Children heal quickly; reduction should be secured early. The orthopaedic surgeon does not have as long to deliberate over a fracture in a child as he does in an adult.

REFERENCES

1. Bright, R. W. and Elmore, S. M.: Physical properties of epiphyseal plate cartilage. Surgical Forum, *19:* 463, 1968
2. Gordon, J. E.: New Science of Strong Materials. London, Penguin Books, 1968
3. Harris, W. R.: The endocrine basis for slipping of the upper femoral epiphysis. J. Bone Joint Surg., *32B:* 5, 1950
4. Hirsch, C. and Evans, F. G.: Studies on some physical properties of infant compact bone. Acta. Orth. Scand., *35:* 300, 1965

2

Injuries of the Epiphysis, Growth Plate, and Perichondrial Ring

Many fractures in children heal well whether they are looked after by a professor in a university hospital or by Robinson Crusoe on a desert island. In these days of spiralling health costs we should ask ourselves whether we are more effective in the treatment of injury than an unflappable granny. But in the injuries to be considered here the doctor does have more to offer than parental peace of mind; intervention can make a world of difference.

EPIPHYSEAL FRACTURES

Fractures of the epiphysis usually involve the growth plate but occasionally occur in isolation. They may be classified as follows (Fig. 2-1): (1) avulsion at the site of ligamentous attachment, (2) displaced osteochondral fragment, and (3) comminuted compression fracture.

Avulsion at the Site of Ligamentous Attachment

The common sites of this injury are the tibial spine, the ulnar styloid, and the bases of the phalanges. The bony fragment retains an adequate blood supply and does not undergo avascular necrosis. If the fragment is displaced, union is rare, because synovial fluid inhibits callus formation. The displaced fragment may block movement or may leave the joint unstable because of functional ligamentous lengthening. These problems justify accurate reduction: closed by choice, but occasionally open by necessity.

Osteochondral Fragments

Osteochondral fragments are most commonly scalped off the distal femur, patella, and radial head. A displaced fragment produces the problems of a loose body and a wound in the articular cartilage. If the fragment is large and from an important part of the joint, it should be replaced and pinned back. If small, it should be removed.

Comminuted Fractures

Comminuted fractures are very unusual because the growth plate acts as a shock absorber. The only fracture of the tibial plateau I have treated personally was in a boy who had just come out of a cast. Disuse osteoporosis had made the epiphysis softer than the growth plate.

GROWTH PLATE INJURIES

The epiphysis is seldom fractured without involving the growth plate. Injuries to the growth plate form perhaps one-third of skeletal trauma in children. The possible consequences of such injuries are: progressive angular deformity, progressive limb length discrepancy,

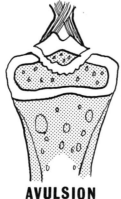 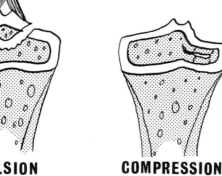 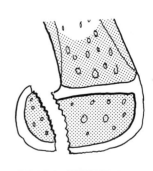

Fig. 2-1. Epiphyseal fractures not involving the growth plate.

AVULSION   **COMPRESSION**   **OSTEO-CHONDRAL**

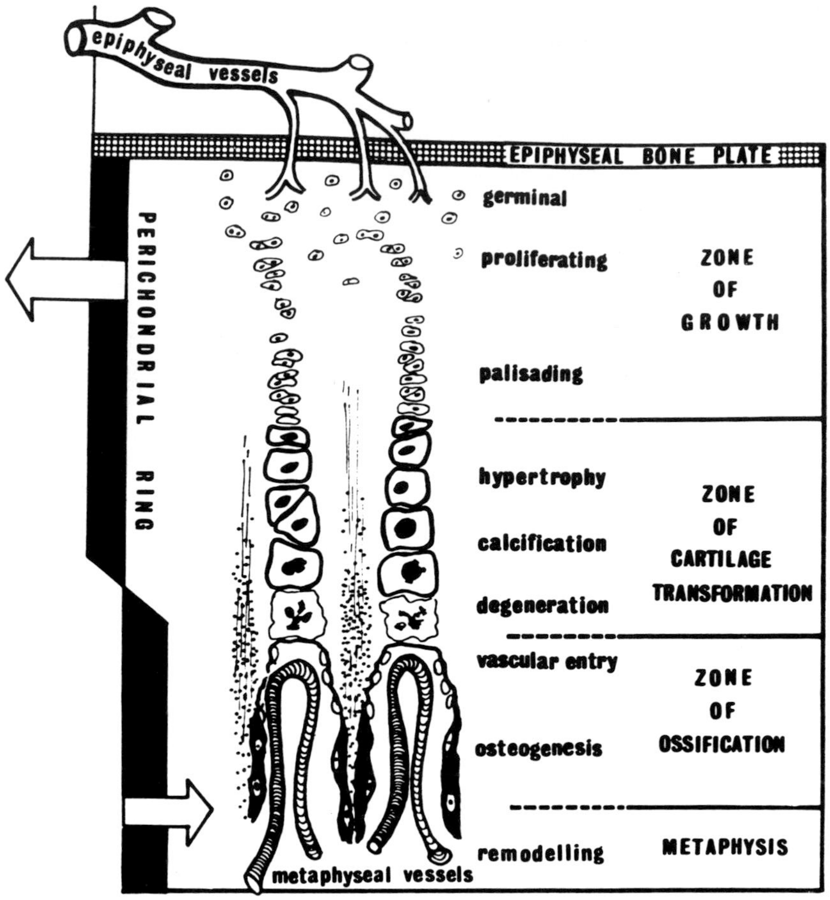

epiphyseal vessels

PERICHONDRIAL RING

EPIPHYSEAL BONE PLATE

germinal	
proliferating	ZONE OF GROWTH
palisading	
hypertrophy	ZONE OF CARTILAGE TRANSFORMATION
calcification	
degeneration	
vascular entry	ZONE OF OSSIFICATION
osteogenesis	
remodelling	METAPHYSIS

metaphyseal vessels

Fig. 2-2. A schematic representation of the growth plate. Separation of the growth plate invariably occurs through the zone of cartilage transformation (Siffert, R. S., and Gilbert, M. D.: Anatomy and Physiology of the Growth Plate. *In* Rang, M. (ed.): The Growth Plate and Its Disorders. Baltimore, Williams & Wilkins, 1969)

and joint incongruity. Although damage to the growth plate has the potential for causing many disastrous problems, in fact the area repairs well, and problems after injury are rare. When growth is disturbed the reason is one of the following:

Avascular necrosis of the plate

Crushing or infection of the plate

Formation of a callus bridge between the bony epiphysis and the metaphysis

Nonunion

Hyperemia producing local overgrowth

The problems and the means of their prevention can only be understood by an appreciation of the anatomy and healing reactions in the growth plate area.

Anatomy

The growth plate is a cartilaginous disc situated between the epiphysis and the metaphysis (Fig. 2-2). The

Fig. 2-3. Blood supply of the growth plate. Damage to the epiphyseal artery destroys the plate. Damage to the metaphyseal artery is unimportant. (Siffert, R. S., and Gilbert, M. D.: Anatomy and physiology of the growth plate. *In* Rang, M. (ed.): The Growth Plate and Its Disorders. Baltimore, Williams & Wilkins, 1969)

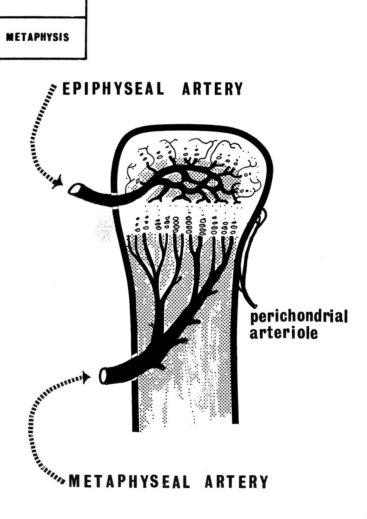

EPIPHYSEAL ARTERY

perichondrial arteriole

METAPHYSEAL ARTERY

germinal cells are attached to the epiphysis and gain a blood supply from the epiphyseal or **E**-vessels (Fig. 2-3). Repeated multiplication of these cells provides the cell population for the rest of the plate. The daughter cells multiply further, secreting a cartilage matrix, and increase in size, thereby producing growth. The matrix calcifies. Metaphyseal vessels enter the cell columns, remove a little matrix, and lay down bone upon the cartilage matrix to form a metaphysis. The invariable plane of separation occurs through the junction between calcified and uncalcified cartilage (Fig. 2-4). A transverse section through the growth plate in this region demonstrates the small amount of structural matrix present, which probably accounts for the relative weakness of the area. The important germinal part of the plate—indeed the greater thickness of the plate—remains with the epiphysis. This plane of separation is bloodless, so that an epiphyseal separation does not produce much swelling.

The blood supply of the epiphysis is important. Dale and Harris showed that there are two fundamental types of epiphysis (Fig. 2-5).

Epiphyses Totally Clad with Cartilage—such as the head of the femur and the head of the radius. Total interruption of the blood supply to the germinal cells

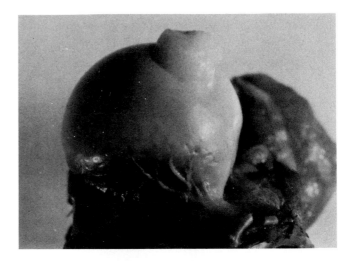

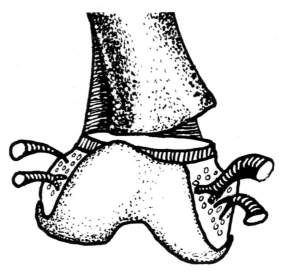

Fig. 2-5. (*Top*) The blood supply of two types of epiphyses. Vessels to the femoral head track in the periosteum just under the synovium. A periosteal tear or a high pressure effusion may cause avascular necrosis. (*Bottom*) Vessels to the distal femur pass through a thick wad of soft tissues.

may follow separation. Avascular necrosis of the plate and epiphysis, and arrest of longitudinal growth naturally follow.

Epiphyses with Soft-Tissue Attachments. When these are separated the soft-tissue hinge will remain attached to the epiphysis, so that the circulation to the epiphysis remains intact. The germinal cells are not injured, and longitudinal growth continues unscathed.

Healing Reactions of the Growth Plate

Dale and Harris have published the most credible description of growth plate separation.[3] The plate separates consistently between the calcified and uncalcified layers of the growth plate. For a week or two the hiatus is filled by fibrin. The plate becomes wider, because

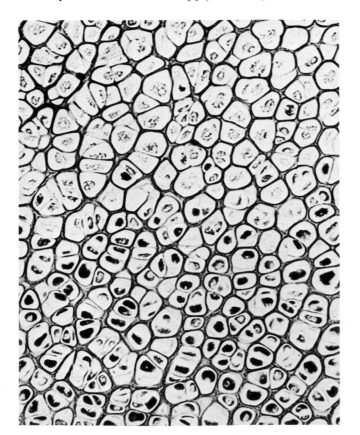

Fig. 2-4. Histology of the growth plate in transverse section through zone of cartilage transformation. The paucity of matrix accounts for the weakness of this zone.

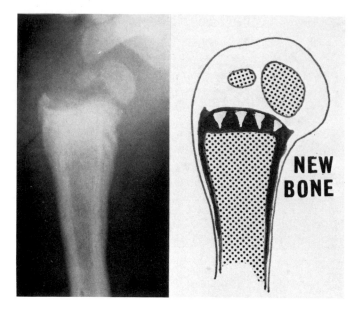

Fig. 2-6.   Healing after growth plate separation occurs by means of new bone formed by the growth plate and by the periosteum.   It can be seen clearly 3 weeks after the initial injury.

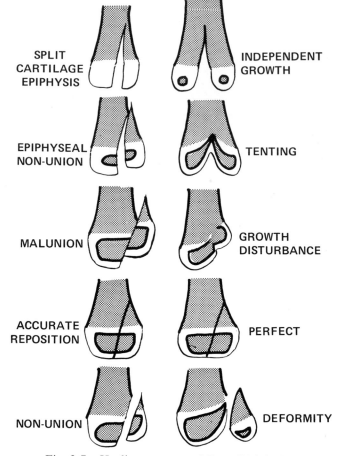

Fig. 2-7.   Healing patterns of Type IV injuries.

growth cartilage continues to be produced without invasion by metaphyseal vessels.   After about 2 weeks, the vessels begin to invade the cartilage columns again. The plate becomes narrower once more, and the healing occurs without leaving a trace.   In this way, the growth plate heals more quickly than a fracture through bone (Fig. 2-6).   The repair of an injury at right angles to the plane of the growth plate shows more variation (Fig. 2-7).

Cartilaginous Epiphysis.   Both parts of the epiphysis continue to grow uninterruptedly, producing a double-ended bone, if they remain displaced. (Siffert)[7]

Ossified Epiphysis.   If the fracture surfaces are not in contact, both fragments continue to grow for some time.   Eventually premature arrest of growth adjacent to the fracture line takes place.

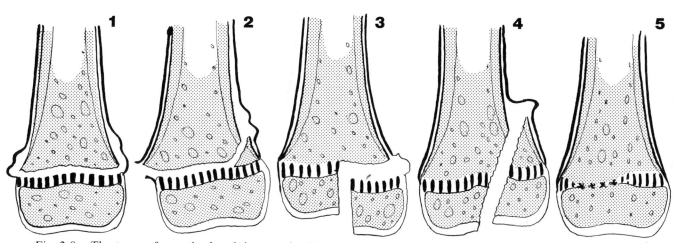

Fig. 2-8.   The types of growth plate injury as classified by Salter and Harris (J. Bone Joint Surg., *45A:* 587, 1963).

If the fracture surfaces are apposed without coaption of the growth plate, a bridge of callus will form between the epiphysis on one side and the metaphysis on the other. This bony bridge is a brake on growth. When the bridge is at the center of the epiphysis, the two outside edges will continue to grow, resulting in tenting of the end of the bone. When the bridge is toward one margin of the growth plate, a progressive angular deformity develops.

If the fracture is accurately reduced so that there is coaption of the growth plate, there will be a small scar at the site of growth plate injury, but this is not sufficient to disturb growth.

Effect of Internal Fixation. Small Kirschner wires passed through the center of the plate do not interfere with growth. If they are passed near the margin of the plate, growth is occasionally disturbed. Threaded pins or screws across the plate act as effectively as Blount's staples.[6]

Salter-Harris Classification of Growth Plate Injuries

The Salter-Harris classification is in general usage.

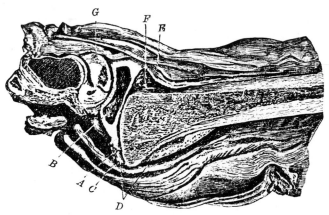

Fig. 2-10. A dissection by Poland of a Type I injury: (*A*) diaphysis of radius; (*B*) carpal epiphysis of radius incompletely ossified; (*C*) flexor tendons displaced forwards; (*D*) pronator quadratus lacerated by anterior margin of end of radial diaphysis; (*E*) periosteum stripped off dorsal aspect of diaphysis; (*F*) blood clot filling space between periosteum and diaphysis; (*G*) scaphoid.

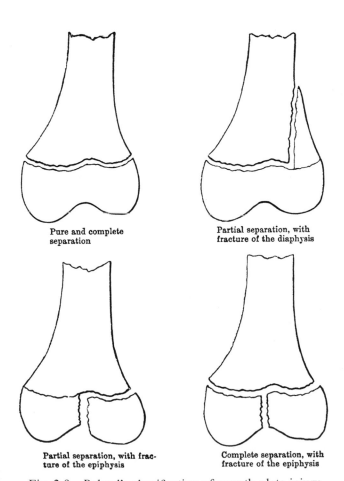

Pure and complete separation

Partial separation, with fracture of the diaphysis

Partial separation, with fracture of the epiphysis

Complete separation, with fracture of the epiphysis

Fig. 2-9. Poland's classification of growth plate injury.

Founded on the pathology of injury, the classification is well-suited to the accurate verbal description of an injury and provides an excellent guide to rational treatment (Fig. 2-8). Most growth plate injuries can be easily classified leaving very few fractures to produce arguments at fracture rounds. The classification should be studied in the original, as it is one of the classic papers in orthopaedics.[5] There have been others. In 1898 Poland illustrated the common variations of separation (Fig. 2-9). Aitkin's classification of growth plate injuries is widely used, although we have not found it as practical as the Salter-Harris.

Type I. In a Type I fracture (Fig. 2-10) the epiphysis separates completely from the metaphysis. The germinal cells remain with the epiphysis, and the calcified layer remains with the metaphysis. If the periosteum is not torn, there is no displacement. The radiograph in these circumstances may be normal, and the diagnosis is made on clinical suspicion. Most parents look on these injuries as sprains, since there is little swelling and little deformity. You will be alerted to them by tenderness over the growth plate and will not be disturbed by the absence of radiological signs. Stress radiographs may be taken if accurate diagnosis is imperative. Diagnosis of separation of an unossified epiphysis is made on clinical signs and on the presence of soft-tissue swelling observed on the radiograph.

When the periosteum is torn, displacement is easily reduced without any satisfying crepitus or the sensation that the fragment is snapping back into position, because the two fracture surfaces are covered with cartilage.

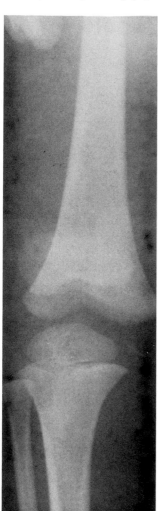 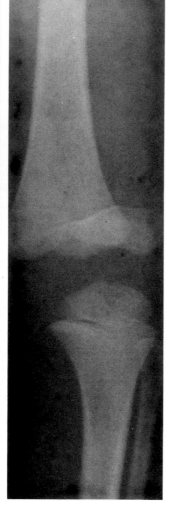

Fig. 2-11. Separation of both distal femoral epiphyses. For 6 weeks this boy, aged 3 years, had been treated with antibiotics and steroids for hectic fever and multiple joint pains. By the time a diagnosis of osteomyelitis was reached, these epiphyses had sequestrated.

Type I injuries are usually the result of shearing, torsion, or avulsion force. Apophyses are usually avulsed.

Pathological Type I injuries occur in scurvy, rickets, osteomyelitis, and disorders associated with hormonal imbalance (Fig. 2-11).

Healing occurs within 3 weeks, and problems are rare (Fig. 2-12). Avascular necrosis of the femoral head is the worst problem to be encountered. Nonunion of a separated medial epicondyle is not uncommon; only rarely does it cause any instability. It is difficult to distinguish between a Type I injury of the growth plate (which has an excellent prognosis) and a Type V injury, in which the plate is crushed, which has a bad prognosis. The history of injury is the best guide; Type V injuries are produced by axial compression. In fact,

Type V injuries are exceptionally rare, so the distinction is not a practical problem.

Type II. The plane of cleavage of a Type II injury (Fig. 2-13) passes through much of the plate before the fracture travels through the metaphysis. The fracture is produced by lateral displacement force, which tears the periosteum on one side and leaves it intact in the region of the triangular metaphyseal fragment.

The fracture is usually easily reduced, and overreduction is prevented by the intact periosteum. The cartilage covered surfaces usually prevent the sensation of crepitus as the fragment is pushed into position. When the radial head is separated, for example, it may be impossible to judge the success of a reduction by clinical means.

Occasionally, the shaft of a bone will become trapped in the button-hole tear of the periosteum. This is most

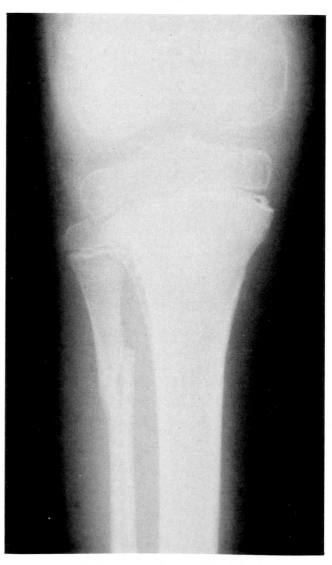

Fig. 2-12. Healing Type I injury. New bone is laid down by the growth plate and subperiosteally. The extent of periosteal stripping and the site of the periosteal hinge are obvious.

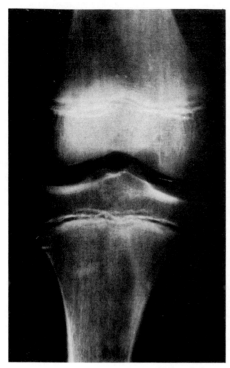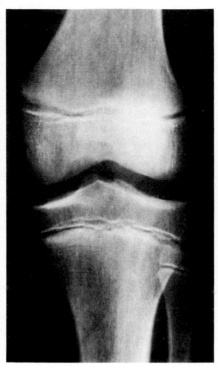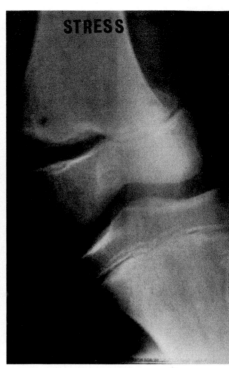

Fig. 2-13. Suppose this 12-year-old-boy came in with a swollen (L) knee that was tender on the medial side. Would you recognize the slight widening of the growth plate? A stress film would have demonstrated a Type II injury.

likcly at the shoulder, if there is a large metaphyseal fragment poking through a small periosteal tear. If the degree of displacement is unacceptable, open reduction may be needed on rare occasions.

Type III. Type III injuries are rare (Fig. 2-14). The plane of separation passes along with the growth plate for a variable period before entering the joint through a fracture of the epiphysis. The fracture is intraarticular and requires accurate reduction to prevent malarticulation. Open reduction may be needed, but the fragment should not be dissected free of its blood supply. The commonest site is at the distal end of the tibia toward the end of growth when the medial half of the plate is closed. Growth disturbances, therefore, are not a problem.

Type IV. The fracture line in a Type IV injury passes from the joint surface, across the epiphysis growth plate, and into the metaphysis (Fig. 2-15). The commonest example is a fracture of the lateral condyle of the humerus. It is an injury for which the doctor can do a great deal. Left alone, this intraarticular injury will produce joint stiffness and deformity due to loss of position, nonunion, and growth disturbance. The fracture must be accurately reduced, usually by open reduc-

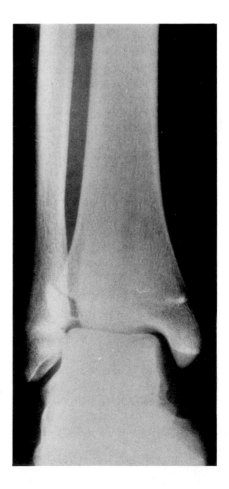

Fig. 2-14. Type III injury of the distal tibia, the Tillaux fracture, in a girl, aged 14. Type III injuries are most likely to occur when most of the plate is closed.

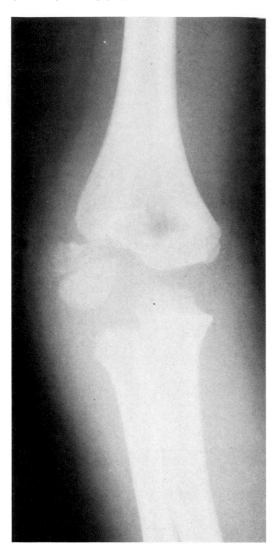

Fig. 2-15.   Fracture of the lateral condyle.   A Type IV injury.

to insure that the plate that looks normal on radiographs, has no sclerosis of the metaphysis and has formed new bone beyond the Harris' line that is the scar of benign injuries.

Guide to the Care of Growth Plate Injuries

Define the Exact Line of the Fracture.   This is usually obvious, but difficult injuries can be very difficult, particularly in the young child with little or no ossification in the epiphysis.   Multiple views, with comparative

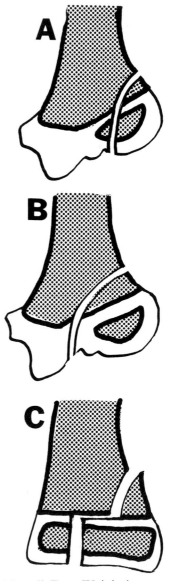

Fig. 2-16.   Not all Type IV injuries are the same.   (*A*) When the fracture line crosses a bony epiphysis, the risk of bony callus bridging the growth plate and causing a growth disturbance is great if accurate reduction is not achieved. (*B*) When the fracture line passes through a cartilaginous epiphysis, bridging is unlikely.   (*C*) A stepped fracture line permits stable closed reduction.

tion and internal fixation, to secure a smooth joint surface, closure of the fracture gap to prevent nonunion, and cell-to-cell apposition of the growth plate to insure that growth is not disturbed.   There are several subvarieties of this injury that are not generally known (Fig. 2-16).

Type V.   Type V injuries, happily, are very rare (Fig. 2-17 to 2-19).   The plate is crushed thereby extinguishing further growth.   All or part of the plate may be affected.   A compression injury of the plate may seem like nothing more than a sprain at first, and only later will the true nature of the lesion be recognized. At other times, a Type I or II injury is obvious initially; then pressure from the most prominent corner of the metaphysis produces a crushing injury, to the chagrin of the surgeon and to the detriment of the patient. Because of this remote possibility, it is wise to follow up all growth plate injuries for 6 months, perhaps a year,

Fig. 2-17. One of the earliest radiographs of a Type V injury was published by Poland in 1898. The growth plate of the radius has closed, and the radius has not grown.

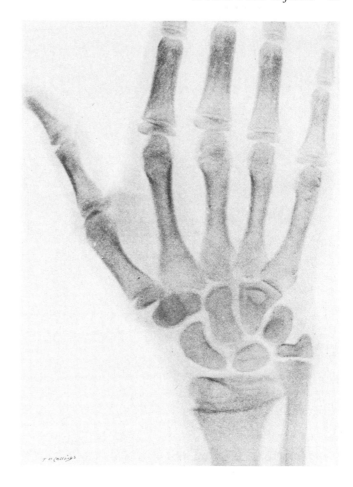

views of the opposite side, may help. (Remember that man is made symmetrical for the purpose of comparison.) Stress films should not be omitted, and arthrography may be helpful. Occasionally, when you suspect a displaced intraarticular fracture but cannot prove it, it is wiser to err in favor of exploration than to rely on your small stock of undeserved miracles.

Classify the Fracture. The Salter-Harris classification is a logical guide to problems that accompany different types of injury.

Treat the Child and the Parents. Reduction should be early and gentle. These injuries unite quickly, so that attempts to correct malposition after a week are liable to do more damage to the plate than good. Repeated efforts at reduction may do nothing more than grate the plate away. If problems are anticipated, they should be communicated to the parents without unduly alarming them, preferably preoperatively.

Open or Closed Reduction? It is usually possible to secure closed reduction of Type I and II injuries. Exact anatomical reduction, though desirable, may be unnecessary, since remodelling will take care of many imperfections. (See p. 22 on remodelling.) Occasionally, soft tissue is interposed (e.g., at the ankle) or the part is so deeply placed (e.g., the radial head) that open reduction will be necessary. Open reduction is also required for

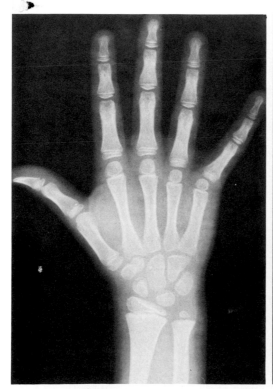

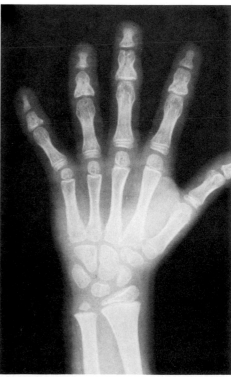

Fig. 2-18. Growth arrest of the phalanges of the (R) hand due to frostbite.

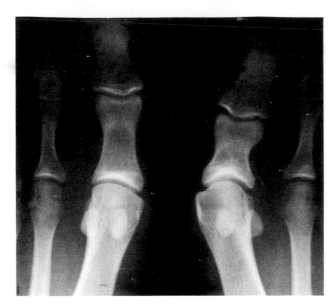

Fig. 2-19. This 14-year-old girl had stubbed her (R) great toe years before. The toe is short due to an old Type V injury of the base of the proximal phalanx.

markedly displaced separations of the medial epicondyle. Stability is easily achieved with a few periosteal sutures, and internal fixation is seldom needed. Type III injuries commonly need open reduction in order to secure a smooth joint surface. Type IV injuries are commonly unstable, and accurate reduction is mandatory. This applies particularly to the lateral condyle of the humerus; it may be possible to reduce this injury, but it is difficult to be sure that it is stable, and almost impossible to be sure, by examining radiographs of a flexed elbow taken through a thick cast, that the position is maintained. For these reasons, open reduction and internal fixation is much safer.

Chondrolysis. A growth plate may be destroyed by infection. This is a theoretical risk in all open fractures and a more practical hazard when open reduction is carried out. For this reason, all Kirschner wires should be buried below the skin, (not left protruding through it) to prevent infection tracking in.

Length of Immobilization. Various rules are invoked. The elbow may become stiff if immobilized for more than 3 weeks. For other joints, we allow 3 weeks for union of an epiphyseal separation, and 6 weeks when we are awaiting bony union.

The Child from Elsewhere General Hospital. Children presenting late with Type I and -II injuries in unacceptable positions should be left after a week, for fear of damaging the plate. Osteotomy should be carried out later if remodelling fails.

Open reduction of displaced Type III and -IV injuries may be better undertaken late than never. Be careful not to devascularize the fragment at the time of replacement. In order to secure better alignment of a Type IV injury the metaphyseal fragment may be peeled off the growth plate and discarded, in order to see that the plate is accurately aligned.

In Conclusion: The majority of growth plate injuries involve little risk of growth disturbance. In a few, simple surgical intervention can make a great deal of difference to the outcome of the injury. Happily, the number of children who have irretrieveable damage is very small.

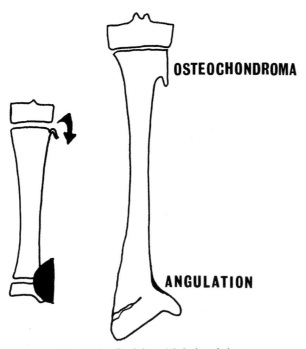

OSTEOCHONDROMA

ANGULATION

Fig. 2-20. Perichondrial ring injury.

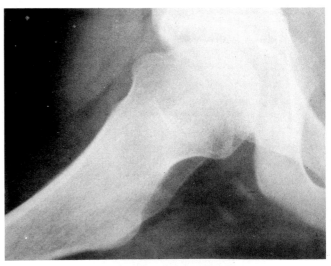

Fig. 2-21. Traumatic exostosis in a boy, aged 18 years. Five years before he sustained multiple injuries. He complained of much pain and stiffness in the (R) hip, but radiographs were normal. He later shows this traumatic exostosis which limited movement and was excised.

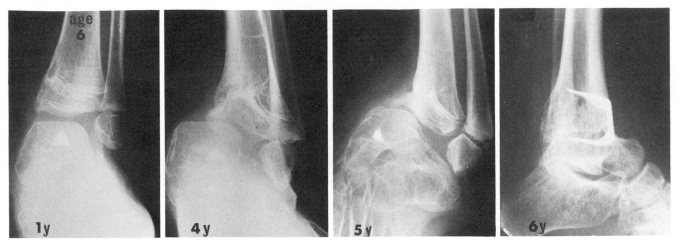

Fig. 2-22. A motor vehicle accident at the age of 5 years removed this girl's medial malleolus. Bony bridging occurred, causing growth arrest. Five years after the accident (at age 10) a tibial osteotomy was performed followed by ankle fusion. She was 6 cm. short. A tibial leg lengthening has left her 0.5 cm. short at the age of 13 years.

INJURIES OF THE PERICHONDRIAL RING

The perichondrial ring encircles the growth plate in the same way that periosteum invests bone. The perichondrial ring appears to regulate the diameter of the growth plate. Injuries are rare but produce characteristic effects (Fig. 2-20).

Displacement of the perichondrial ring produces a traumatic exostosis, clinically and experimentally[4] (Fig. 2-21).

Removal of the perichondrial ring permits bony bridging between the epiphysis and metaphysis. Fracture callus joins the epiphysis to the metaphysis leading to progressive angular deformity.

The perichondrial ring is most commonly removed by a lawn mower "scalping" the medial side of the ankle (Fig. 2-22). The surgeon usually replaces the lost skin by split-thickness grafts. A progressive varus deformity follows. Before repeated open wedge osteotomies are carried out, the grafted area must be replaced by a full-thickness flap. Bright, confronted by this unenviable program carried out experimental work.[2] The injury was easily produced in experimental animals and was invariably followed by deformity. Noting that the deformity was due to fracture callus joining the epiphysis to the metaphysis he found (in experimental animals) that he could prevent the ingress of callus by placing silicone rubber cement over the exposed growth plate. Progressive deformity did not occur. Confronted by partial plate closure, you should consider resection of the bony bridge and implantation of silicone rubber.

REFERENCES

1. Aitken, A. P. and Magill, H. K.: Fractures involving the distal epiphyseal cartilage. J. Bone Joint Surg., *34A:* 96, 1952
2. Bright, R. W.: Surgical correction of partial epiphyseal plate closure in dogs by bone bridge resection and use of silicone rubber implants. J. Bone Joint Surg., *54A:* 1133, 1972
3. Dale, G. C. and Harris, W. R.: Prognosis in epiphyseal separation. An experimental study. J. Bone Joint Surg., *40B:* 116, 1958
4. Rigal, W. M.: Diaphyseal aclasis. *In* Rang, M. (ed.): The Growth Plate. Edinburgh, E. & S. Livingstone, 1969
5. Salter, R. B. and Harris, W. R.: Injuries involving the epiphyseal plate. J. Bone Joint Surg., *45A:* 587, 1963
6. Siffert, R. S.: The effect of staples and longitudinal wires on epiphyseal growth. An experimental study. J. Bone Joint Surg., *38A:* 1077, 1956
7. Siffert, R. S. and Barash, E. S.: The potential for growth of experimentally produced hemi-epiphyses. J. Bone Joint Surg., *48A:* 1548, 1966

3

Fracture Care Is a Game of Chess

Each fracture type, like each piece in a chess set, can move only in a certain number of ways. Are you going to win or lose? Obviously you cannot win if you do not know the moves of each fracture piece, but even after you have mastered this, and you are playing several games at once, it is easy to be outwitted. In this chapter a few of the obvious traps are identified.

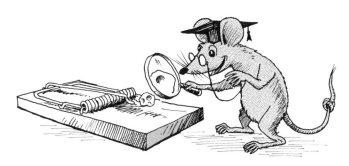

TRAPS TO HAPPY RELATIONSHIPS

The injured child and the alarmed parents are impressed—positively or negatively—by your initial behaviour. If you ignore the parents, palpate the fracture directly, and then shout your opinion to the parents above the screams of the child, you have created the wrong impression. Every time you see the child there will be screams; every time you speak to the parents it will seem as if they do not understand what you say.

Remember that even if you have to be convinced that there is a fracture, the child and the parents have already made up their minds. They have dropped whatever they were doing, left children with neighbors, and are trying to remember if they locked the front door. Be gentle, interested, and compassionate. Shake the parents by the hand and introduce yourself. Ask them what happened and ask a few questions to discover what they feel about it all. Then ask the child to point to the painful place instead of discovering it yourself by palpation. Watch the digits being moved actively before touching the child just enough to feel the pulse and test sensation. Splint the limb before sending the child for a radiograph; fractures are painful. Instruct x-ray technicians never to take films of unsplinted fractures

(Fig. 3-1). The opportunity to make a good start should not be wasted.

TRAPS TO DIAGNOSIS

Failure to make the correct diagnosis sets treatment off in the wrong direction; a significant proportion of

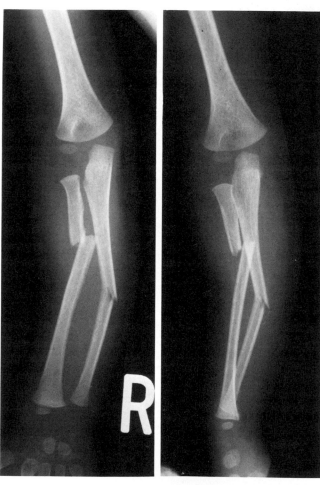

Fig. 3-1. This child was sent to x-ray for "AP and lateral of the forearm." The arm was not splinted. The elbow is seen in the AP projection in both views. The technician has twisted the wrist, moving the arm through the fracture site. Peace lovers always splint the arm and move the x-ray machine and not the limb.

18

the children who have poor results owe it to this initial error.

Fractures are easily *missed* because of the presence of growth cartilage. There is no tell-tale fracture line to be seen in growth cartilage. Growth plate injuries that are unstable but undisplaced provide a trap. For example, separations of the epiphyses of the upper tibia, lower femur, and lateral malleolus yield normal radiographs (apart from soft-tissue swelling) if there is no displacement (Fig. 1-1). Stress films will reveal these. Separation of the lateral malleolus is so common that we are content to diagnose this on suspicion.

Separation of Unossified Epiphyses. In infancy, the upper and lower ends of the humerus and the upper end of the femur may be separated. In older children the unossified epiphyses at the sternal end of the clavicle may mimic a sternoclavicular dislocation. These injuries are easily missed or mistaken for dislocations when the epiphysis is in its preradiographic existence (Fig. 14-8).

When reduction is attempted, soft crepitus will be appreciated. Arthrograms offer a tempting diagnostic aid but usually represent a further source of uncertainty. Arthrography of an unfamiliar joint in a child is not helpful.

Some Injuries Do not Show on Standard Views. Minimal displacements of the lateral and medial condyles may not be apparent on standard anteroposterior and lateral radiographs. Oblique radiographs provide the answer (Fig. 3-2). Oblique radiographs are essential in all ankle injuries.

Always include the joint above and the joint below (Fig. 3-3). Do not miss a dislocated hip for weeks while treating a femoral shaft fracture. Always be certain that the radial head is not dislocated in fractures of the forearm. Remember that two fractures sometimes occur in the same limb; it is the proximal one that is overlooked (Fig. 3-4).

Radiographs May Show the Injury but the Observer Does not Recognize It. Displaced epiphyses may not be instantly obvious when one side alone is radiographed. Separation of the medial epicondyle is the classical example. Always radiograph the opposite limb when in doubt (Fig. 3-5).

The fracture line may be obscured by overlapping bone. Only the observer who has the injury in mind will recognize it. The Tillaux fracture of the ankle is a good example (see Fig. 20-9).

Overdiagnosis. At the beginning everyone mistakes growth plates on radiographs for fractures, but this usually passes. Poorly centered films produce strange appearances, e.g., a radiograph centered on the mid-humerus and taken at short distance gives a good imitation of a shoulder dislocation.

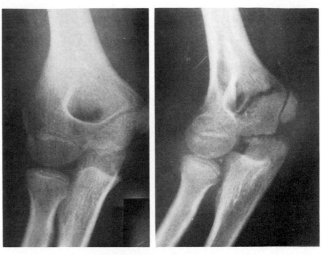

Fig. 3-2. The standard anteroposterior and lateral roentgenograph show nothing more than soft-tissue swelling. Only when an oblique film is produced can the fracture of the medial condyle be appreciated.

Some Fractures Do not Conform to a Standard Pattern. Occasionally, the nature of the injury cannot be recognized with certainty, especially when the fracture fades into growth cartilage or is of an unusual type. Order additional views (Fig. 3-6). Sometimes post-reduction films will clarify things.

Standard Radiographs May not Show the Degree of Displacement. Two radiographs taken at 90 degrees to

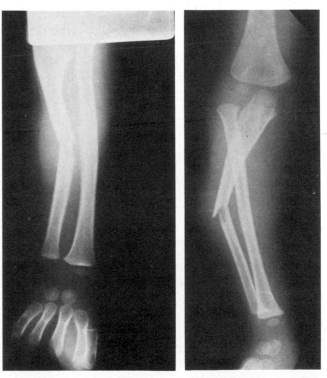

Fig. 3-3. Always include the joint above and below. You will often be tempted to accept the left film. Always insist on the second.

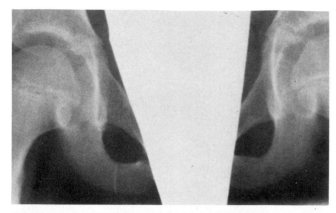

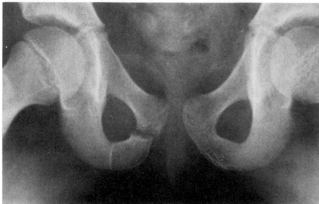

Fig. 3-4. A shield obscured this fracture of the pubic ramus the first time around.

each other may still be at 45 degrees to the plane of maximal displacement (Fig. 3-7).

Greenstick fractures of the upper tibia commonly appear to have a trivial degree of deformity. Always have an AP radiograph of the whole *extended* tibia and femur to determine the degree of valgus; it is usually unacceptable.

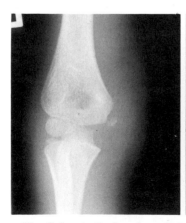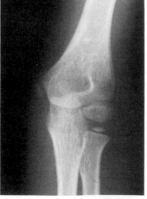

Fig. 3-5. A displaced medial epicondyle produces much soft-tissue swelling that is obvious to the clinician. The x-ray appearances may be much less convincing unless comparison is made with the normal elbow. (Boy, aged 7.)

Think of the Soft-tissue Injury. Injuries to blood vessels do occur. Volkmann's contracture rarely follows elbow injuries today because everyone guards against it. Problems are common with high tibial fractures and midtarsal injuries because arterial injury, though common, has not received the same amount of publicity (Figs. 3-8, 3-9).

Clinical Judgement Will Never Be Superseded. If there is every clinical indication of a fracture but the radiographs do not show it, have further appropriate films taken. Talk to the radiologist, and challenge him to demonstrate the fracture. Most radiologists welcome the opportunity to order appropriate films as a change from reading endless films that have been ordered by others.

TRAPS BETWEEN YOU AND CORRECT TREATMENT

When the small number of possible moves is considered, it is a wonder that there is any difficulty in deciding which to select. Yet put a case up at rounds and there will always be somebody who would have done something else. To some extent this is because perfect methods do not exist. Every method has drawbacks; which do you want to take on? Which are acceptable?

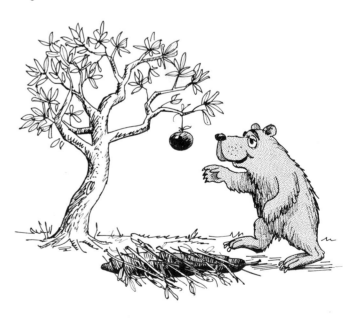

The choice of treatment may be difficult because the results of children's fractures, though obviously much better than corresponding fractures in adults, are not well documented. Children do not usually return to the surgeon more than once after the cast is removed. On many charts at our hospital the last ambiguous note reads "movement returning well, see in 2 months." We are not unique. Few surgeons can produce a good set

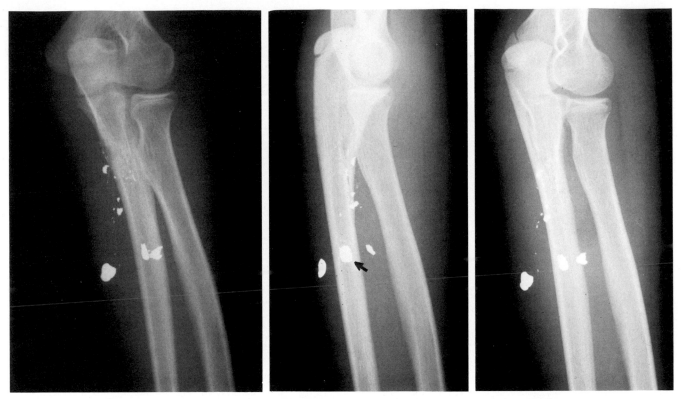

Fig. 3-6. The entry wound was on the medial side of the elbow. Where is the fragment marked with an arrow?

of films to demonstrate remodelling though the word is on the lips of all. When ex-patients are recalled for review, all kinds of things come to light that had been either unnoticed or hidden. Children are uncomplaining about minor imperfection; for example, a child with a congenital synotosis of the radius and ulna will pass for normal for several years. It is my impression that a corresponding degree of disability following a fracture easily goes unnoticed.

The key to successful treatment in children's fractures is a clear understanding of what remodelling will accomplish and what it will not.

Remodelling

The scene is a young resident talking to an elderly orthopaedic surgeon:

E.O.S.: But why did you reduce that fracture? It would remodel.

Y.R.: But it is a beautiful reduction. Anyhow, how do you know for sure that it would remodel?

E.O.S.: Seen a lot of them do it, that's how.

Y.R.: What about that child in the clinic today who didn't? She was in my mind when I reduced this child's fracture.

E.O.S.: Knowing who will and who won't is what you learn with experience.

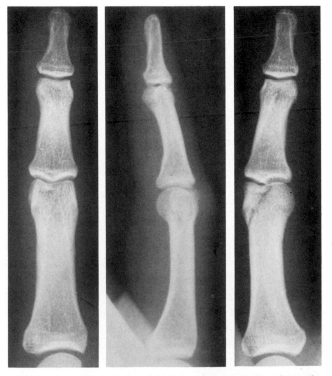

Fig. 3-7. Two views at right angles may not show the maximum degree of displacement. Three views may. The fragment in Figure 3-6 is intramedullary.

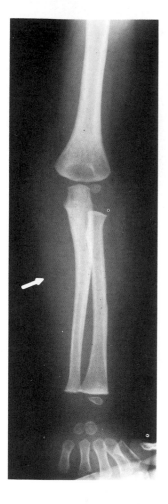

Fig. 3-8. (Left) This 1-year-old child sustained a wringer injury. There are no fractures. The swelling and mottled pattern in the soft tissues indicate extravasation of blood.

Fig. 3-9. (Right) The appearance of this boy's arm after a baby car fracture tells more than his radiograph. Vascular repair did not help.

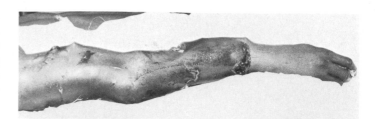

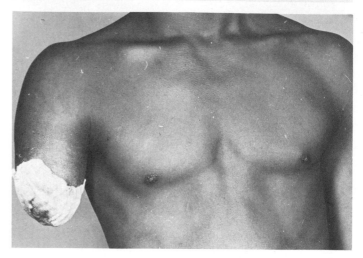

A few general principles may help:

Remodelling will help:

1. Children with 2 years or more of growth ahead of them.
2. Fractures near the ends of bones.
3. Deformity in the plane of movement of a joint.

Remodelling will not help:

1. Displaced intraarticular fractures.
2. Fractures in the middle of the shaft of a bone which are grossly shortened, angulated, or rotated.
3. Displaced fractures with the axis of displacement at right angles to the plane of movement.
4. Displaced fractures crossing the growth plate at right angles.

Remodelling is largely a process of rounding off the bones on radiographs. In fractures of the shaft of a bone the periosteum drapes one side of the bone, and this gradually fills in. On the other aspect the bone is bare of periosteum, and these sharp ends are eroded. The result is that the fracture looks less obvious. This does nothing for the alignment, angulation, and rotation of the fracture site. Near an epiphysis the growth plate can become realigned (Fig. 12-45).

In a supracondylar fracture that has healed with posterior displacement the shaft acts as an anterior bone block. Movement is restricted until, with growth, the joint moves away from the bone block. The range of movement increases, therefore, with growth.

Most parents are vaguely dissatisfied with the surgeon who puts much faith in remodelling. At the wrist, where this problem comes up most frequently, the bones are just under the skin, and malposition shows. It is our habit to reduce these injuries whenever possible, partly to avoid the risk of further displacement within the cast, and partly to avoid long looks from the parents. There are occasions when it is wiser to await remodelling than to reduce the injury, even though reduction is possible. Metaphyseal fractures and epiphyseal separation about 2 weeks old tend to react badly to attempts at reduction. Heterotopic ossification and growth plate damage are possible sequelae. Poor anesthetic services constitute another reason for accepting remodelling as a basic treatment. Anesthesia is a definite risk in emergency work. If a child aspirates in the course of reducing a trivial greenstick fracture, it is tragic. There is much to be said for dosing children with these trivial fractures with intravenous diazepam and reducing the fracture quickly while the cast is setting.

Another area in which the extent of remodelling is important is in fractures of both bones of the forearm. Striking remodelling can be seen on radiographs, but it is my impression that this does not help the range of pronation and supination. Any rotatory deformity persists. In other words, remodelling of fractures of

Fig. 3-10. An appalling cast. The interior is lumpy and the thickness uneven.

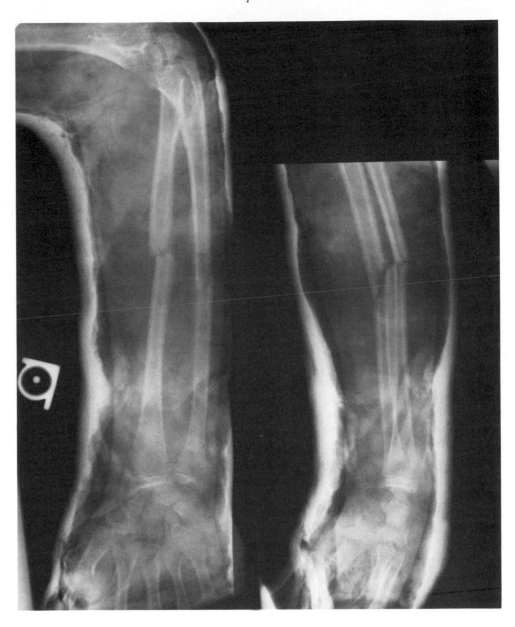

both bones of the forearm consists only of rounding off the bone ends on radiographs and is of no clinical value (Fig. 1-11).

Overlap on radiographs becomes less obvious with the passage of time. After fracture about 1 cm. of overgrowth can be expected in a long bone, so that shortening is lost in the remodelling process. The importance of overlap in fractures that are treated in casts is that reduction may be unstable. So long as rotatory and angular alignment have been preserved while the fracture heals, the result will be good.

These principles should help you to decide whether or not to correct deformity in a fracture. But if you accept slight malposition you do not want to lose position any further in the cast—which brings us onto the next question.

Casting Without Tears

It may seem callous to you to look at fracture care as a game of chess, but looking at the casts that pass through a clinic make it clear that compassion is not guide enough. Skill is required to avoid common losing gambits such as this: an undisplaced fracture is encased in a lumpy, loose, unmolded cast. A few days later the edge of the cast is digging into the skin and has to be trimmed away; this is a sign that the cast is beginning to slip down. A little later a window is cut because the cast rubs where it touches; the fracture has displaced (Fig. 3-10).

Applying a cast to a conscious child, particularly a small chubby child, needs cunning. Get everything ready before having the child in the room; we keep

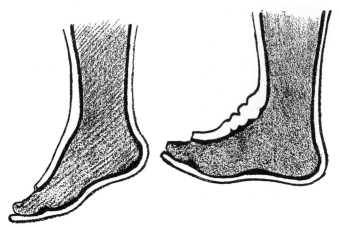

Fig. 3-11. Joints should be held in the correct position when plaster is applied to avoid pressure sores produced by wrinkles in the cast. The cast was applied with the foot in equinus, and then the position was corrected. (Calot, R.: Indispensible Orthopaedics. London, Balliere, Tindall & Cox, 1914)

scissors chained to the table, since this seems to be the only way to make them constantly available. Bring in the child and mother "to put a bandage on." Most children love to have a bandage on. Don't make the child lie down—he will surely scream and fight. Let him sit or stand. Always use padding. For children who are chubby put on Friar's balsam first to glue the padding and cast on. Roll the padding on evenly and snugly, particularly at the top where the cast always tends to become loose. Don't do this in silence. Use patter like a magician, to distract them from what you are doing. I usually talk to mother when the child is uncommunicative and ask if she has ever seen a cast go on before, recount how the plaster was first mined in Montmartre where there are extensive catacombs you can visit now. That Antonius Mathysen, a Dutch military surgeon, invented plaster bandages in 1851, though the Arabs long before used to put the limb in a box and fill it with liquid plaster. Rather heavy etc., etc. Standard patter has a great advantage over animated conversation, because the quality of the cast is inversely related to the quality of the conversation.

Wrap the plaster around evenly up and down, overlapping by half a bandage width so that the thickness of the cast is even. If you are putting on an above-elbow cast, hold the arm flexed to 90 or 100 degrees. Do not hold it flexed less than a right angle and then correct the position as the plaster is setting. It produces a ridge first and a plaster sore later. Similarly the position of the ankle and knee must be right before the first turn of plaster goes on (Fig. 3-11).

After applying one or two rolls of plaster the cast should be smoothed and shaped before more reinforcing

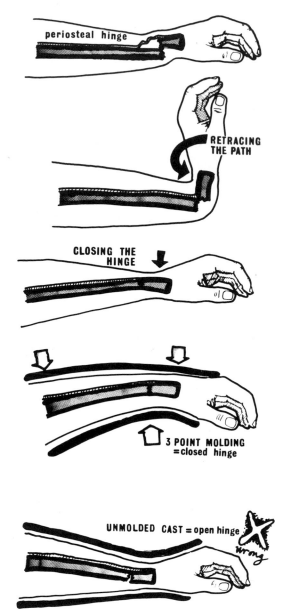

Fig. 3-12. *Three-point pressure casting.* (*A*) Displaced fracture—the hinge prevents reduction by traction. (*B*) Retracing the path. (*C*) Reduced—the hinge prevents over reduction. (*D*) A cast with three-point molding holds the hinge closed and the fracture reduced. (*E*) An unmolded cast may make the arm look straight, but it allows the hinge to open.

plaster is applied. In subsequent chapters the details will be considered. As the cast reaches the consistency of wet cardboard the time to mold has come. Use the flat of the hand or the thenar eminence, not the fingertips. The cast should not look like a limb, because you are trying to hold the bones, not the mobile muscle bellies and subcutaneous fat. Use three-point molding, so well described by John Charnley in *The Closed Treatment of Common Fractures* (Fig. 3-12). Many people try to use two-point molding—squeezing the cast at the site of the fracture—which does nothing for the fracture but effectively occludes the circulation.

When the cast has hardened, the edges should be neatly turned back to ensuring that the fingers have a full range of movement at the M.P.J., and then enough plaster should be applied, depending on your assessment of the character of the child, to forestall breakage. Draw the fracture and write the date on the cast using an indelible pencil so that, when the notes you have carefully made are lost, treatment can continue. Finally give mother a "plaster care sheet" telling her not to let the cast get wet, how she should recognize swelling of the limb inside the cast, and an appointment to come for a cast check the next day.

If your first cast is a good one, well-shaped and strong, it is unlikely that another will be required.

But some fractures will require reduction.

Did You Call that a Manipulation or a Reduction?

For the majority of children's fractures good alignment may be achieved by manipulation or by traction.

When Should Open Reduction be Employed?

There are situations where an open reduction is indicated *only when a closed reduction fails.* Fractures of both bones of the forearm in teenagers, fractures of the tibial spine, and fractures of the radial neck fall into this group. Some surgeons will operate on overlapping metaphyseal fractures of the distal radius and fractures

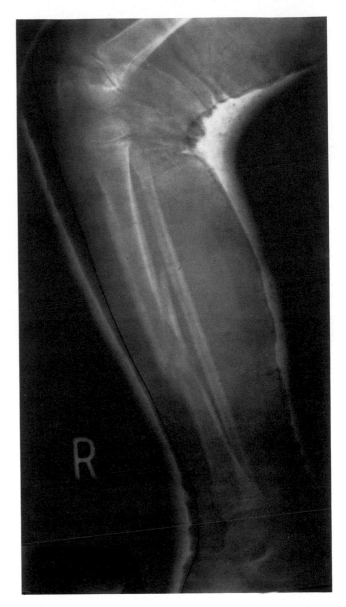

Fig. 3-14. The swelling has subsided and the cast is loose. A black line marks the surface of the skin. Always look at the fit of the cast on the radiograph.

of the proximal humerus, but it has been my experience that, armed with the correct technique of manipulation, open reduction is unnecessary. Open reduction is said to be hazardous in cases of epiphyseal separations that present late because of the danger of growth plate damage: osteotomy after healing is to be preferred.

Open reduction and internal fixation should be the *first choice* in displaced intraarticular fractures such as those of the lateral condyle of the humerus and femur, of the olecranon, and of the patella. Other fractures will also benefit from this approach, e.g., fracture dislocations of the talus and acromioclavicular fracture dislocations. Children with prolonged decerebrate ri-

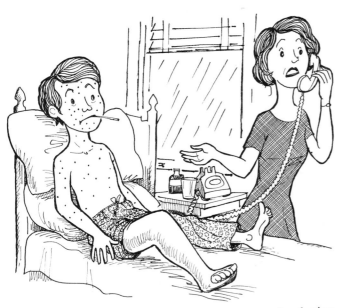

Fig. 3-13. Poor follow-up is a common cause of malunion.

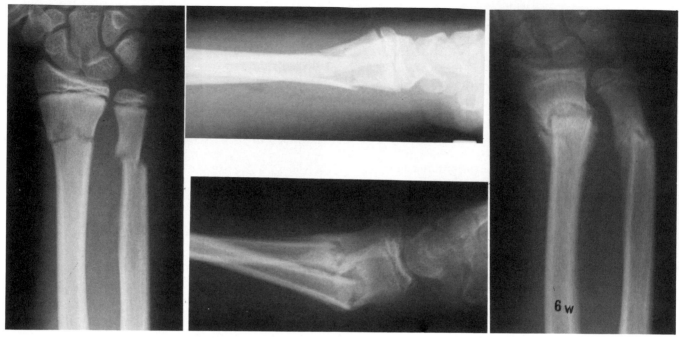

Fig. 3-15. A minimally displaced fracture of the distal forearm. He broke his cast and did not attend for follow-up. He heals with angulation. The new bone under the dorsal and radial hinges can be seen. These fractures require carefully molded casts to prevent this problem.

gidity and multiple injuries may benefit from nailing a fracture of the shaft of the femur.

TRAPS ARISING DURING TREATMENT

The general public are curiously stupid about fractures. They will believe, for example, that a nerve palsy first noticed after a cast is applied is due to the surgeon's manipulation and was not merely overlooked before the fracture was set. The public believe that if a fracture slips at 2 weeks and needs remanipulation that it is the surgeon's poor cast that has permitted slippage. They believe that the calcaneus limp, universal after the cast comes off a child with a fracture of the tibia, represents some error in treatment. They will think these things if you do not tell them about these events before they attract the parents' attention. *Try to tell the parents your plan for the total care of their child at the initial emergency consultation.* Repeat it later.

The wise surgeon should acquaint parents ahead of time with all the problems that are likely to occur. Certainly before he himself takes on treatment. In the 18th century, Heister stated that very clearly: "The surgeon should be very cautious offering his prognosis concerning fractures to avoid being called a knave or a fool."

The traps arising during the course of treatment can be avoided by adhering to the following principles.

1. Use Your Working Knowledge of the Various Complications to Look Deliberately for Them. Recognize nerve palsies before reduction. Recognize unstable fractures so that you apply casts that are paragons of molding. Recognize situations where your manipulation may fail so that the operating room is prepared for open reduction. Do not allow a child to wake up from a general anesthetic until you have radiographic proof that the fracture is in a satisfactory position. Remember that the acceptability of a reduction is inversely related to the ease with which you can alter the position.

2. Children are Only Uncooperative when There is Something Wrong. Regrettably, children are unable to tell you that skin, nerve, or muscle is undergoing necrosis. Instead, they weep or call for their mother or hide their head. Often reassurance works well and aspirin even better. Don't be fooled; split the cast widely or adjust the traction immediately. You do not want to have the experience that will enable you to talk about Volkmann's ischemic contracture at medical meetings.

Remember that pain goes when tissue dies; if you put your head in the sand until the pain goes away you will be too late. For the fracture surgeon hysteria does not exist until after the fracture has united.

3. Ensure that Your System of Follow-up Does not Permit Patients to be Lost (Fig. 3-13). Each year a few children do not return to our clinic for about a month after the fracture has been reduced. When they do appear and the radiograph on the viewing box shows malunion, this will be the moment that a colleague will wander into your clinic. Nothing you say will wholly extract you from this situation. Avoid it by calling back all fracture patients who fail to keep appointments.

4. Recognize a Loose Cast. A loose cast will allow a fracture to slip. If you can put your hand inside, if the cast telescopes up and down, if the radiograph shows an air gap (Fig. 3-14), change the cast.

Assess the quality of the cast on the radiograph. A cast that only fits in places should be replaced.

5. Recognize the Earliest Signs of Slip. When a fracture angulates slowly it is a sign that the cast is not maintaining three-point pressures. Change the cast to a better one to avoid gross angulation later (Fig. 3-15).

6. Talk to the Parents. If parents are a nuisance it is always your fault. You have not told them what to do or what to expect. Parents object to insufficient orders and not to too many. If you ask them to check the color of the digits every hour for the first night after reduction most parents would do this without complaint. But if a child refractures the arm during karate practice one day after coming out of a cast they will blame you. Tell them about cast care and your arrangements for cast repair. Tell them of the likely problems at the outset: the likelihood of remanipulation, stiffness, deformity, bumps of obvious callus, hairy legs in teenagers, limp. Warn them about growth arrest and avascular necrosis if these are real hazards, but do not tell everyone with an epiphyseal separation that this is a hazard, because it is not.

4

Fractures with Vascular Damage

On the battlefield arterial injuries come quickly, and the decision to expose the artery is already partly made. The amputation rate is only 13 percent because of prompt expert repair. For *closed* fractures with arterial damage the amputation rate is up to 50 percent because of late diagnosis.

The maximal permissible interval between injury and repair is about 6 to 8 hours, depending on the degree of arterial occlusion, the state of the collaterals, and shock. These 6 to 8 hours may pass quickly while the patient is given narcotics and a doctor is found to split the cast. The doctor *always* realizes there is trouble but seems unable to act immediately and decisively, hoping that the situation will miraculously improve. Slowly he comes to appreciate that hope is not enough and calls for an arteriogram or transfers the case to another hospital. Every minute should count, because invisible changes are taking place in the muscles and nerves of the limb. Yet in all the patients we have cared for, hours have been frittered away. Successful care comes from a high index of suspicion and early arterial repair. Successful care produces a normal limb; delay, a Volkmann's contracture or a gangrenous limb.

PHYSICAL SIGNS

Unfortunately, in the Emergency Room, a child with a fracture with ischemia is not startlingly different from a child with a simple fracture. A crying child, with his limb swathed in splints and bandages, and surrounded by distraught relations is not easily viewed with cold, clinical detachment. A quick squeeze of a protruding digit or nail bed for capillary filling is often considered sufficient to demonstrate an intact circulation. Demonstrate the fallacy of this sign next time you operate. Inflate the tourniquet before the limb is exsanguinated. Squeeze the digit: capillary return is still present. This test only indicates that blood is present in the limb, and not that it is circulating.

THE THREE FACES OF ARTERIAL OCCLUSION

If occlusion is not recognized on admission there is usually a considerable delay before anyone notices it. A child's ischemic pain may be borne stoically by the staff and attributed to fracture pain or clouded by opiate. Pulses are hidden by cast or traction so that observation is difficult. Remember that a splinted limb should be painless. *Pain after reduction should be attributed to ischemia until proven otherwise.* A special trap is painless ischemia in a child with a nerve palsy.

Complete Occlusion

The pulse is absent, the veins are empty, and in the course of an hour or two the limb becomes white and cold. Failure of nerve conduction produces glove and stocking anesthesia and paralysis. After a few more hours, rigor mortis results in the muscles shortening, and attempts to overcome this are painful. Pain is extreme. Later the skin becomes marbled, and gangrene follows.

Incomplete Occlusion—Compartment Ischemia

Ischemia of muscle, called Volkmann's ischemia (Fig. 4-1), is compatible with an intact pulse and adequate peripheral circulation. The first signs are pain in the muscle and pain on stretching the muscle. For this reason, we do not give any analgesic to children with fractures that have a reputation for vascular problems. If the flow in the main artery is reduced, there may be sufficient flow to maintain a pulse and distal circulation, but not sufficient to maintain perfusion through the muscle. The muscle becomes hypoxic and swells within a closed fascial compartment. Arterial inflow, capillary through-flow and venous outflow become occluded. The outcome of muscular ischemia is a Volkmann's contracture.

Compensated Occlusion

Not uncommon is the child with a supracondylar fracture who has an adequate distal circulation but no pulse (Fig. 4-2). The extremity may be a little cool, but there are no signs of nerve or muscle ischemia. Despite occlusion of the major artery, the collaterals maintain an adequate circulation. (The same effect is seen after a Blalock operation.) Apart from worrying and ordering an hourly check on sensation and movement, there is nothing special to do. Arteriography and exploration are meddlesome. Within a few weeks the pulse returns, and I have yet to see a child with claudication.

Sites of Fracture Associated with Vascular Damage

While any fracture carries the hazard of vascular damage, the problem is most likely in supracondylar fractures, elbow dislocations, fractures of the shaft of the femur, especially the distal one-third (Fig. 4-3), fractures of the proximal tibia, grossly-displaced fractures of the ankle and talus, and mid-tarsal dislocations.

The Nature of the Arterial Lesion

The incidence of arterial damage, as distinct from ischemia, in fractures is not known. As one mother of a child with arterial damage put it, perhaps all children with fractures should have an arteriogram. Only by this radical experiment would we know the incidence of arterial damage.

Lesions in Discontinuity. There is complete transsection of the vessel.

Lesions in Continuity. *Intimal lesions.* Intimal tears and contusions can only be diagnosed with confidence by arteriotomy. The distal part of the vessel is empty and stringlike. The condition is indistinguishable from spasm until intima is inspected.

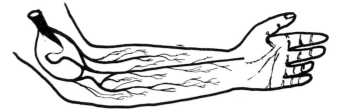

Fig. 4-2. Compensated occlusion. Anastomotic channels maintain perfusion at low pressure and sufficient to sustain the tissue but insufficient to produce a pulse at the wrist. The pulsations have been abolished but the flow remains. If an eponym had been attached to this condition it would be diagnosed frequently.

Spasm. Traction has been shown experimentally to produce spasm. Application of this observation has reduced the incidence of Volkmann's ischemia in fractures of the femoral shaft (see p. 176). However, in the

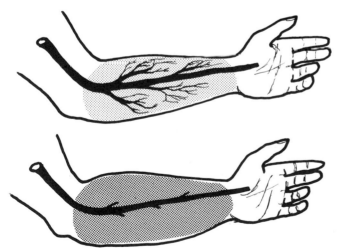

Fig. 4-1. Volkmann's ischemia. (*A*) Normally the pressure in the brachial artery is 120 mm. Hg. Muscle is perfused at a pressure of 30 mm. Hg. (*B*) Muscle ischemia. If the pressure within the muscle compartment is raised above 30 mm. Hg, muscle will not be perfused, but the radial pulse is *not necessarily* occluded.

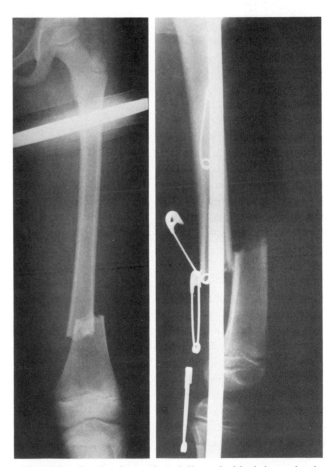

Fig. 4-3. In the hour that followed this injury the leg became cold, white, anesthetic, and weak. The pulse was absent. After the fracture was reduced under general anesthesia the veins became full, the foot warm and pink. The pulse did not return for several weeks. The femoral artery passes through the adductor opening at this site, where it is liable to injury.

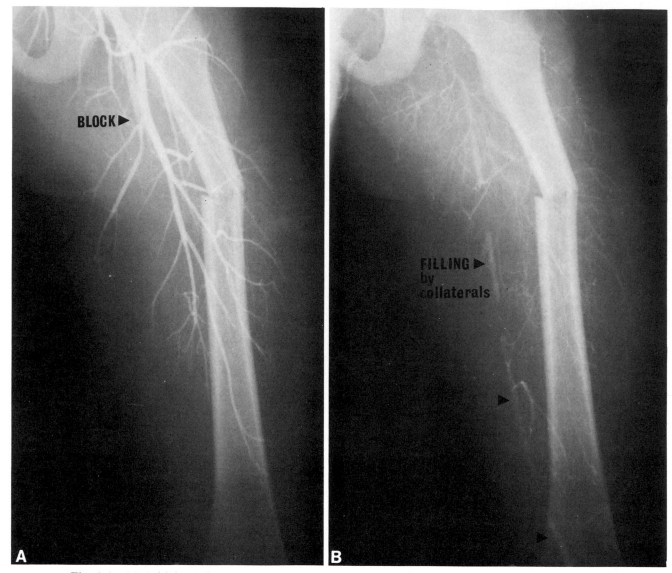

Fig. 4-4. (*A*) Initial arteriogram made 15 hours after injury shows a complete block in the superficial femoral artery. (*B*) At a later phase the superficial femoral artery fills slowly (*cont. on facing page*)

past, the importance of spasm has been greatly overplayed at the cost of many limbs.

Compression. The commonest causes of ischemia are undoubtedly tight casts and deformity at the fracture site. Release the cast or align the limb, and the circulation comes bounding back. Kinking and stretching of vessels has been convincingly demonstrated after high tibial osteotomy.

Thrombosis. Prolonged occlusion due to any cause will produce propagating thrombosis.

MANAGEMENT

Prevention

Traction, tight casts, excessive flexion of a swollen elbow, and hypotension all produce ischemia in the absence of an arterial injury at the time of fracture. Be vigilant, be quick, and be decisive. If you are lucky, removing bandages, bivalving the cast, and placing the limb in a dependent position may be enough to improve circulation. If you are the resident, get on and do this, don't call your chief first, however precious the patient or the reduction.

Treatment of Ischemia

If the circulation does not improve in 5 minutes, you must make very many preparations to take the child to the operating room immediately. As soon as diagnosis of ischemia is reached, it is obviously a matter of extreme urgency, and you must not be put off by any other service commitments nor by anesthetists telling

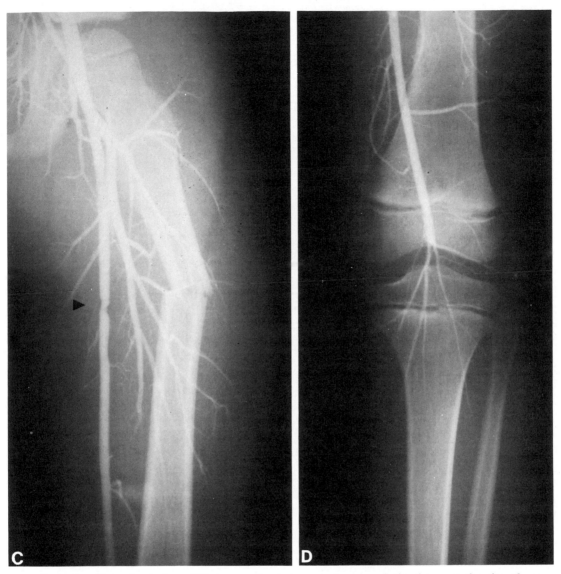

through collateral arteries. (*C*) A second arteriogram shows an intimal tear at the site of the arrow. (*D*) Ischemia is due to a clot at the popliteal trifurcation.

you that the child has a full stomach. You should carry out surgery with the help of a vascular surgeon. However, in civilian practice vascular surgeons do not have much experience with this problem, and you should not look to him to make all the decisions. His greatest experience is in the treatment of vascular disease in the elderly.

Treatment may include:

Arteriography. Arteriography is only of value if it can be carried out immediately: do not waste time rounding up staff. Arteriography always takes at least an hour, whatever you are told, and in most cases *this time could be better spent relieving ischemia.* It will demonstrate the site of occlusion, although it will probably not disclose the type of lesion. The site of occlusion is usually opposite the fracture site. Arteriography may be of medicolegal value. In one recent case, I

suspected that the cause of ischemia may have been tight bandaging, however, the arteriogram showed an intimal tear opposite the fracture site.

Jim, aged 8, was used to bicycles with "back pedal" brakes. He went down the hill on his friend's bike so quickly that he was unable to master the brakes on the handlebars. Jim hit a truck, fracturing the left femur. The circulation was unremarkable and he was placed in traction. The following morning the leg was found to be white, anesthetic, and cold. An arteriogram showed obstruction of the superficial femoral artery (Fig. 4-4A). At a later phase the distal part of the artery filled slowly through collaterals (Fig. 4-4B). Had distal run-off been better, the artery would have filled better through the collaterals. The appearances indicate a block in the femoral artery with a distal compartment syndrome.

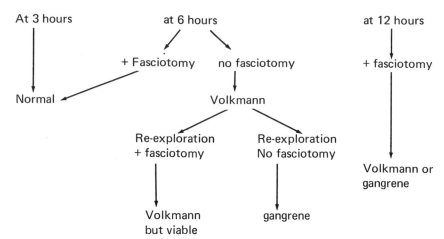

Fig. 4-5. Expectations of arterial repair for complete ischemia.

A femoral arteriotomy in the groin was carried out; Fogarty catheters were passed beyond the popliteal artery, and the clot was removed. Subcutaneous fasciotomy of three compartments of the leg was carried out. The skin became warm and pink, but the pulse did not return.

Thirty-six hours later the circulation deteriorated and the leg looked like white marble. It looked like the end. Another arteriogram (Fig. 4-4C) showed an intimal tear at the fracture site and a block at the popliteal trifurcation (Fig. 4-4D). The leg was laid open through a Henry approach from groin to ankle. The medial head of the gastrocnemius and the tibial attachment of the soleus were divided to reveal the entire vascular tree. After excision of the damaged section of the femoral artery, Fogarty catheters were passed under vision to the ankle through the anterior and posterior tibial arteries.

The artery was anastomosed. All four compartments were decompressed (revealing the inadequacy of subcutaneous fasciotomies). The skin was left open. The circulation was no better. Myringotomies were carried out, and the boy began a series of dives in the hyperbaric chamber. Heparin was administered. After each dive the color of the foot improved.

The back of the leg was closed with skin grafts at 5 days. The fracture was managed in a hip spica throughout because it was longitudinally stable. At 8 weeks the fracture was united and the cast was removed. Dressings were still needed because dead muscle was extruding. He began walking in running shoes.

Six months after injury Jim had anesthesia from mid-calf downwards and about 30 degrees of equinus. A year later sensation had returned but paresthesiae were a problem. A posterior release was performed and neurolysis of the posterior tibial nerve. The skin grafts were excised. The paresthesias disappeared immediately. He walks normal distances but with a marked limp, because most of the muscle below the knee has been destroyed.

This is a typical story. Ideally arterial damage should be recognized early and repaired before irreversible complications occur.

Exploration, Fasciotomy, or Both? Fasciotomy alone is indicated when you have no doubt that the artery is intact and that a compartment syndrome alone requires decompression. The circulation to the digits must be normal. Anterior compartment syndrome complicating a mid-tibial fracture is an example.

Exploration of the vessel is indicated in all other circumstances. If the lag between injury and repair is more than 4 to 6 hours, repair should be followed by complete fasciotomy of all compartments, including the carpal tunnel. Muscle that has been ischemic will swell when the circulation is restored. If you omit fasciotomy the circulation will soon wane again.

Treatment of the Arterial Lesion. Direct inspection is the only certain way to determine the nature of the lesion. For this reason we expose the vessel widely through one of Henry's extensile exposures. The effectiveness of repair can be judged, the extent of muscle damage can be discerned, and wide fasciotomy may be carried out.

Lesions in continuity. When the artery is constricted at the level of the fracture an intimal tear or contusion is most likely. A segment of artery is excised between bulldog clamps. The proximal end is flushed out. The distal part is dilated and cleared of thrombus with a Fogarty catheter, which is pushed down to the wrist or ankle through each major branch of the artery. These vessels are flushed with heparinized saline to clear any loose thrombus. Back flow should be seen. End to end suture is undertaken if this can be done without tension; otherwise, insert a reversed saphenous graft.

When an artery remote from the fracture site becomes narrow, spasm is the cause. Insert a Fogarty catheter through a proximal arteriotomy to dilate the artery and remove clots. Wash out until back flow is seen, and then close the arteriotomy.

NOTE: Papaverine and segmental dilation are ineffective, outmoded, and a waste of time.

Lesions in discontinuity. Excise the segments, wash out, and anastomose or graft.

Fasciotomy. Subcutaneous fasciotomy is quick and easy. It leaves little scar and does not decompress the deep flexor compartments (Fig. 4-6). For this reason open fasciotomy is mandatory. In the leg, all four compartments must be opened—anterior, peroneal, superficial, and deep posterior. Anterior and posterior incisions are used. Fasciotomy-fibulectomy has been advised in adults but is likely to produce a growth deformity of the ankle in children. In the arm the deep flexors require decompression.

Do not excise any muscle at this time. It is impossible to distinguish the sick from the dead. After arterial repair and fasciotomy distal pulses should become palpable and the veins should fill. The skin can never be closed after fasciotomy, because the muscle has swelled. Cover the extensive wound with tulle, and rejoice that compression is relieved.

Care of the Fracture. Is internal fixation the ideal method? The Vietnam experience suggests that it only adds to morbidity because of infection and nonunion. Our experience is very small, but for children who have not been injured on the battlefield we favor internal fixation whenever possible, because traction may pull the anastomosis apart and does not fit into a hyperbaric chamber, and because a cast prevents examination of the entire limb.

Postoperative Heparin. Subsequent thrombosis may ruin an initially good result; use heparin. As the circulation improves, the ends of severed vessels may begin to bleed and require tying off. This is more likely than bleeding due to carefully controlled heparin administration.

Hyperbaric Oxygen. The effect of hyperbaric oxygen can be dramatic in children. If this facility is available, it should be employed. As soon as the patient has regained consciousness following exploration, he should start a course of dives. A myringotomy is usually required in children to prevent ruptured ear drums, and an ear, nose and throat surgeon should be encouraged to do this whilst you are exploring the artery. It is only a minute's work. Do not be disappointed if the limb does not pink up after the first dive. Order a minimum of three dives before coming to any decision.

Complications. Because thrombosis affects 20 percent of repairs, the circulation must be closely watched in the intensive care unit. At the first sign of failure the vessel must be explored once again and the thrombus removed.

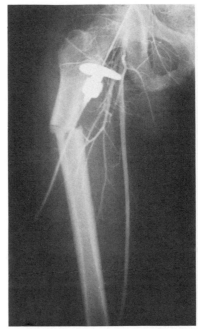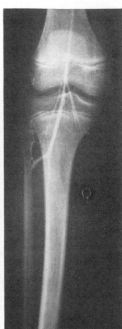

Fig. 4-6. This girl fell out of a tree. She almost died during the next 12 hours because of hypotension from a ruptured spleen and a hemothorax. The fractured femur was placed in skin traction. The combination of muscle hypoxia due to hypotension and somewhat tight bandaging produced a white, anesthetic leg. Arteriogram shows no damage at the fracture site but complete vascular occlusion caused by compartment compression. All compartments were opened, and the arteries were dilated with Fogarty catheters.

Note-Keeping and Public Relations. Parents of children in whom ischemia is noticed late usually believe that this catastrophe is somebody's fault, and often they are right. These cases usually go to litigation. Keep scrupulous notes; every time you see the child, record your findings and note the time. Put down everything, nothing is too insignificant to note. In all probability, you will rely on these notes in court. You or your colleague will need all the help that only pages and pages of notes will provide.

At every stage you would be wise to take photographs, and to request your colleagues' advice. Not only may this be helpful, but their written notes may be useful as well. If the case is referred to you, you should keep in touch with the original doctor. Do not jump to the conclusion that it is all his fault. Do not write inspired opinions about the quality of his care. If you do, you will usually be wrong, and certainly damage not only his reputation but also your own. If the question of negligence arises in your mind, you will be wise to notify your Medical Protective Society.

The Aftermath

In a few days, you will know whether a normal limb

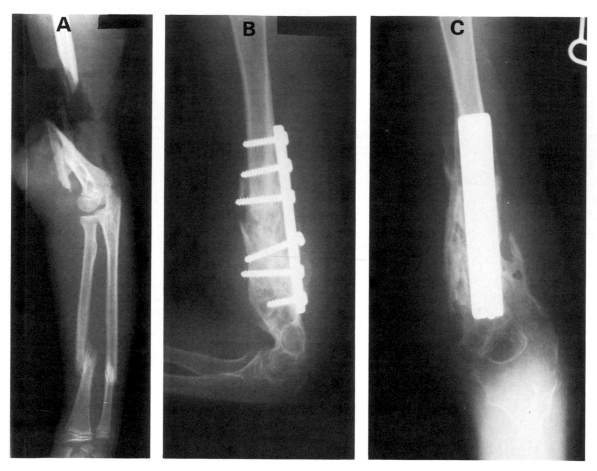

Fig. 4-7. (*A*) A spin drier in a laundromat produced this injury. (*B, C*) Two years later. (See text)

may be expected or whether amputation or reconstruction will be required. The reward of early repair will be a normal limb. Wet gangrene usually requires early amputation and secondary suture. In children it is worth skin-grafting a stump in order to preserve length, and, in particular, to save a knee joint.

RECONSTRUCTION OF A DAMAGED LIMB

After a week the fasciotomy bed is formed by young granulations on living muscle; a skin graft should be performed to cover the defect. When there is much necrotic muscle, this must be removed by dressing changes and excision before a skin graft is used to cover the defect. Usually necrotic muscle separates through a sinus in the graft for several weeks.

While the limb is anesthetic and the fracture un-united, it is wrong to try to correct contracture very energetically. Pressure sores and screams are the only results. Discourage the effects of gravity aggravating the contracture, and allow the physiotherapist to prevent joint stiffness, but no more. As sensation returns, pain-

ful, tingling, hyperesthesia may be a problem. If the incident of ischemia is short-lived, producing only neuropraxia, sensation returns within a week or two. Severe ischemia may result in axonotmesis, so that sensation returns at the rate of 1 inch a month, or not at all.

Leg. When the fracture is united, a below-knee brace with a sheepskin liner in the boot may be needed to control the paralyzed ankle, discourage contracture, and protect the anesthetic foot. Walking definitely wards off contracture. If the child is laid up in bed for any reason, the contracture will increase dramatically in a few days if frequent stretching is not carried out.

Arm. Keep the fingers and wrist splinted to prevent flexor shortening as much as possible.

In the succeeding months reconstruction will be required. In the arm excision of the infarct and tendon transfers are indicated. The leg is simpler because contractures can be released by tendon lengthening.

A triple arthrodesis may be necessary later to stabilize the foot. However, in children, I have been surprised by the remarkable degree of muscle power than can return, even when large volumes of muscle are known to have been destroyed. Some children come to amputation late because a stiff, deformed, anesthetic foot is heir to repeated trophic ulcers. The amputation flap should be specially fashioned to preserve the area of skin with sensation. This should be mapped out accurately, using a pen, immediately before operation.

THE SEVERED LIMB

A severed limb is a challenge most of us could do without. My only experience was with a boy who twisted his arm off in a laundry wringer, perhaps the commonest cause of this injury today (Fig. 4-7). Four hours after the accident, he was admitted to hospital with the arm hanging on by three bruised nerves and a strip of skin. He had a circumferential wound around the elbow at the site of a humeral fracture, and fractures of the radius and ulna. His vessels were completely severed. The vascular, orthopaedic, and plastic surgeons joined together to repair the arm. The distal vessels were flushed with heparin and saline until they ran clear. This helped identify the vein. The humerus was shortened slightly, and fixed quickly with a plate. Next the large veins were repaired with a saphenous graft. The artery was repaired with saphenous graft, and blood flow was established again about 6 hours after the injury. The radius was held with an intramedullary Kirschner wire, and this provided the opportunity to carry out a fasciotomy. The skin was partly closed with sutures and partly with "silon" sheet. The boy was transferred to the hyperbaric oxygen chamber on anticoagulants. To our surprise, he moved his fingers the following day and had no edema. He showed no sign of ischemic contracture; indeed, the hand became perfect. The humeral fracture required grafting for nonunion, and then he regained full elbow movement.

The results of replantation of limbs depends particularly on nerve regeneration. The procedure is more likely to succeed in children than adults and if the limb is only partially severed as in the case described above. Reattachment is worthwhile for uncrushed injuries up to about 6 hours from time of severance.

The Chinese have recently popularized microvascular techniques for replacing severed limbs and severed digits. Such striking results have been demonstrated that it would seem useful for large centers to have one or two people on staff to whom these problems may be referred.

In closing, remember that some limbs with vascular damage are so severely injured initially that immediate amputation is the right answer.

BIBLIOGRAPHY

Ernst, C. N. and Kauffer, H.: Fibulectomy-fasciotomy. J. Trauma, *11:* 365, 1971

Galasko, C. S. B.: Spin dryer injuries. Brit. Med. J., *4:* 646, 1972

Haas, L. M. and Staple, T. W.: Arterial injuries associated with fractures of the proximal tibia following blunt trauma. South. Med. J., *62:* 1439, 1969

Makin, G. S., Howard, J. M., and Green, R. L.: Arterial injuries complicating fractures or dislocations: the necessity for a more aggressive approach. Surgery, *59:* 203, 1966

Mustard, W. T., and Simmons, E. H.: Experimental arterial spasm in the lower extremity produced by traction. J. Bone Joint Surg., *35B:* 437, 1953

Rich, N. M., Baugh, J. H., and Hughes, C. W.: Acute arterial injuries in Vietnam: 1,000 cases. J. Trauma, *10:* 359, 1970

Rich, N. M., Metz, C. W., Hutton, J. E., Baugh, J. H., and Hughes, C. W.: Internal versus external fixation of fractures with concomitant vascular injuries in Vietnam. J. Trauma, *11:* 463, 1971

Rorabeck, C. H., Macnab, I., and Waddell, J. P.: Anterior tibial compartment syndrome: a clinical and experimental review. Can. J. Surg., *15:* 249, 1972

Seddon, H. J.: Volkmann's contracture: treatment by excision of the infarct. J. Bone Joint Surg., *38B:* 152, 1956

———: Volkmann's ischemia in the lower leg. J. Bone Joint Surg., *48B:* 627, 1966

Steel, H. H., Sandrow, R. E., and Sullivan, P. D.: Complications of tibial osteotomy in children for genus varum or valgum. Evidence that neurological changes are due to ischemia. J. Bone Joint Surg., *53A:* 1629, 1971

Thompson, S. A. and Mahoney, L. J.: Volkmann's ischemic contracture and its relationship to fracture of the femur. J. Bone Joint Surg., *33B:* 336, 1951

White, J. C.: Nerve regeneration after replantation of severed arms. Ann. Surg., *170:* 715, 1969

5

Fractures in Special Circumstances

Most fractures run a predictable course. Sometimes there are special circumstances that cannot be ignored. In this chapter, a potpourri of these conditions will be described.

THE BATTERED CHILD

Although assault has been a criminal offense for centuries when directed towards adults, it has only in the last hundred years been considered an offense when directed against children. The first action brought on behalf of a battered child took place in New York City in 1870. Mary Ellen was being beaten daily by her parents. Attempts to correct this situation by appeals to the police and District Attorney's office were unsuccessful. Eventually an action was brought by the American Society for Prevention of Cruelty to Animals, which succeeded because Mary Ellen was certainly a member of the animal kingdom and was being cruelly used.

Today child abuse is a major pediatric problem affecting about 225 children per million of population. Two to 3 percent of abused children die; the mortality rate of battering is equal to that of leukemia.

Each year The Hospital for Sick Children in Toronto treats about 100 battered children. The frequency of child battering is three times as great as that of congenital dislocation of the hip, or of clubfoot.

Recognition of Battering

Battered children may come to hospital with head injuries, or visceral injuries, or fractures, or bruises, or with all of them. The special features are as follows:

Multiple Injuries Over a Period of Time. Some fractures are new and some are old. Infants commonly sustain Type I epiphyseal separations. If these are manipulated every day, a characteristic appearance is produced (Fig. 5-1). A skeletal survey is mandatory; it may show healed rib fractures with more recent limb injuries (Fig. 5-2).

Though these radiographic appearances are diagnostic and much used as illustrations, it should be realized that they are unusual. *Most* battered children have fractures indistinguishable from those produced by a motor vehicle (Fig. 5-3).

Evasive Explanations. "He must have fallen out of his crib." "He fell downstairs three days ago." Considerate parents bring their children right away when

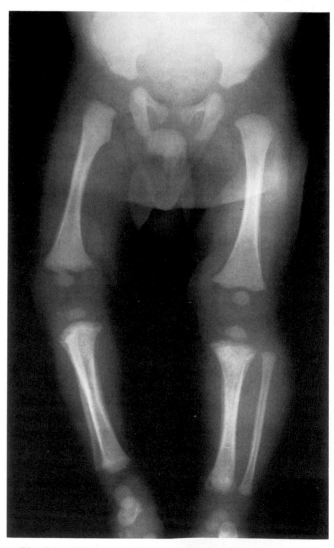

Fig. 5-1. The corner fracture, the ring of new bone at the growth plate, and subperiosteal new bone are characteristic of child abuse of the chronic variety. Boy aged 18 months.

Fig. 5-6. Pathologica
ture through a bone cyst
aged 12. Despite cui
and bone grafting twic
cyst has recurred. Thou
bone has not fractured
the cyst remains a threa

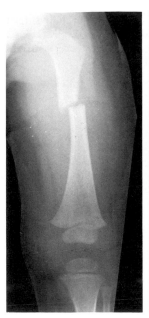 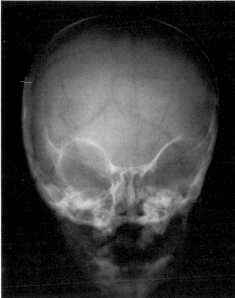 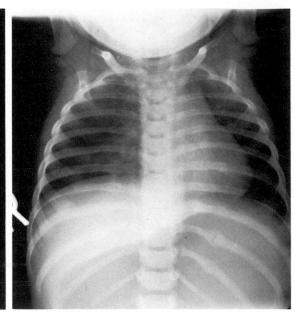

Fig. 5-2. The femoral fracture is fresh. If it were the only injury it would not raise the radiologist's suspicion. However, skull and healing rib fractures make the diagnosis of child abuse certain.

cious explanation.
were the culprits; wh
found out (Fig. 5-4).
cases where infants v
these killings were di

PATHOLC

By definition, a pa
weak bone of abnorm
causes of pathology.

Local Bone Lesions

Simple Bone Cyst.
upper humerus are
displacement is the r
made on the radiolc

The presence of th
ing, and the fractur
present. Because th
uncomplicated, and
whether the bone w
to function normall
fracture before offe
operation should be
a fracture, in order
site.

Neer found that
three refractures aft
had some deformity
of 42 did not com
advocates surgery in
reoperation because
should be carried c
avoid an unsightly s

Bone cysts occasio

they are hurt, and they are sure of the cause of injury. In fact few children who fall do themselves any harm. Levin studied 100 infants who fell (and these were only the falls that alarmed mother) and not one gave cause for concern.

Admission Desired. Mother is generally the guilty party, and father has known about it. When the child is obviously hurt, father wants the child admitted.

Lack of Tenderness. Parents are gentle as they handle an injured child. "Battering" parents handle him like a sack of potatoes and are oblivious of his cries. Once in an interview I asked the parents, "Is he a good boy?" "No, he is very bad." "What do you do when he is bad?"

Father grabbed the boy's arm—his thumb fit exactly a large bruise on the boy's arm—and shook his fist at him.

History of Previous Obvious Injuries. Some children are already known to the Children's Aid Societies because of family problems. Others have been seen in emergency departments before. This information is difficult to obtain but sometimes emerges later.

Management

A high index of suspicion is warranted. Statistics indicate that 10 percent of all injuries in children under the age of 2 years are due to battery, and 25 percent of all fractures in children under the age of 3 years. The doctor should approach all fractures in this age group as due to battery until he has been convinced

otherwise. In Ontario and many other places the doctor is required by law to inform the Children's Aid Society whenever he has a *suspicion* of child abuse. This law protects not only the child and siblings from further injury but the doctor from legal proceedings.

Whether or not the injury itself demands admission, the child should be admitted for protection and to provide time for investigation. The family must be understood; the child must be examined and tested to exclude scurvy, rickets, bleeding disorder, pseudarthrosis of the

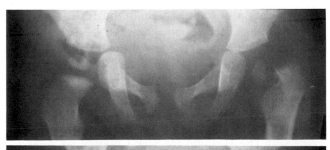

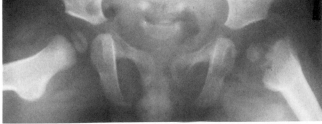

Fig. 5-3. Separated upper femoral epiphysis. Knowledge of the family background raised the family doctor's suspicions. Boy aged 11 months.

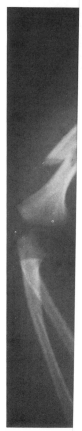

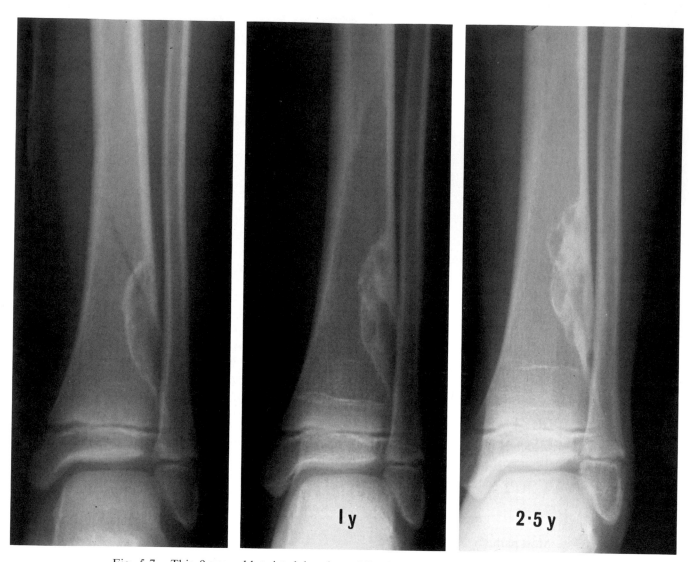

Fig. 5-7. This 9-year-old twisted her leg while skating. The fibrous cortical defect obliterates first at the fracture line and later the whole defect becomes filled with new bone.

tibia and b
in a strange
the parents
sel. The s
cumstances
able to alle
munity res
and may pt
an organiza

If a child
be charged
home; but
child is bet
ent home,

Social w
to refer ca:
doubt. At
cases to a
Children's
been forme
treatment
doctor has
ist," and w
velop.

The Battei

A 6-wee

no special care. The fracture usually spells the end of ambulation, however (Fig. 5-9).

Cerebral Palsy. Fractures in children with cerebral palsy are uncommon. Their bones are strong. It is only after immobilization in the cast that they become weakened enough to fracture. Routine care is generally effective. However, in bedfast patients, particularly those with contractures and convulsions, there are frequent fractures. Very simple methods of treatment are needed for these patients, because pressure sores are difficult to avoid.

Spina Bifida and Paraplegia. Diagnosis is often delayed when a fracture occurs in an anesthetic part of the lower limb. The surgeon is confronted with a swollen, hot, red limb in a child with a slight fever—symptoms that simulate acute osteomyelitis. This clinical picture is not peculiar to spina bifida; it may occur in

a battered child or a stoic who walks on a fractured ankle. Fracture is very common after operation and cast immobilization; supracondylar and trochanteric fractures of the femur are so common after hip surgery that I warn the parents to expect them.

Rapid healing is the rule. Commonly, hyperplastic callus is seen (Fig. 5-10). There is no single explanation for the massive volume of callus; repeated movement, unspecified neural influence on bone formation, and hyperphosphatemia are possible reasons.

Treatment should be simple and carefully supervised. Remember that a child with a shunt should not be put head-down in traction. Overriding is seldom a problem because of flaccid paralysis. It is important to maintain alignment and rotation correctly. We generally use bulky dressings for a period of 2 weeks, in order to avoid the problem of pressure sores. An early return to brace-wearing for the tibia, or a well-padded weight-bearing cast, is advised in order to prevent further disuse osteoporosis and a succession of fractures.

General Bone Disease. Fractures in osteopetrosis and osteogenesis imperfecta are common. Displacement is usually slight, and there is much to be said for simple splinting. Air splints have been advocated for osteogenesis imperfecta (Figs. 5-11, 5-12).

FRACTURES IN SPECIAL GROUPS OF PATIENTS

Head Injuries with Long Bone Fractures

When a child is hit by a car, Waddell's triad of injuries is commonly produced. A child's femur is at the level of the bumper; his trunk is at the level of the hood; he may receive a blow to the head on landing on the road (Fig. 5-13).

Fractures of the femur and the shaft of the humerus can be difficult to manage in restless, recumbent children. If the head injury is minor and expected to clear in a day or two, the fracture should be immobilized by simple splinting in a Thomas leg- or arm splint until routine methods may be employed. Fat embolism may be blamed for prolonged unconsciousness if this is not done.

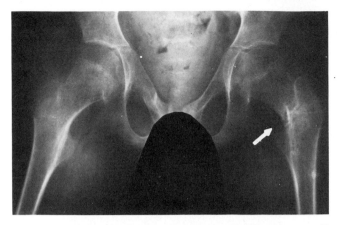

Fig. 5-9. At 10 years of age Laurie was barely able to walk because of muscular dystrophy. He was seen 2 weeks after sustaining this fracture. It had not displaced and he was nursed at home. The fracture healed *in situ,* but he did not walk again.

When decerebration is likely to be prolonged beyond a few days, we use 90-90 traction for the femur, or intramedullary fixation, depending on the degree of restlessness and the extent of other injuries. Fracture of the shaft of the humerus is treated by vertical skeletal traction through the olecranon.

Fluorothane "shakes" when anesthesia is discontinued makes the bones overlap. If you add extra weight to the traction to prevent this, be sure to remove them in a short time, so that a traction injury to the nerves will be avoided when the shakes stop.

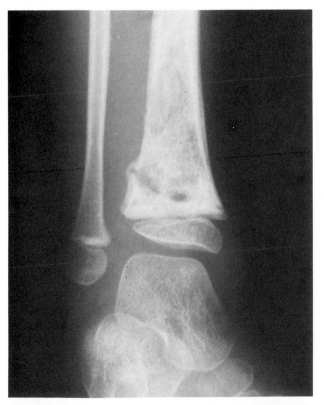

Fig. 5-8. Healing osteomyelitis should be protected to prevent fracture. Girl aged 3½ years.

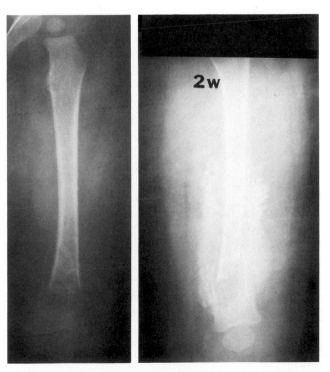

Fig. 5-10. Hyperplastic callus in paraplegia due to meningomyelocele in a child aged 1 year.

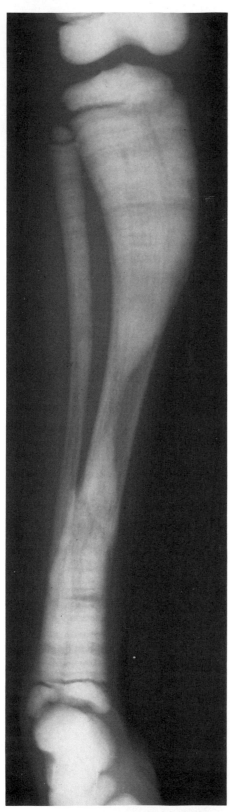

Fig. 5-11. Fracture due to osteopetrosis in a girl of 8 years. This family of affected children sustain frequent fractures.

Fractures in the Newborn

The literature is full of birth injuries of every type,

a sad reflection on obstetric care. We see very few nowadays, except in babies with fragile bones or with contractures. Any injury may be produced: long bone fractures are easily recognized, but separations of unossified epiphysis present a challenge to diagnosis. Truesdall, in 1917, analyzed 33,000 deliveries for skeletal injury and found 85 injured children. These were no greenstick fractures, and only 10 percent were epiphyseal separations. The humerus and clavicle were most commonly fractured, and a Velpeau bandage controlled these well. Fractures of the midshaft of the femur accounted for 12 percent, and traction was required to prevent gross overriding and anterior angulation (Fig. 5-14).

Spinal cord injury may be produced by longitudinal traction, resulting in "floppiness." Radiographic changes are usually absent. This is discussed further in the section on spinal cord injuries.

Hemophilia

A well-controlled hemophiliac today is free of crippling deformities and can lead quite an adventurous life. Fractures present no special problem if cryoprecipitate is administered. Fractures heal at the normal rate.

The child should be admitted and a careful watch kept for a few days. While the fracture may produce no problems, the neighboring joint may have been injured slightly at the time of fracture; one boy with no circulating A.H.G. had repeated hemoarthrosis of the knee following cast immobilization for a fracture of the tibia.

A greater risk than fractures, which provoke immediate attention, is a slow bleed into a closed compartment, which results in Volkmann's contracture. This obviously demands urgent decompression.

Renal Osteodystrophy and Rickets

Children waiting for a kidney transplant may develop profound osteodystrophy. A slow slip of the upper femoral epiphysis should be pinned as soon as it is noted. Dialysis is no bar to anesthesia (Figs. 5-15, 5-16).

STRESS FRACTURES

The commonest sites of stress fracture in children are the upper third of the tibia, the lower half of the fibula, followed by metatarsal, rib, pelvis, femur, and humerus. They are particularly common in the spring when children become active after a winter of inactivity. The radiographic appearance may be confused with a neoplasm or an infection, but the distinction is usually clear. If the diagnosis is in doubt, serial radio-

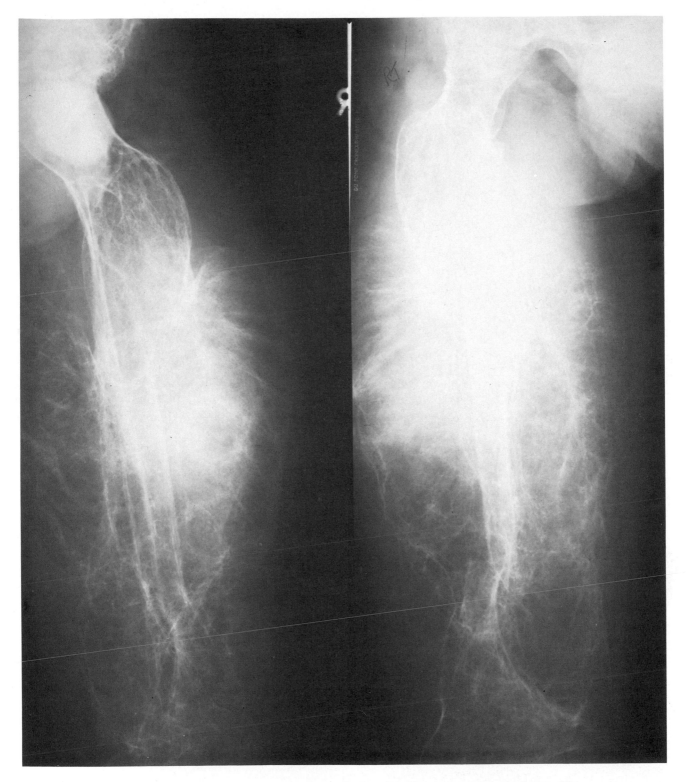

Fig. 5-12. An extreme example of hyperplastic callus in osteogenesis imperfecta. This phenomenon has only been noted in association with dislocation of the radial head.

graphs should be obtained over a short period of time (Fig. 5-17). A bone scan will demonstrate a stress fracture earlier than a radiograph.

Abstinence from sport may be sufficient treatment, but a cast is helpful if a child is wild, if pain is marked, or if the fracture looks as if it may become complete. All stress fractures of the femoral neck should be immobilized.

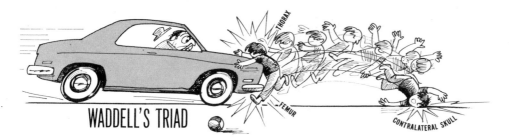

Fig. 5-13. Waddell's Triad of injuries in children.

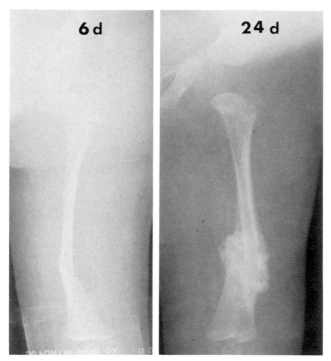

Fig. 5-14. There was difficulty bringing down the leg in this breech delivery.

LUCKY BREAKS

In a child with fixed deformities a fracture will sometimes provide a serendipitous opportunity for straightening the limb (Fig. 5-18).

SECOND-HAND CASES

Both mother and father come in. "We are very concerned, doctor. Joe broke his arm and we took him to Elsewhere General Hospital where they set it. He came out of the cast last week. Now look at it. He can't move it, and it is not straight."

The care of a healing fracture is quite different from that of a fresh fracture. You will need the tact and delicacy of a diplomat—qualities not usually first in the orthopaedic firmament—and the skill of a technocrat. The choice lies between awaiting natural improvement, late osteotomy, or immediate correction.

Diplomatic Considerations

Everyone treating fractures will leave some patients

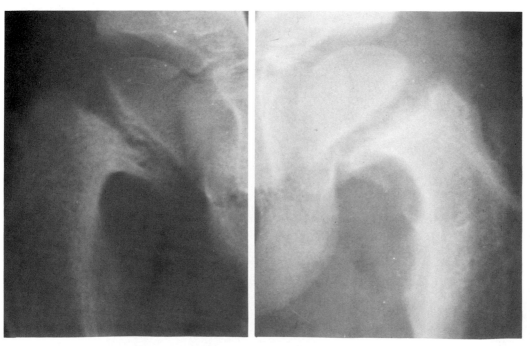

Fig. 5-15. Leon was on dialysis at the age of 14. Control of his metabolic bone disease had become increasingly difficult. These radiographs were taken because he developed a waddling gait. The hip was pinned *in situ;* he has had a renal transplant and he has a good functional result.

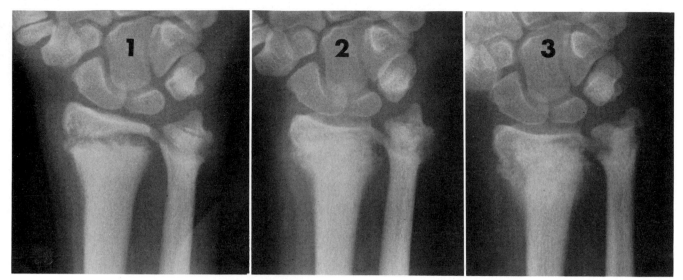

Fig. 5-16. (*1*) Vitamin D-resistant rickets. This child was receiving insufficient vitamin D. (*2*) A slight fall produced a pathological epiphyseal separation. The dosage of vitamin D was increased. (*3*) At 2 months the separation has healed.

with crooked limbs (though some doctors have more than others). Therefore do not deride the other doctor; rather, communicate with him. Seek the reason. Perhaps the child was not brought for follow-up examination, or he may have repeatedly broken the cast.

Most parents have no concept of the difficulties of fracture care, and when these are explained they may lose their anger, especially if you offer a positive course of future action.

Technical Considerations

When a limb comes out of a cast, muscle wasting and stiffness detract from its appearance. Ask yourself: will it improve, stay the same, or get worse? Several factors should be taken into consideration.

Age of Patient. In the young, remodelling is more effective, but the effects of growth disturbance are more harmful.

Age and Site of Fracture. Between 6 weeks and 3 months after the accident, when most of these problems present, it is not difficult to refracture the bone, either by closed means or by drill osteotomy. Secondary changes are few, and normal anatomy can be restored.

Angulation. Angulation in the plane of joint movement will improve spontaneously. Valgus, varus, and rotatory malunion should be corrected, but generally, there is no urgency about this, and osteotomy may wisely be postponed to the school vacation. However, a forearm angulation should be corrected as soon as possible, because remodelling and secondary joint changes adversely affect late repair.

Shortening. Excessive shortening is most common in the femur, owing to overlapping or angulation. One inch of discrepancy is dramatic in a 3-year-old, but improvement can be expected because of postfracture overgrowth, and increase in height. If the final discrepancy will be more than 1 inch, drill osteotomy should be performed and the child put in steep traction to bring the leg out to length.

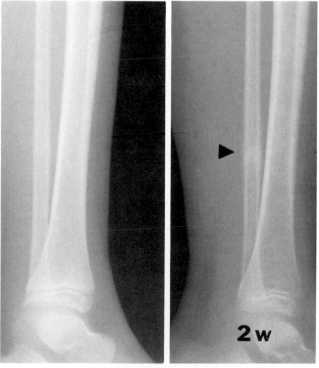

2w

Fig. 5-17. A short history of localized pain accompanied by bone tenderness made a stress fracture the most likely diagnosis in this 5-year-old. Initial films were normal; 14 days later the diagnosis was confirmed.

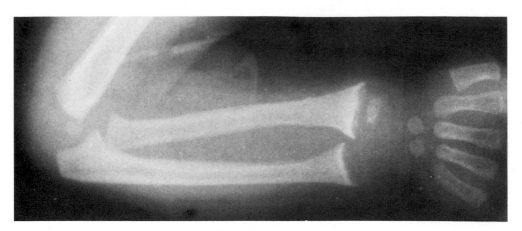

Fig. 5-18. A lucky break: the buckle fracture of the distal radius brought to light this 11-month-old child's rickets.

Growth Plate Disruption and Joint Surface Irregularity. It is difficult and dangerous to try to shift a Type I or II injury after a few days. Remodelling is very effective, and if this is not sufficient, a late osteotomy is indicated. Malunited displaced Type IV injuries only become worse with time and should be replaced at open operation at almost any time. Callus must be removed, and the joint surface realigned without depriving the fragment of its blood supply. Un-united lateral condylar fractures at the elbow are probably best left alone after a few months.

BIBLIOGRAPHY

Battered Child

Adelson, L.: The battering child. J.A.M.A., *222:* 159, 1972

Kempe, C. H. and Helfer, R. E.: Helping the Battered Child and His Family. Philadelphia, J. B. Lippincott, 1972

Levin, quoted in Editorial: Infant Fall Out. Can. Med. Ass. J., *108:* 130, 1973

Van Stolk, M.: The Battered Child in Canada. Toronto, McClelland & Stewart, 1972

Bone Cyst

Neer, C. S., et al.: Treatment of unicameral bone cyst. J. Bone Joint Surg., *48A:* 731, 1966

Cerebral Palsy

McIvor, W. C. and Samilson, R. L.: Fractures in patients with cerebral palsy. J. Bone Joint Surg., *48A:* 858, 1966

Hemophilia

Kemp, H. S. and Matthews, J. M.: The management of fractures in hemophilia and Christmas disease. J. Bone Joint Surg., *50B:* 351, 1968

Newborn

Truesdell, E. D.: Birth Fractures and Epiphyseal Displacements. New York, Hoeber, 1917

Nonossifying Fibroma

Drennan, D. B., Fahey, J.S., Maylahn, D. J.: Fractures through large nonossifying fibromas. J. Bone Joint Surg., *54A:* 1794, 1972

Poliomyelitis

Robin, G. C.: Fractures in poliomyelitis in children. J. Bone Joint Surg., *48A:* 1048, 1966

Renal

Shea, D. and Mankin, H. J.: Slipped capital femoral epiphysis in renal rickets. Report of three cases. J. Bone Joint Surg., *48A:* 349, 1966

Spina Bifida

Eichenholtz, S. N.: Management of long bone fractures in paraplegic patients. J. Bone Joint Surg., *45A:* 299, 1963

Handelsman, J. E.: Spontaneous fractures in spina bifida. J. Bone Joint Surg., *54B:* 381, 1972

Korhonen, B. J.: Fractures in myelodysplasia. Clin. Orthop., *79:* 145, 1971

Stress Fracture

Devas, M. B.: Stress fractures in children. J. Bone Joint Surg., *45B:* 528, 1963

Engh, C. A., Robinson, R. A. and Milgram, J.: Stress fractures in children. J. Trauma, *10:* 532, 1970

6

Soft-Tissue Injuries

Hugh G. Thomson, M.D., M.S., F.R.C.S.(C), F.A.C.S.

An orthopaedic surgeon should know how to manage soft-tissue injury. Orthopaedics is more than the treatment of a specific condition involving bones; it is the care of a patient with a bone problem in a soft-tissue envelope.

Sometimes a consultation with an associate is necessary in the treatment of your patient. Indeed, Sir Harold Gillies believed that the sign of a good consultant was that he was prepared to consult!

It is the purpose of this chapter to outline the detailed management of some soft-tissue injuries. The excellence of fracture treatment or the outcome of an orthopaedic operation could be considered proportional to the excellence demonstrated in the management of the overlying soft tissue, be it an open or closed injury.

The soft-tissue envelope is subject to various types of injury. Assigning the wound to the correct category is the most important single step for you to take. For example, a clean laceration produced with a scalpel does not damage the margins of the laceration and will heal by primary intention after suture; whereas a laceration produced by heavy pressure with a blunt object devitalizes skin edges, destroys some soft tissue, and requires more elaborate treatment. Soft-tissue injuries may be classified in many different ways, based on the elements of cutting, abrading, burning, crushing, and tearing.

HEMATOMA

A hematoma, whether produced by blunt trauma or a fracture, seldom requires more than cleaning of the overlying skin and masterful inactivity. But a loculated hematoma within the subcutaneous or deep tissue, while unusual, should alert the surgeon to the risk of local or diffuse infection, avascular changes in the skin, nerves, and muscles, and the possibility of an underlying blood dyscrasia. All these influence a program of treatment. Conservatism, observation, and investigation are the keynotes of the treatment routine.

A Small Hematoma is unlikely to require treatment. It may give rise to a zone of regional fibrosis with skin tethering or puckering for as long as 6 to 12 months after the injury. The parents should be warned of this possibility, because it will temporarily compromise the cosmetic appearance of the clinical result.

A Large Tense Hematoma may require evacuation if there is impending skin necrosis or impending Volkmann's ischemia. Otherwise it may be left to resorb, or it may be aspirated after it has liquefied. When surgical evacuation is necessary, the incision should be placed as far from the hematoma as access will permit and preferably just off and parallel to a skin flexion crease. The hematoma can then be approached subcutaneously or subfascially and evacuated. A modified pressure dressing over tulle gauze should be applied. There is controversy about whether drainage, irrigation, or both should be used; what type of tube and for how long? A flat, compressible, malleable catheter without irrigation has served me well. The catheter should be removed 36 to 48 hours after incision and drainage. Antibiotic treatment prior to drainage is certainly worthwhile in the presence of a fracture but is less strongly indicated for an isolated soft-tissue injury.

FAT FRACTURE

The commonest cause of a fat fracture is a sharp, nonlacerating force; it can overlie a bone fracture (Fig. 6-1). The phenomenon is rare and usually late to appear, with an interval of several months between injury and initial observation. It is almost impossible to foresee this clinical entity, and this causes more problems than anything else. The patient and his relatives cannot be prepared for this phenomenon.

A fat fracture is probably due to shearing through the fat, superficial fascia, and (on occasion) deep fascia. This creates a diastasis in the fat compartment and a degree of fat necrosis due to the original compression-contusion force. As resolution occurs, the proximal edge is elevated, and the distal edge is usually flattened. This unsightliness is difficult to improve. It can be attempted with fat, fascial-, and even muscle rotation flaps through a curved marginal incision. This and other types of local augmentation are fraught with potential complications. Therefore, it is important to assess accurately the functional and esthetic disability the

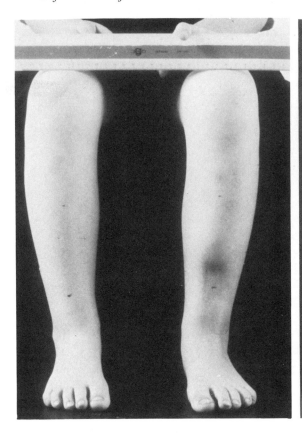 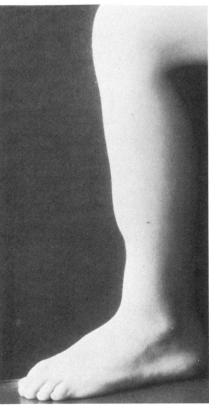

Fig. 6-1. Anteroposterior and lateral views of lower tibial fat fracture 2 years after injury. Notice the gravitational fullness of the proximal portion!

patient is experiencing. For example, there is relatively little disability when this problem involves the buttock, whereas involvement of the anterior tibia of a girl is a different matter. You must remember that for most reconstructive surgery the patient and surgeon always must make a trade, and here the trade is a large incision in a previously unscarred area. Is it worth it to the patient?

FOREIGN BODY PENETRATION

From time to time surgical procedures are frustrating to the operator. However, very few can appear so simple yet result in such overwhelming frustration as the removal of a foreign body. The presence of a foreign body is usually heralded by a simple puncture wound and is therefore disarming. Its absence cannot be assumed from a negative roentgenogram. The history, location, wound appearance, and palpation are usually enough to assist in the presumptive diagnosis. Conservative management and wound observation are appropriate when a puncture wound exists alone and the history and clinical and roentgenographic examinations are negative and there is no other indication to explore the area. If the index of suspicion is higher and one or more positive findings are present, then wide exploration of the wound is necessary. Don't try to probe the wound. It is useless! Don't pull out the foreign body. This is a convenient trap. Even if it is smooth metal it may have carried clothing or other foreign material with it. The area must be operatively and adequately explored. In most cases this requires fluid and mechanical debridement followed by primary closure of the wound. An image intensifier can be very helpful if the initial roentgenograph is positive.

LACERATION

Is it a tidy or an untidy wound? Your management depends on this easy distinction. A wound is tidy if: (1) it is to be repaired within eight hours after injury; (2) it was made by a sharp object, whether from within or without; and (3) it has no gross evidence of contamination by bacteria or foreign bodies. In other words, a tidy wound resembles a surgical wound. An untidy wound has ragged edges, disrupted soft tissues with areas of impending necrosis, and obvious foreign body contamination. Any wound that has remained open for more than 8 hours should be considered untidy.

At the initial examination, examine the patient for signs of divided vessels, tendons, and nerves. Then cover the wound with a sterile dressing. While the patient is still awake, inquire about allergies to antibiotics that you may want to administer while the patient is anesthetised. Either tetanus toxoid or immune globulin should be used to protect against tetanus.

Fig. 6-2. (*A*) Simple laceration of upper extremity. Note
the widely spread wound,
which gives the appearance of
tissue loss! (*B*) Subcutaneous
closure of superficial fascia and
fat with absorbable suture. If
using subcuticular suture, a
two-layer closure of this zone
is necessary, as shown.

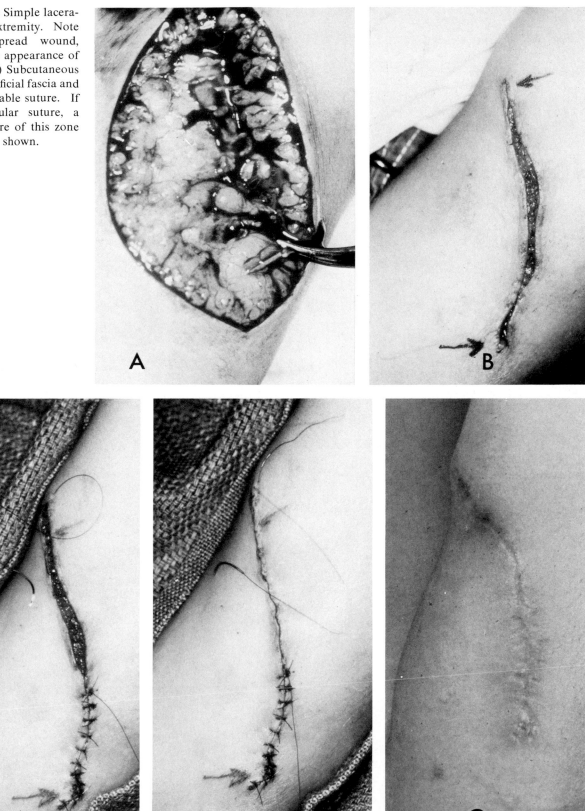

Fig. 6-3. (*A*) Use of interrupted and subcuticular closure for the wound shown in Fig.
6-2. (*B*) Closure complete. (*C*) Three months later; scar showing "railroad tracks" in area
closed by interrupted sutures.

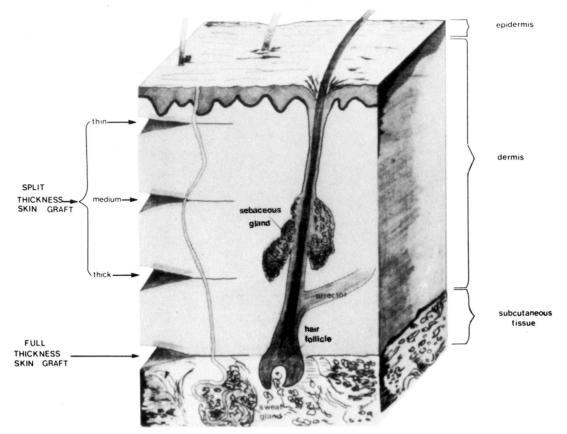

Fig. 6-4. This drawing demonstrates the levels at which different skin grafts are cut.

Simple Tidy Laceration

Initial care of the wound requires regional antiseptic preparation up to its margins and profuse fluid irrigation (normal saline, Ringer's solution), with or without antibiotics, in its depth. Almost without exception I prefer to irrigate the wound at this point with a dilute solution of bacitracin (10,000 u. in 500 ml. saline). Surgical debridement should be relatively conservative but influenced by site, depth, and type of injury. Judicious excision of skin and subcutaneous margins, necrotic tissue, and previously unseen foreign bodies should be carried out.

It is often difficult to determine if a wound on an extremity is deficient of skin and soft tissue. As a matter of fact, almost all lacerations on the extremities give this appearance (Fig. 6-2A). This is due to the circumferential tension the skin exerts around a cylinder and the important sheathing effect of the superficial and deep fascia, which is lost when lacerated. These factors coupled with local wound edema complicate the clinical picture. If a wound is closed under undue tension, ischemia of the wound margins is assured, with obvious complications. Therefore, a decision must be made early. Is there tissue loss, or is the wound edema so great that primary direct closure is unwise? Must some

other means of closure be considered? Using two skin hooks crossed on each other can be helpful in this decision. If slight tension on the hooks approximates the edges, the primary direct closure is unlikely be a problem. Don't test this tension using toothed thumb forceps. They do not provide the proper perspective, and at the same time they tear the skin margins.

Direct Closure

The deep closure should be carried out with absorbable, interrupted, and inverted sutures. Polyglycolic acid sutures provide excellent support to the deep structures owing to their prolonged tensile strength (Fig. 6-2B).

Prior to actual skin closure, it is important to anticipate the late contracture of the mature wound. If the wound lies at right angles to any flexion crease, it will create a significant contracture problem. Therefore, anticipating this problem may save your patient another operation. This can be accomplished with a simple Z-plasty or Z-plasties in tandem. Remember: the angles of the arms of the Z should rarely exceed 60 degrees. (This principle must also be remembered when closing elective incisions.)

The best way to close the skin margins continues to be a matter of controversy (Fig. 6-3). Remember that the patient will always have a scar, and your responsibility is to provide the least noticeable scar. Should you use interrupted cuticular sutures or continuous subcuticular sutures? This is a matter of personal preference. The major advantage of subcuticular suture is the elimination of "railroad-tracks," which are so common with interrupted sutures. Wound infection is almost inevitable if interrupted sutures are left under a plaster cast for weeks or months; removal always causes some discomfort. Subcuticular sutures usually overcome these problems. On the other hand, interrupted sutures are suited to irregular wounds, to wounds that have been grossly contaminated, and to areas such as the face favoring early suture removal. When a wound becomes infected unexpectedly it is helpful to remove a few sutures.

Skin Graft Closure

Direct edge-to-edge closure of all wounds is not always possible. The most useful alternative is a skin graft. The thickness of the skin graft depends on the needs of the recipient site (Fig. 6-4). A free full-thickness skin graft is rarely used to close a tidy traumatic defect. It is usually reserved for an elective procedure under more optimal conditions. The thinner the skin graft, the better its chance of survival in any environment. Therefore use a split-thickness skin graft to replace traumatic skin deficits. Although a split-thickness graft is more likely to "take," it is more susceptible to contracture, to hyperpigmentation, and to instability. It does not provide insulating skin coverage. A full-thickness graft provides stable cover and is less liable to contracture and pigmentation.

A skin graft can be obtained with a variety of instruments ranging from a basic straight-bladed knife to a rapidly oscillating gas turbine blade (Fig. 6-5). This latter type of dermatome has more universal application, because it requires relatively little experience and because the thickness of the graft can be readily changed any time during its operation. Try to become adept with one instrument only!

The care of the skin graft and the donor site is critical:

1. Place the skin graft in a gauze moistened with Ringer's lactate. Store it in a separate basin to lessen the chances of it being discarded!

2. Place Ringer's lactate sponges over the donor site, which will be covered by a petroleum jelly tulle gauze at the end of the operation.

3. When wound toilet has been completed and the recipient site prepared, the graft is laid, glistening side down, into the defect.

4. Long marker sutures attach the periphery of the

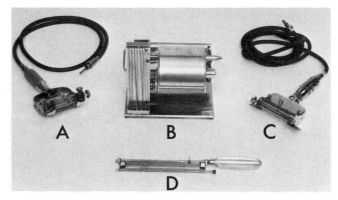

Fig. 6-5. Dermatomes: (*A*) Brown electric, (*B*) Reese drum, (*C*) Hall Turbine, and (*D*) Cobbett knife.

graft to the margin of the skin defect. These sutures should hold the graft under even tension, which is comparable to the tension of the skin prior to its removal from the donor site. This is why you must insert the marker sutures on one margin first and then stretch the graft before inserting the other marker sutures (Fig. 6-6).

5. Noncutting quilting sutures are placed through the graft into the bed (when anatomically possible) and tied over a piece of silence cloth (moleskin) to tether the skin graft to the recipient bed (Fig. 6-7).

6. Hematoma from nonspecific oozing can be prevented by making small incisions in the skin graft using a No. 11 blade (Fig. 6-8).

7. The long marker sutures are tied over a bolster of cotton waste with tulle gauze as an interface between graft and bolster.

8. Immobilization of the part for 5 to 7 days is important to lessen hematoma and shearing of the graft, and permit maturation of the new endothelial channels.

If these principles are followed carefully, skin graft coverage should never pose a difficult hurdle for you.

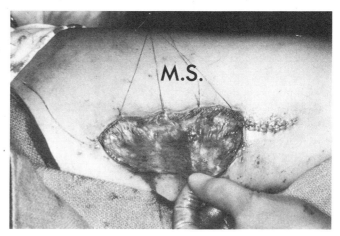

Fig. 6-6. Skin graft techniques: Marker sutures (M.S.) in place with traction applied to the skin graft.

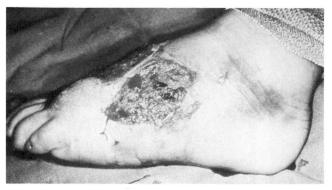

Fig. 6-19. The immediate vascular response after escharectomy and fasciotomy. (Note increased swelling compared with Fig. 6-18.)

the tissues are thinned in the zone of compression and appear white and avascular (Fig. 6-18A). Bones may be fractured by the crushing force (Fig. 6-18B). *These extremities should be surgically decompressed as soon as possible* (Fig. 6-19). Local escharectomy-fasciotomy will cause the clinical appearance to change with resultant edema, venous congestion, and possible additional infarction. The use of sympathetic blocking agents, anticoagulants, coupled with antisludging parenteral therapy, local hyperoxygenation, and even hyperbaric chamber dives are all controversial—singly or in combination. All too often the injured limb is salvaged only to leave the patient with a hypoesthetic extremity, which may require late amputation.

AVULSED FLAPS

Simple Avulsion

Sharp avulsion of a soft tissue flap (whether produced by a bale hook and associated with fracture of both bones of the forearm or by a meat hook tear) is not complicated by crushing, friction-burning, or additional shearing force on the skin flap. It is important to realize that, in general, this flap is a viable structure. The variables determining survival of the skin flap are: vascular supply of the general region; whether the flap is based proximally or distally; proportions of the avulsed flap (length-to-base ratio); depth of the plane (such as dermis-fat, fat-fascia, fascia-muscle); and scything and ragged skin edges.

If there is no doubt concerning the survival of the flap, it can be replaced and atraumatically sutured. A three-sided flap has a tendency to bulge after suture when the wound contracts, pulling the flap up in a "pout." This can be corrected at a later date by simply breaking up the scar line with a few carefully placed **Z**-plasties.

On occasion there is no doubt in your mind concerning the survival of the flap, but it is replaced only to

become edematous, blue, and blistered in 3 to 5 days due to infarction (Fig. 6-20). It should be excised across the base, and a free split-thickness skin graft should be used to cover the defect.

If in your opinion, the flap has a 50-50 chance of survival, it is sutured. Both the patient and the relatives should know the reason for your decision, and you should be prepared to look at the flap within 5 to 7 days. If it is infarcted, it should be excised and replaced with a free split-thickness skin graft (Fig. 6-21).

If some or all of the criteria for viability have been violated and the flap is assured of subsequent infarction, primary wound closure should be obtained. This can be done by total excision of the flap at its base, removing a split-thickness skin graft from it, discarding the remnants, and resurfacing the defect. However, if it is so severely compromised, it is probably better to throw the whole flap away and obtain a free skin graft from an elective donor site, such as the high lateral thigh or buttock region. Remember free split skin grafts have a great propensity to survive on almost all living tissue and particularly on periosteum.

Complex Avulsion with Exposure of Vital Structures

A sharp penetrating object, such as a fence spike, may tear up a nonviable flap and expose deep vital structures. Amputation of the avulsed flap is completed, and immediate local or distal pedicle flap coverage is applied over the repaired deep structures (Fig. 6-22). This will encourage primary skin healing as well as providing adequate protection for the repaired deep structures.

DEGLOVING INJURIES

Partial Degloving

This type of injury may appear to be a broad-based

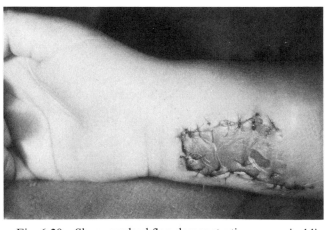

Fig. 6-20. Sharp avulsed flap demonstrating cyanosis, blistering, and early evidence of total infarction, even though proximally based.

Fig. 6-21. (*A*) Large broad-based flap undermined by injury at deep fascial level and thought to be viable. Obviously this opinion (the author's) was incorrect. (*B*) Ten days later after wide excision and free split-thickness skin graft.

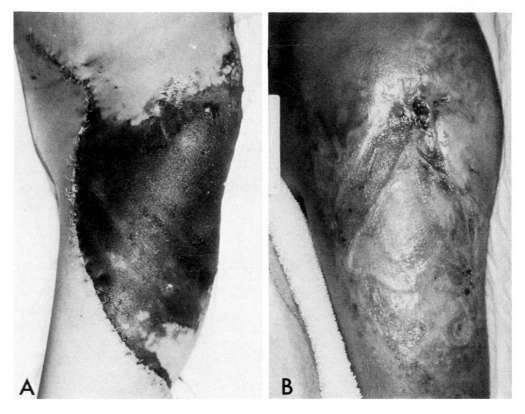

flap or even a simple looking laceration. The wound is often disarming at first sight, but on sterile examination the operator's whole hand and forearm can be passed up and around the cleavage plane. There is shearing at the fibro-fatty fascial interface with tearing of communicating veins. The decision to save or replace the skin is important to the fate of the underlying tissue; primary wound healing must be achieved (Fig. 6-23).

If evidence of crush and contusion is judged to be

Fig. 6-22. (*A*) Sharp avulsion of distally based infarcted flap with transsection and repair of brachial artery and median nerve. (*B*) The flap was excised and the wound was closed with a primary thoracic tube pedicle flap.

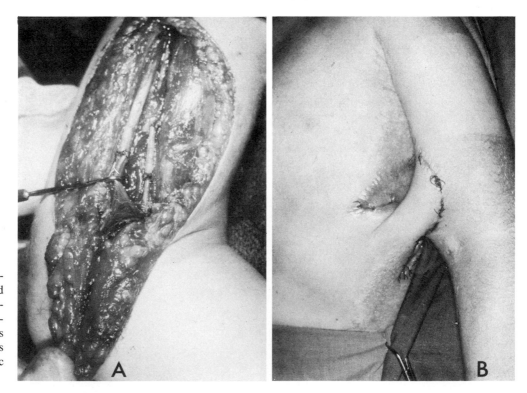

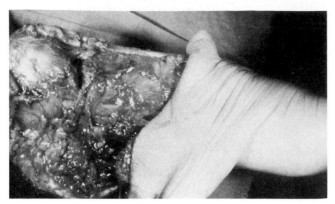

Fig. 6-23. Degloving of foot with exposure of ankle joint.

minimal considering the mechanism of injury, the lack of abrasion, ecchymosis, and avascular white zones, then the degloved tissue is replaced after fluid and mechanical debridement; suction drainage is used for 36 hours.

If the wound shows minimal crush and contusion but is abraded or "friction burned," as can occur in a rope-tow or water ski injury, then the abraded superficial wound requires attention as well as the deep injury. This takes the form of deliberate brushing to remove all foreign material and prevent traumatic tatooing. It is necessary to use some form of tulle gauze or antibiotic ointment to prevent a purulent coagulum from forming. This dressing should remain intact for 7 to 10 days, the required time for reepithelialization.

A truck tire may produce severe injury. Not only is a large flap raised, but severe ecchymosis and abrasions are in evidence, plus some scattered white areas as well as a general duskiness to the flap. Removal of the flap is imperative. When removal is necessary, it must be complete. If you are going to have a defect, then a big one is no worse than a small one. If the wound bed can be made suitable with muscle-fascial rotation flaps over any fracture fragments, a skin graft is an ideal cover (Fig. 6-24). Formal plaster immobilization above and below the wound is important. A window is made immediately in the plaster to provide access to the skin graft area for both observation and dressings.

Some degloving injuries are very complex. If a small or large area of specialized soft tissue has been degloved or torn away and a specialized covering is required, a free split-thickness skin graft may not be the ideal coverage for primary wound closure. In these cases consideration must be given to the use of local, regional, or distant skin flap coverage. This type of tissue can ultimately supply a good milieu for nerve regeneration and tactileognosis. It also provides flexibility to the tissues, and there is less tendency to contract or hyperpigment. It does bring an independent blood supply, permitting joints to move freely, bone to regenerate, and reconstructive surgery to be done later (Fig. 6-25).

Total Degloving

Total degloving may be (1) simple—in which no vital subcutaneous structures are exposed, (2) complex—in which important structures are bared and cannot be covered with split thickness skin grafts, or (3) unsalvageable.

Simple Total Degloving. The patient who presents with total degloving of an unspecialized area that does not expose vital structures has a simple problem. Careful wound toilet under operating room conditions and wound closure are required. The degloved skin is rarely brought into the hospital. Because a large circumferential area may be involved, free split-thickness skin grafts alone are adequate to provide closure (Fig. 6-26).

The high thigh or buttock of the contra or ipsilateral sides (as governed by associated injuries) should be the donor sites. The grafts can be obtained rapidly with a power dermatome. The grafts should be gently spiralled around the circumferential defect. This lessens the intrinsic contraction of the graft and the effect of the shortening of the scar at the skin graft juncture. It is important to realize that there are many methods of achieving primary wound closure, but the simplest is often the best. The use of split-thickness skin grafts supports this concept. Remember that skin grafts can always be excised at a later date and replaced by a more ideal type of skin coverage.

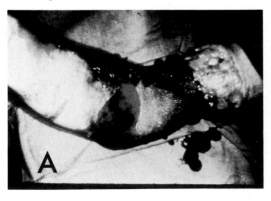

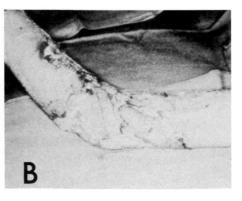

Fig. 6-24. (*A*) Extensive degloving of the upper arm and elbow with obvious infarction and associated supracondylar fracture. (*B*) Ten days after internal fixation of fracture and primary free split-thickness skin graft.

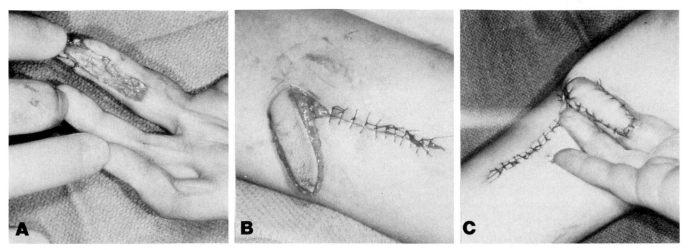

Fig. 6-25. (*A*) Partial degloving of specialized surface. (*B*) Cross-inner arm pedicle flap, (*C*) After primary direct closure of donor site and insertion of flap.

A fingertip amputation is another common example of this type of injury: the tip can be replaced as a composite graft in the form of a free full-thickness skin graft. This injury is usually the exception to the previous rule, because the tip is usually brought into the

Emergency Department. As with all other avulsed and degloved skin, the operator's management must be influenced by the degree of intrinsic skin injury and the expired time. If this is minimal and the wound tidy, it is worthwhile replacing the defatted free composite

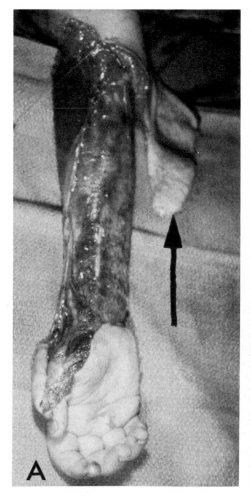

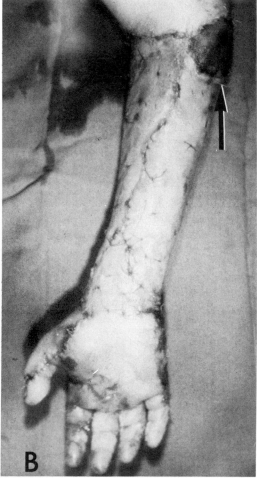

Fig. 6-26. (*A*) Total circumferential degloving of the forearm with a residual attached skin flap. (*B*) Ten days after primary free split-thickness skin graft. (Arrow shows that even residuum of replaced flap is infarcted.)

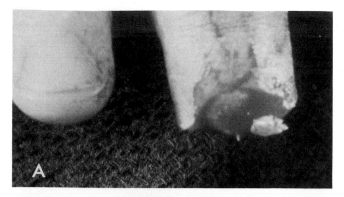

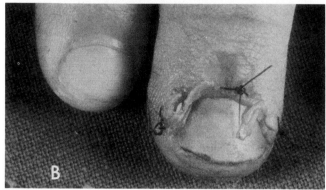

Fig. 6-27. (*A*) Total avulsion of fingertip showing phalangeal tuft. (*B*) Ater defatting and replacement as a free full-thickness graft (nail left attached as a splint).

graft (Fig. 6-27). All the principles of skin grafting must be applied, even more than with a split-thickness graft. A free composite graft must obtain a good vascular supply within 48 hours, as it will not survive on a plasma clot. This means the graft must be treated with even greater respect, and the recipient site must be better than with the free split-thickness graft.

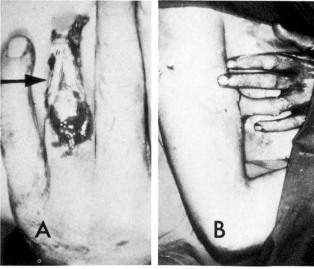

Fig. 6-28. (*A*) Total degloving of the distal phalanx and exposure of tendon and joint (*arrow*). (*B*) Three weeks after cross-arm tube pedicle insert.

Complex Total Degloving. An extensive area of degloving which exposes tendon, joint, cartilage, and bone may not be amenable to a simple skin graft. This limits the available methods for primary wound closure. It may be possible to close the defect with a large pedicle flap from the contralateral extremity. This could include an entire leg and thigh. Occasionally, another fracture site in the same injured leg can be used as a false joint to permit soft-tissue coverage for a more important injury on the same extremity. There is no doubt that if the articular cartilage, joint, bone, and tendon can be covered with vital skin, there is more assurance of their survival. Sufficient flap tissue may not be available because of the size of the wound area or the mechanical difficulty of moving the flap to the wound. If this is the case, then the important dogma of primary wound closure must be abandoned. In its place must be substituted a delayed primary skin graft. The wound is fastidiously debrided, and as much local fat-fascial tissue or even muscle is mobilized to cover the tendon, joint, cartilage, and bone. A tulle gauze dressing is applied, with or without topical antibiotic. The initial dressing should be changed 3 days after the wound debridement, and daily thereafter for a total of 7 to 10 days, depending on how rapidly granulation tissue forms. When the granulations appear receptive, a split-thickness skin graft is applied. A few minor modifications in skin graft technique must be considered with this type of procedure. Granulation tissue bleeds readily and may cause a hematoma that will elevate the graft and cause its demise. Therefore, fixation sutures cannot be inserted into the wound margins; rather they are inserted into the skin surface wide of this zone. For the same reason, no deep fixation quilting sutures can be used. All other rules must be followed stringently.

The avulsed skin can be replaced only occasionally as a free full-thickness skin graft, because the skin itself is usually so severely injured. On rare occasions the totally degloved area is small, and specialized circumferential coverage is needed, (for example in the finger; Fig. 6-28). Coverage can be achieved in these injuries

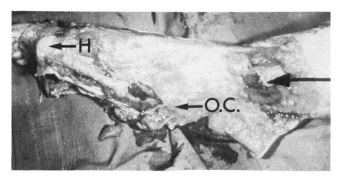

Fig. 6-29. Unsalvageable right foot. Note fractures and partial amputation of hallux (*H*) and os calcis (*O.C.*).

with a cross-arm tube pedicle from the medial aspect of the upper arm. This tissue is ideal, as it is thin and soft and the donor site scar is relatively hidden. The donor site can be closed directly edge-to-edge or with a skin graft, depending on the required width of the pedicle flap. The flap is separated, and the wounds are closed in 3 weeks.

The Unsalvageable Degloved Extremity

This type of limb injury is usually associated with a degloving of both skin and soft tissues, including nerve, vessel, tendon, and muscle, as well as multiple fractures and open joints (Fig. 6-29). This is probably the most difficult injury to deal with, particularly for the novice. It provides a tremendous hurdle because amputation is required. If you are torn with indecision, then it is imperative to obtain a colleague's opinion in the Operating Room and have this second opinion documented. Even if you are not racked with indecision, consultation is a good idea. It is important for you, for the patient, and for medicolegal purposes. When the decision to amputate is delayed, it becomes psychologically more difficult for the patient and relatives to accept and leads to many useless salvage operations and heartbreak. On the other hand, and much in your patient's favor, is the ease with which children can adapt to a prosthesis.

COMMON COMPLICATIONS

Hypertrophic Scars

The hypertrophic scar is red and raised, with linear shortening along its length. It always remains within the confines of the original wound. It is frequently confused with the rare keloid. The main significance to your patient is the fact that the hypertrophic scar will improve with time and certainly will improve if properly revised. This is not true with the keloid. An incision or wound crossing at right angles to a flexion crease will always develop a hypertrophic scar unless initially revised. This is not always technically possible. You will find that the Z-plasty is your closest ally for early or late revision of this problem (Fig. 6-30). It entails an elliptical excision of the scar and the elevation of the two Z-plasty flaps which are interposed. Remember: in order to lengthen the scar on an extremity, you are gathering soft tissue *in a circumferential direction.* Therefore, beware of the flaps being too large and the angles greater than 60 degrees. It is better to make two or more Z-plasties in tandem gathering a little circumferentially with each rather than one very large Z-plasty. Make sure they are *in* tandem and not *out!*

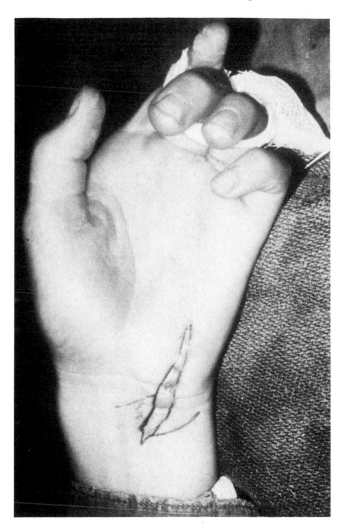

Fig. 6-30. Hypertrophic scar at right angles to wrist flexion crease. Elliptical excision and a single Z-plasty is proposed as a solution to the problem. Had it been done initially, it would have prevented this problem.

Linear Tightness

In time, the juncture point between wound margin and a skin graft will cause linear tightness. It may form a hypertrophic scar, but the treatment is the same. If 12 months have elapsed since the skin graft was inserted, the graft itself can be used in the formation of the Z-plasty in the revision (Fig. 6-31).

Donor Site Scarring

Until you become experienced in handling the dermatome equipment, the most common complication that will plague you is the appearance of the donor site. It may be ugly and raised with patchy hypertrophic scars because the skin graft is too thick or because the donor site became infected secondarily. To avoid these problems, the site of the donor area should be the high thigh or buttock region. If the area of skin graft is

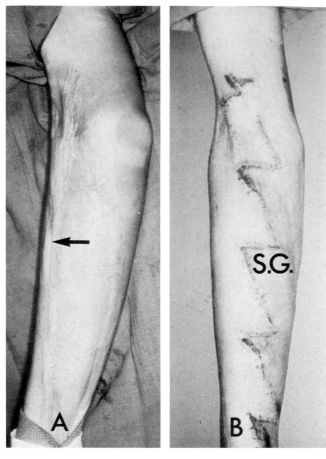

Fig. 6-31. (*A*) Postfasciotomy skin graft juncture (*arrow*) showing linear tightness, particularly in antecubital fossa. (*B*) Serial or in-tandem **Z**-plasties incorporating the skin graft (S.G.) can be used to correct this problem.

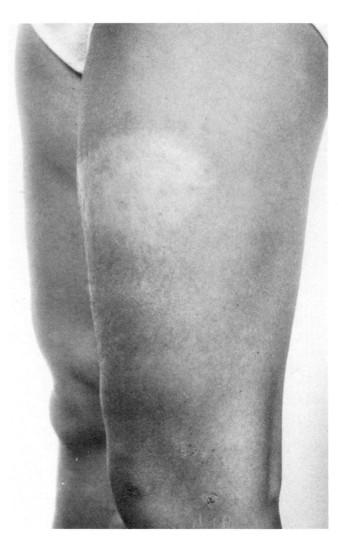

Fig. 6-32. Hypopigmented and slightly raised donor site scar on anterior thigh. The graft was elective and could have been taken anywhere!

extensive, use the other side as well, or, if you need still more skin, advance down to the mid-thighs or "miniskirt level." *Using the anterior thigh or abdomen as a donor site is inexcusable* (Fig. 6-32). When you begin to obtain your skin graft, *take a small sample of skin and stop.* Feel the graft and look at the bed. If the graft feels thin and the edges are not curling, you are doing fine. If the donor bed is finely stippled with bleeding you can proceed, but if the graft is thick and curling and if the donor bed bleeds from a few large widely separated points you are too deep. Stop! When a thin graft has been removed, a nonshearing, antiseptic tulle gauze dressing should be applied to the donor site to lessen potential destruction of the new epithelium by friction and infection.

Skin Graft Contraction

One of the inevitable features of skin grafting is the intrinsic contraction that accompanies maturation. The thinner the graft, the more significant the contraction. The skin graft will have an accordion-pleated tight ap-

pearance which should lessen with time. An involved joint can be progressively subluxated or even dislocated by this phenomenon (Fig. 6-33). Revisionary correction must be carried out long before this point is reached,

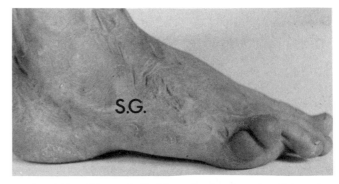

Fig. 6-33. Skin graft (S.G.) contracture causing dislocation of metatarsophalangeal joints.

and it can be done with another skin graft insert or an interposed local pedicle flap.

Skin Graft Hyperpigmentation

Hyperpigmentation is esthetically displeasing (Fig. 6-34). The thinner the skin graft, the more pigmentation can be anticipated. If this condition requires treatment, the skin graft is excised and replaced with a full-thickness skin graft or local flap. However, there will still be an element of hyperpigmentation with the replacements.

SUMMARY

In this chapter I have outlined the important principles which should be applied to the treatment of common problems that you will encounter. This style of presentation was chosen to provide a quick reference, but it is not detailed enough to provide all the problems and solutions that will confront you. Remember this is the age of specialization and fellowship. When in doubt, take comfort by consulting with one of your professional associates.

RECOMMENDED READING

Cannon, B., and Constable, J. D.: Reconstructive surgery of the lower extremity. *In* Converse, J. M. (ed.): Reconstructive Plastic Surgery. vol 4. Philadelphia, W. B. Saunders, 1964

Douglas, D. M.: Wound Healing. Edinburgh, E. & S. Livingstone, 1963

Limberg, A. A.: Design of local flaps. *In* Gibson, T. (ed.): Modern Trends in Plastic Surgery. vol. 2. London, Butterworths, 1966

Mc Gregor, I. A.: Fundamental Techniques of Plastic Surgery. ed. 5. Edinburgh, Churchill Livingstone, 1972

Mustarde, J. C.: Plastic Surgery in Infancy and Childhood. Edinburgh, E. & S. Livingstone, 1971

Paletta, F. X.: Pediatric Plastic Surgery. vol. 1. Trauma.

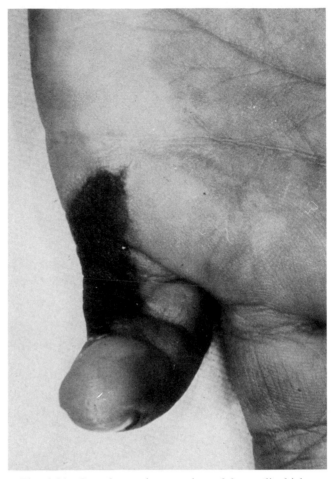

Fig. 6-34. Late hyperpigmentation of free split-thickness graft used to close a skin defect on the little finger.

St. Louis, C. V. Mosby, 1967

Peacock, E. E., and van Winkle, W.: Surgery and Biology of Wound Repair. Philadelphia, W. B. Saunders, 1970

Rank, B. K., Wakefield, A. R., and Hueston, J. T.: Surgery of Repair as Applied to Hand Injuries. Edinburgh, E. & S. Livingstone, 1968

Stark, R. B.: Plastic Surgery. New York, Harper and Row, 1962

7

Chest and Gastrointestinal Tract

Sigmund H. Ein, B.A., M.D.C.M., F.A.A.P., F.A.C.S., F.R.C.S.(C)

Accidental injury is the commonest single cause of death in children over 1 month old. Among Canadian children accidents outnumber all other causes of death combined.

At The Hospital for Sick Children in Toronto the number of accidents treated has increased by 2,000 each year between 1960 and 1967. A study of the records of 20,000 accidental injuries treated in 1967 brought forward a number of interesting facts. Accidents were commonest in June, July, and August and least common in February and December. Most accidents came for emergency treatment between 4:00 P.M. and 8:00 P.M. Sixty percent of the accidents had occured at home, and 10 percent at school. One quarter of the children were between 2 and 3 years old, and almost half were not yet attending school.

Automobile accidents account for half the admissions, and falls were next in frequency. Falls down stairs were commonest and a quarter of children so injured were less than 2 years old. Slides proved to be the most dangerous piece of playground equipment. Less than 1 percent of the children admitted to hospital died. One third of deaths could be attributed to accidents involving transport, including bicycles. More than half the children injured while riding in cars were under 5 years old; many had been thrown against the dashboard in sudden stops. Seat belts would have prevented many of these injuries. One half of one percent of children had been physically abused by their parents or other adults.

This unhappy picture has an optimistic side; children involved in trauma tolerate major reparative surgery surprisingly well, heal quickly, and in general have vigorous powers of recuperation. They rarely suffer from pulmonary, thromboembolic, or cardiovascular complications, so that convalescence is rapid except when there has been irreparable tissue loss or neurologic damage.

INITIAL CARE OF SEVERE INJURIES

Hospitals should have a special room equipped for resuscitation, to which a severely injured child can be taken directly from the ambulance. Put him on a radio-lucent stretcher so that he need not be moved for radiography. The doctor in Emergency looks over the child quickly and deals with any respiratory difficulty until the anesthetist arrives. External hemorrhage can be controlled with a pressure pad. Clothes are cut off as necessary, and a quick inventory of the injuries is made. A call is put out for all the specialty services likely to be needed.

A detailed history of the accident can wait until the situation is under control. Assume that all victims of major accidents have multiple injuries. Most children injured in road traffic accidents have a head injury, some degree of blunt trauma to the trunk, and a limb fracture (usually of the femur).

The immediate examination seeks to determine the presence of (in descending order of importance):
1. Respiratory difficulty
2. Major hemorrhage
3. Depression of the state of consciousness
4. Shock
5. Internal injuries
6. Fractures
7. Superficial soft tissue injuries.

This order of priorities varies, depending on the circumstances and experience of those examining the child. Several of these assessments can be carried out simultaneously. As soon as respiratory difficulties have been relieved and hemorrhage has been controlled or countered by transfusion, the remainder of the examination can proceed with less haste. The specialty service responsible for the care of the most pressing injury should take charge. Confusion can only be prevented by having one man, not a committee, in charge of the patient. Very often this is the general surgeon.

There is often a conflict between making a complete evaluation and starting treatment. Patients rarely need to be rushed to the operating room—perhaps only when a pupil dilates quickly or when the abdomen becomes distended with blood before the surgeon's eyes.

Airway

Unconscious patients should be transported lying on the side to reduce the chance of aspiration. A clear airway is vital. An anesthetist will maintain the airway expertly, but do not wait for his arrival before providing aid. Remove vomitus and debris by pharyngeal suction, and pass a large nasogastric tube to empty the stomach. Aspiration pneumonia adds insult to injury. If these measures are ineffective, pass an endotracheal tube. (An oral airway is useless; immediate tracheostomy is rarely indicated). If respiratory difficulties persist after a good airway has been established, look for signs of tension pneumothorax.

Shock

Although neurogenic mechanisms may initiate and potentiate posttraumatic shock, one must always assume that clinical shock is due to blood loss. Fractures and lacerations seldom deplete the blood volume sufficiently to produce shock, so it should always be attributed to intrathoracic or intraabdominal hemorrhage. Abrasions and bruises on the trunk are the outward signs of internal injury.

When shock is suspected, blood is taken for emergency cross-match, and an amount equal to the patient's blood volume (approximately 10 percent of the body weight in grams) is urgently requested. At the same time the hemoglobin and hematocrit can be determined. The only other blood test which may be useful is serum amylase. Elevation usually indicates pancreatic injury. Serum electrolytes are unnecessary at this time.

Rapid transfusion may be needed; use a large-bore catheter or cut down as the intravenous route. Choose the site carefully. Infused blood should reach the heart before escaping from the circulation, so when intraabdominal injury is suspected use an arm vein. Do not set up the transfusion on a limb with a fracture. While awaiting blood, use lactated Ringer's, normal saline, or concentrated human albumin as a volume expander. Dextran may interfere with future cross-matching or cause capillary bleeding and, sometimes, renal tubular necrosis.

The time needed for the most rapid blood typing, grouping, and cross-match, should not exceed 30 minutes. Immediate transfusion of O-negative blood is seldom warranted and can cause transfusion reactions. When blood is transfused in quantities approaching the child's blood volume certain precautions should be taken. The transfusion set should incorporate a small pore filter to remove debris that may produce "posttransfusion lung." The blood should be warmed as it passes through the tubing. For every 100 ml. of blood transfused, the child should be given 5 ml. of 8.4 percent sodium bicarbonate and 1 ml. of 10 percent calcium gluconate. The serum electrolytes should be checked. Depletion of coagulation factors and platelets can cause continued bleeding. Ask the hematologist for assistance.

Direct estimation of blood loss and circulating blood volume are not always satisfactory guides to therapy. The volume and speed of administration are judged by the color of the child, the blood pressure, urinary output, and, to a lesser extent, by the hemoglobin and hematocrit.

No analgesics, in *any* amount, should be given, because they may confuse the clinical picture, produce respiratory depression, and mask concealed injuries, thereby postponing treatment for several hours.

Unconsciousness Confuses the Picture

Head injuries frequently accompany injuries of the trunk and extremities. The apparent seriousness of the head injury should not distract attention from other injuries. A combination of head and abdominal injuries is four times as likely to cause death as a head injury alone. Coexisting chest injuries and major fractures do not affect the mortality rate from head injuries.

Head injury alone does not produce shock; another cause must be found. However shock may depress the level of consciousness.

Head injury does not cause a rigid abdomen (unless rigidity is generalized throughout the body) and does not cause ileus. The signs of an abdominal injury in an unconscious patient may include hypotension, abdominal rigidity, ileus, and restlessness on palpation.

Radiography

For most patients there is time to make a detailed assessment and obtain radiographs *after* resuscitation. The patient with multiple injuries with an inadequate airway, or a malfunctioning intravenous transfusion must not be left in the semi-darkness of a radiography department.

Most patients require radiographs of the skull, chest, abdomen, and one or two limbs. The lateral film of the skull should include a lateral view of the cervical spine. The abdominal radiographs should include the pelvis. Ideally the chest and abdominal radiographs should be taken with the patient upright to show fluid levels, but when the child is unconscious or too sick, lateral decubitus views will suffice. Radiographs of the chest and abdomen on admission are necessary as a baseline for the interpretation of any subsequent radiological changes.

Urological Investigation

The kidneys are frequently injured in abdominal trauma; this will be discussed in Chapter 8. Suspicion of injury is much commoner than injury requiring treatment. Bruises or abrasions on the trunk, hematuria, and a fracture of the pelvis should suggest a urological injury requiring investigation.

The unconscious child with abdominal injuries should be catheterized and the catheter left in.

After Resuscitation

Once the vital signs have stabilized and the injuries are identified the patient can be moved to the operating room or the Intensive Care Unit (ICU). In the ICU the neurological, respiratory, abdominal and limb status are systematically determined. Frequent examinations are needed, because signs of visceral injury develop insidiously. Further fractures may be noticed.

Some children go straight to the operating room for craniotomy or reduction of a fracture. If the blood pressure becomes difficult to maintain and the abdomen becomes distended while the child is under anesthesia, you should suspect intraperitoneal bleeding of massive proportion. The diagnosis is confirmed by the finding of blood that does not clot on aspiration of the lower quadrants. Immediate laparotomy is necessary.

CHEST INJURIES

Some chest injuries are so serious that patients do not always live through them; others are so minimal that they are missed. Severe respiratory difficulty demands examination for signs of tension pneumothorax in which the simple insertion of a needle into the pleural cavity may be life-saving.

Closed chest injury may produce few outward signs or be overshadowed by other injuries. The surgeon may be unaware of serious lung damage until there is gross impairment of respiratory function, by which time there may be uncertainty whether the cause is anesthesia, fluid overloading, aspiration, or trauma.

In every patient with multiple injuries a search for chest injuries should be made. Look for signs of rib fractures and subcutaneous emphysema; auscultate the chest, and request an upright chest radiograph because pleural fluid cannot be seen on supine films. Blood gases should be obtained if there is any respiratory impairment.

Children with any signs of chest injury should be observed in ICU for a few days. Obtain daily radiographs and blood gases, because abnormalities may not show for a few days. Clinical deterioration is always heralded by a decrease of P_{O_2} and an elevation of P_{CO_2}.

The child's chest wall is more flexible than that of an adult, so the chest contents can be injured even though the ribs are not fractured. Indeed, the mortality of closed chest injuries is higher in children without fractures than in those with fractures. Simple rib fractures, so common in adults, are unusual in children.

Rupture of the Diaphragm

A ruptured diaphragm, while not common, will often produce immediate symptoms. The rupture is usually on the left, and a chest radiograph shows bowel in the left pleural cavity. Immediate laparotomy is required to repair the rent in the diaphragm, to prevent strangulation of the herniated bowel, and to treat any associated intraabdominal injury such as a rupture of the spleen.

Lung Contusion

Lung contusion, the commonest major chest injury in children, usually presents insidiously. Seldom sought and often associated with other injuries, a lung contusion may go unrecognized without a routine chest radiograph to show the fluffy infiltrates of perivascular and peribronchial parenchymal hemorrhage. Initially a child with a lung contusion and no fractures may be completely asymptomatic. Occasionally bloody sputum or frank hemoptysis will bring the condition to light. A few children go on to develop "traumatic wet-lung" syndrome with increasing tachypnea, dyspnea, mild cyanosis, and wheezes and rales at both bases. The child becomes apprehensive. Mucus, serum, and blood fill the bronchial tree.

The diagnosis should be reached before this stage by serial radiography and repeated blood gas determinations. Endotracheal intubation for toilet and ventilatory support should be undertaken. Cultures should be obtained and antibiotic administered. Inhalations may loosen secretions. Bronchoscopy is occasionally helpful. Most lung contusions resolve within a week or two, leaving no sequelae.

Pneumothorax, with or without hemothorax, may result from any lung contusion. In a simple pneumothorax air enters the pleural cavity slowly through a laceration of the surface of the lung. In a tension pneumothorax air is pumped into the pleural cavity under pressure, because the laceration behaves like a valve. The mediastinum is shifted so that this type of pneumothorax is very dangerous. The emergency treatment has already been mentioned.

The accumulated air and blood must be removed with a large intercostal tube connected to an underwater seal and suction. In children the tube should be inserted in the anterior axillary line in the fifth or sixth intercostal space so air and fluid can be removed without damaging the major vessels, which are very close to the infraclavicular area. A Heimlich flutter valve attached to the distal end of the chest tube works immediately and allows time for setting up the underwater suction. If the flutter valve is to be used for several days, it must be kept clear of blood clots and serum.

The efficiency of the drain can be assessed by repeated radiographs taken in the upright or in the lateral position to allow fluid to layer out. The chest drain can be removed in a few days when the air leak has sealed and the lung has expanded. When ventilation is maintained with a respirator the air leak may persist; the drain should remain in position until mechanical ventilation is discontinued.

Traumatic Asphyxia, a result of crushing chest injury, is infrequent but obvious. Severe cyanosis, engorgement and ecchymosis of the face, neck, and upper part of the trunk and subconjunctival hemorrhage are characteristic. Most children with this injury, bad as it looks, make a complete recovery. Those who die immediately probably do so from more serious associated injuries.

The underlying pathophysiology is a temporary obstruction of the superior vena cava and a comcomitant increase in intratracheal and intrapulmonary pressure. The injury occurs in people who take a deep breath, hold it, and brace for the crash.

Children with traumatic asphyxia must be observed in ICU while 40 percent oxygen is administered; this will provide good oxygenation and assist absorption of any residual air trapped in the mediastinum and pleural cavities. These children are initially agitated and disoriented, but any loss of consciousness is usually due to concomitant head injury. The cerebral irritability probably results from minor intracranial ecchymoses and edema. However, all these signs and symptoms recede within a few days. Neurologic sequelae are rare. Major pulmonary and mediastinal hemorrhage, pulmonary edema, pneumothorax and pneumomediastum are more serious and require ventilatory assistance, chest drains, and diuretics.

Subcutaneous Emphysema may result from injury of the tracheobronchial tree within the mediastinum, injury of the bronchi, puncture of the lung by a fractured rib, a chest drain or a penetrating injury of the chest wall.

Rupture of the trachea usually results in a quick death. Bronchial tears within the mediastinum give rise to subcutaneous emphysema of the head and neck—a puffball appearance—and a functionless lung. A tear beyond the reflection of the pleura is suggested by a continuing pneumothorax unrelieved by a chest tube or even by suction. When the site has been located by bronchoscopy, the tear must be repaired.

The commonest cause of subcutaneous emphysema is a pneumothorax due to a fractured rib. The air may track from clavicle to scrotum producing an alarming appearance, but, because the air can spread, no vital structures are compressed. Once the pneumothorax is treated the emphysema gradually disappears.

Flail Chest is uncommon. Even when multiple rib fractures occur, paradoxical movement is seldom sufficient to hinder respiration. Intermittent positive pressure ventilation by means of an endotracheal or tracheostomy tube is the most effective treatment of the unstable chest wall.

Penetrating Chest Injury is so dramatic that signs of damage to thoracic viscera are sought immediately. Wounds usually cause a pneumothorax and a hematoma of the lung. Penetration of the heart, great vessels, and abdomen is possible. Cardiac tamponade threatens life and demands paracentesis as first aid followed by immediate exploration.

As an emergency measure the pneumothorax may be relieved by inserting a chest drain through the wound. Air leak around the tube can be prevented by petroleum jelly gauze packing. Most patients who reach hospital can be adequately treated with débridement, closed tube thoracostomy, and blood replacement.

Surgical intervention should only be considered when there is a brisk continuous flow of blood from the chest tube and the volume of blood transfused exceeds the child's estimated blood volume.

Lung laceration, the commonest source of hemorrhage, can be easily controlled with a large catgut suture at thoracotomy. Resection is rarely necessary. Repair of a major vessel is preferable to ligation. Direct pressure is the best method of immediate control. The hole in the vessel is then isolated with a finger or vascular clamp until occluding tapes can be applied above and below allowing repair of the laceration with a graft or suture.

The keys to the successful treatment of chest injuries in children are early recognition of problems and a well-staffed intensive care unit.

ABDOMINAL TRAUMA

A review of 200 cases of blunt abdominal trauma seen and operated at The Hospital for Sick Children, in Toronto, between 1955 and 1965 has produced several interesting facts. Seventy-five percent of the injured were boys. Most of the injuries occured during the summer and early fall. Car accidents, direct blows (including athletics), and falls caused 85 percent of injuries. The kidney, spleen, or liver had been ruptured in 75 percent of patients. In addition to the abdominal injury, 45 percent of the children had one or more other injuries: fractures (25 percent), craniocerebral (20 percent) and thoracic (15 percent). More than one important abdominal structure was damaged in 10 percent. The mortality rate was 12 percent.

Although only a small percentage of children with multiple trauma suffer intrathoracic and/or intrabdominal injuries requiring exploration, many have minor injuries that present difficult diagnostic problems. Initially, a diagnosis can only be reached in the most obvious cases. For the remainder careful initial examination and frequent reexamination is required.

Initial Management

It is wise to pass a nasogastric tube in any child whose abdomen is not completely soft and scaphoid to relieve gastric dilatation, which is commonly present. This, in itself, will often make the child more comfortable, reduce the chance of vomiting and aspiration, and make abdominal examination much easier. Connect the tube to suction and irrigate periodically to ensure patency. Gastric dilatation, the hallmark of abdominal trauma in children, may be due to neurogenic shock, ileus, or crying. Insert a large-bore intravenous catheter into a vein in the arm—not the leg.

Much has been written about the unreliability of physical signs in abdominal injuries. The most useful signs are shock, tenderness, guarding, rigidity, and increasing girth. The site of tenderness is a guide to the site of injury. Rectal examination should be carried out in all children. Penetrating wounds may be overlooked unless every square inch of a child's abdomen and back is examined. Blood at the urethral meatus and hematuria should be looked for.

In addition to radiographs, isotope scans may assist in the diagnosis of ruptures of the spleen and liver. The value of peritoneal tap is controversial because a small amount of blood in the abdomen is not necessarily a reason to operate; false negatives are common.

Definitive Care

Nonoperative Care. Children with trauma to the trunk should be admitted to an intensive care unit. The majority improve with time, a nasogastric tube, and intravenous fluid. When gastrointestinal function returns after a few days the tubes are removed. As soon as a child has progressed from clear fluids to a regular diet and is eating and stooling normally he can be transferred to the appropriate service for treatment of residual injuries. If he has none he can be discharged from hospital with an appointment to return in 2 weeks.

Operative Care. The indications for operation are
1. Shock occuring after resuscitation, particularly when associated with increasing abdominal girth
2. The presence of free intraabdominal gas
3. Gradually increasing abdominal pain, tenderness, and rigidity

Intraperitoneal Hemorrhage

Solid viscera are more commonly ruptured than hollow organs because solid viscera are relatively fixed in the abdomen and are subject to shearing forces; the ribs, normally protective, can become agents of injury.

Intraperitoneal hemorrhage, the result of a ruptured viscus is manifested by shock, abdominal distension and tenderness and by a falling hemoglobin.

Ruptured Spleen

The commonest cause of intraperitoneal hemorrhage is rupture of the spleen. The speed and volume of bleeding determines the clinical picture and the treatment. Only a few children bleed so suddenly and massively that immediate surgery is mandatory. A few develop unexpected abdominal distension and hypovolemia under anesthesia while the orthopaedic surgeon is treating a limb fracture. The majority of children are immediately suspected of a ruptured spleen when they present with mild shock, pallor, complaints of left shoulder tip pain, left upper quadrant tenderness, and guarding. In children the ribs are commonly intact. The left kidney is nearby and the possibility that it also may be injured should not be overlooked. Start intravenous infusion and measure the abdominal girth repeatedly with a tape. Blood should be administered if hypotension is present or if the hemoglobin falls below 10 gm./100 ml.

At The Hospital for Sick Children we do not operate on every child thought to have splenic rupture. A review of our cases by Simpson supports the view that bleeding usually stops and the tear heals. Our indications for splenectomy are massive initial hemorrhage, hemorrhage that continues after initial resuscitation (recognized by increasing abdominal girth, hypovolemia, and a falling hemoglobin) and delayed hemorrhage. Children treated nonoperatively are maintained on intravenous fluid and nasogastric suction in the intensive care unit where vital signs can be frequently monitored. At the slightest signs of deterioration laparotomy and splenectomy are undertaken. Children treated nonoperatively should be observed in hospital for 7 to 10 days, and activities should be restricted at home for several weeks.

When the diagnosis is in doubt, an isotope scan of the spleen is helpful because it may show a filling defect due to hematoma or laceration. Four-quadrant tap frequently misleads the surgeon, but when the child is unconscious, under anesthesia and cannot complain of abdominal pain, a tap may have a place in diagnosis.

Splenectomy in a child of any age with a previously normal spleen does not diminish resistance to grampositive infections.

Ruptured Liver

Rupture of the liver is the next commonest cause of intraperitoneal hemorrhage. While the features are similar to those of splenic rupture, the risk of morbidity and mortality is greater. The spectrum of liver injury is wide. At the one end are minor lacerations of no clinical significance which may be noted at laparotomy after trauma. At the other end are massive transsections of the liver that cause death at the scene of the accident or in the operating room.

The indications for laparotomy are the same as those for rupture of the spleen. When bleeding is rapid, several large-bore intravenous routes with pumps should be established immediately in the arms. Order blood (equal to twice the patient's blood volume) at once, hurry the child to the operating room, and place him on a cooling mattress.

When the abdomen is opened the blood pressure may plummet to zero as the tamponading effect of the intraperitoneal blood is lost. The pressure will remain very low until hemorrhage is controlled. Many children are lost at this stage because of bleeding from hepatic veins that have been torn from the inferior vena cava. To obviate this problem a large-bore catheter may be introduced into the heart through the long saphenous vein at the groin. The catheter can be used both as a "stent" to occlude the inferior vena cava (when tapes are passed around it above and below the liver) and as a central venous route.

Severed veins require repair or ligature. Transsected devascularized liver should be removed, and the base closed with large sutures over-sewn with omentum. Bleeding lacerations require a few large sutures; those that do not bleed should be left alone.

The postoperative course may be stormy. The child may be jaundiced for a week or two, and chemical indices of liver function may take several weeks to return to normal. Meanwhile the patient will require extra sugar, proteins, and Vitamin K_1. Infections and bleeding from the operative site are matters of concern. The liver will regenerate a new lobe in 3 to 6 months; the progress of regeneration can be observed by liver scans.

Traumatic hemobilia, the result of a central contusion (that seldom requires exploration) may occur 4 to 6 weeks after liver injury. Hemobilia is due to a fistula between the bile-collecting and vascular systems of the liver. The child appears to have recovered from his injury when suddenly he has biliary colic accompanied by severe upper gastrointestinal hemorrhage. Hepatic angiography will show the lesion which is best treated by selective hepatic artery ligation or, failing this, by lobectomy.

Other causes of intraperitoneal hemorrhage include tears of the mesenteric and large retroperitoneal vessels.

Retroperitoneal Hemorrhage

In many cases of blunt abdominal trauma there is some degree of retroperitoneal hemorrhage, but this is usually of no clinical significance. It is helpful if retroperitoneal hemorrhage can be distinguished from intraperitoneal hemorrhage, because the former tends to tamponade to a halt and does not lend itself so readily to operative correction. Retroperitoneal hemorrhage due to renal, spinal, and pelvic injuries can often be recognized on an abdominal radiograph and one-shot intravenous pyelogram (IVP).

Minor degrees of retroperitoneal hemorrhage produce ileus and are best managed by nasogastric suction and intravenous fluids for a few days until bowel function returns. The problems arise when hemorrhage is continuing or massive. Despite repeated transfusions, anemia develops and abdominal girth may become enormous. Ileus is compounded by duodenal obstruction due to hematoma. The wise surgeon sits on his hands in this situation, because when such a massive hematoma is opened, brisk venous bleeding begins from multiple sites that cannot be identified in the distorted, stained tissues. Even when IVP shows one kidney functioning and one without function, there is still no necessity to explore the kidney. On the one hand, repair is seldom possible, and on the other, function may be temporarily suppressed only to return again when the hematoma resorbs. Transient prehepatic jaundice may accompany resorption.

Exploration should only be considered when there is the suspicion of a large laceration of the inferior vena cava that causes the abdomen to fill before the surgeon's eyes. Venography may help to confirm this. When the peritoneum is opened massive hemorrhage and shock will follow, so have plenty of blood at hand. Press on the tear with a finger to control hemorrhage, because tapes above and below do not halt collateral flow through the lumbar veins. The laceration should be patched and over-sewn, because ligature will produce gross edema and even gangrene. Unfortunately, whatever is done is often fruitless.

Retroperitoneal hemorrhage due to pelvic fracture is (contrary to common belief) usually slight; in only a few cases is transfusion required for pelvic blood loss alone. Urologic injury should be looked for. The question of exploration for hemorrhage associated with pelvic fractures only arises in desperate circumstances, after a child has been transfused by an amount equal to his blood volume. Massive hemorrhage, the result of disruption of a major vessel, may be suspected if a sacroiliac joint is disrupted and a femoral pulse is absent. In addition, the child may have a degloving injury around the hips and miscellaneous other injuries. For operation, two suckers and several liters of blood should be available. If tying a single large vessel stops the hemorrhage, this will be fortunate. Usually many small vessels must be packed. Packs should be soaked in a bacteriostatic solution to diminish the risk of infection and secondary hemorrhage. The packs should be removed a little at a time, after soaking, beginning on the fifth day.

Bowel Injuries

The usual site of rupture is near the fixed attachments of the small bowel (the ligament of Treitz and the ileo-cecal valve). The abdomen will be tender and somewhat distended with decreased bowel sounds at first. As time passes, signs of peritonitis will appear. In the unconscious patient there is a special need to look for these signs in order to make an early diagnosis. Fever, leukocytosis, and free intraperitoneal gas on upright or lateral decubitus radiographs are usually present. At laparotomy every inch of the bowel should be examined for injury to it and to the mesentry. Injuries cannot be felt, they must be seen. There may be more than one injury. Damaged small bowel should be treated by resection and anastomosis. Tears in the mesentery should be closed to prevent obstruction. Perforated colon should either be exteriorized *or* repaired, drained and kept empty with a temporary proximal colostomy.

Duodenum and Pancreas

Bicycle handlebars are a notorious cause of intra-abdominal injuries, particularly of the pancreas and duodenum. Both may be injured simultaneously. Upper abdominal bruising, pain, and guarding should raise the suspicion of injury. An immediate serum amylase determination is necessary for the detection of pancreatic injury (repeated at 24 hours if normal) and an upright radiograph of the abdomen for free intra-peritoneal air or the "double bubble" appearance of duodenal obstruction.

The duodenum may be ruptured or it may contain a subserosal hematoma. Barium introduced into the nasogastric tube will differentiate hematoma from rupture. Extravasation indicates rupture requiring immediate laparotomy and repair. The advocates of the nonoperative treatment of subserosal hematomata suggest that a long feeding tube be passed into the jejunum under flouroscopy.

Pancreatic injury may produce signs similar to those of duodenal rupture which increase as enzymes leak out to produce peritonitis. We have no way of distinguishing between bruising and complete transsection.

When the history suggests that the injury is mild, nonoperative management is wise. The management of major injuries is controversial. Some surgeons manage these cases conservatively, if necessary with hyper-alimentation, so long as the child's condition is not deteriorating. Others advocate immediate laparotomy because the best treatment for a transsected pancreas is removal of the tail and drainage. A torn duct should be repaired. However at operation bruising may obscure the extent of injury and make it impossible to recognize a divided duct. Because of these difficulties, pancreatic pseudocyst can develop a few weeks after injury, even when the pancreas has been explored. Injuries of the pancreas and duodenum may be overlooked when laparotomy is undertaken for some more obvious injury, so the lesser sac must always be opened and inspected.

Penetrating Injury

Stabbing and gunshot wounds are unusual in children. There is no place for probing abdominal wounds in the emergency department, however innocent they may appear. As soon as the child's general condition is suitable, all wounds should be explored under general anesthesia. If there are obvious signs of intraperitoneal hemorrhage or free air, laparotomy is mandatory, but opinions vary on the value of laparotomy when there is no sign that the peritoneum has been entered. Some surgeons have injected a mixture of blue dye and contrast material through a rubber catheter inserted as far as possible into the stab wound and held in place with a purse-string suture. A radiograph will show if the contrast material enters the peritoneum. This has been useful as a method of distinguishing patients requiring laparotomy from those requiring nothing more than debridement.

Gastrointestinal Hemorrhage

The pathogenesis of upper gastrointestinal hemorrhage after injury is still obscure. Hemorrhage may present as hematemesis, shock, or melena. A wide-bore nasogastric tube is passed and irrigated with iced saline every 1 to 2 hours to empty the stomach. Antacid (1 to 2 oz.) is left in the stomach after irrigation. Blood is cross-matched. If the child has been receiving steroids or aspirin, discontinue them.

Successful conservative treatment should be continued for a week to reduce risk of a recurrence. If hemorrhage necessitates transfusion of more than the child's blood volume, operation is required. The best procedure is still a matter of debate. Good results have been obtained from gastrotomy and ligation of bleeding points followed by pyloroplasty.

RECOMMENDED READING

1. Douglas, G. J., and Simpson, J. S. The conservative management of splenic trauma. J. Pediat. Surg., *6:* 565, 1971

2. Haller, J. A., and Donahoo, J. S.: Traumatic asphyxia in children: pathophysiology and management. J. Trauma., *2:* 453, 1971

3. Jones, P. G.: Trauma in childhood. *In* Jones, P. G., (ed.): Clinical Pediatric Surgery. Bristol, John Wright & Sons Ltd., 1970

4. Jordan, G. L., Jr., and Beall, A. C., Jr.: Diagnosis and Management of Abdominal Trauma in Current Problems in Surgery. Chicago, Year Book Medical Publishers, 1971

5. Kilman, J. W., and Charnock, E.: Thoracic trauma in infancy and childhood. J. Trauma., *9:* 863, 1969

6. Moseley, H. F.: Accident Surgery. 3 vols. New York, Appleton-Century-Crofts, 1964

7. Naclerio, E. A.: Chest Injuries. Physiologic Principles and Emergency Management. New York, Grune & Stratton, 1971

8. Quinby, W. C., Jr.: Fractures of the pelvis and associated injuries in children. J. Ped. Surg., *1:* 353, 1966

9. Stremple, J. F., Mori, H., Lev. R., and Glass, G. B. J.: The stress ulcer syndrome. Current Problems in Surgery, April 1973

10. Welch, K. J.: Abdominal and thoracic injuries. *In* Mustard W. T., *et al* (eds). Pediatric Surgery. ed. 2. vol. 1. Chicago, Year Book Medical Publishers, 1969

11. Wilson, C. B., Vidrine, A., Jr., and Rivers, J. D.: Unrecognized abdominal trauma in patients with head injuries. Ann. Surg., *161:* 608, 1965

12. Wood, M.: Penetrating wounds of the vena cava. Recommendations for treatment. Surgery, *60:* 311, 1966

8

Genitourinary Trauma in the Pediatric Orthopaedic Patient

Martin Barkin, M.D., B.Sc. (Med), M.A., F.R.C.S.(C), and J. F. Schillinger, M.D., F.R.C.S.(C)

Trauma is the commonest cause of death in the pediatric age group (17/100,000). Major genitourinary trauma, however, is relatively rare. When it does occur, it is usually associated with multiple severe injuries or a preexisting urinary tract abnormality. Death is more commonly due to non-genitourinary injury rather than the genitourinary injury *per se*.[7]

There are certain features of the child's urinary tract that distinguish it from its adult counterpart and result in somewhat different manifestations of injury.

1. The bladder tends to be intraabdominal rather than intrapelvic, and therefore *intra*peritoneal extravasation of urine is slightly less rare in children than in adults.

2. The retroperitoneum is extremely thin, and severe injuries of the kidney may produce intraperitoneal extravasation of blood and/or urine that can make the diagnostic abdominal tap deceptive.

3. The vessels in the pediatric age group are more elastic, and vascular injury is more likely to produce intimal tear and thrombosis rather than pedicle avulsion.[3]

4. The elasticity of bone increases the incidence of greenstick fracture and decreases the incidence of sharp spicules producing secondary penetrating injuries.

5. Since congenital anomalies may be present, relatively minor trauma may be associated with signs, symptoms, and injury of an inordinately severe nature. Fifteen percent of children presenting to an emergency department with signs of severe renal injury come after minor trauma associated with a preexisting congenital abnormality such as hydronephrosis or cystic disease.[5] Figure 8-1 demonstrates a copious blood clot collecting in the renal pelvis of a hydronephrotic kidney that ruptured after a fall from a tricycle.

INITIAL MANAGEMENT OF THE TRAUMATIZED CHILD

The first obligation of the casualty officer is the immediate assessment and correction of conditions that are immediately life-threatening, such as obstructed airway, massive hemorrhage, expanding hematoma of the central nervous system, sucking wounds of the chest, and tension pneumothorax. An adequate infusion should be placed into the circulatory system, and volume replacement should take place immediately, with guidance by central venous pressure monitoring.[1]

The subsequent discussion is confined to the genitourinary aspects of the patient's injuries.

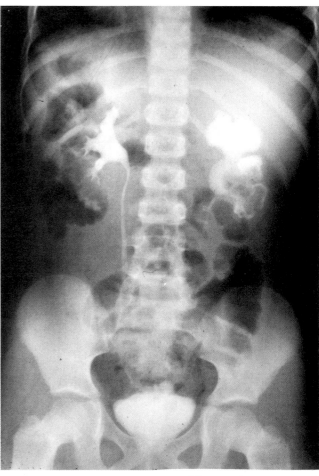

Fig. 8-1. Intravenous urogram of 8-year-old girl who fell from a tricycle. The left kidney is hydronephrotic due to ureteropelvic junction obstruction. The filling defect in the lower pole is a blood clot secondary to renal injury.

PRESENTATION AND DIAGNOSIS OF GENITOURINARY INJURIES

Children with multiple injuries and those with fractures to the lower ribs or pelvis should be examined for genitourinary injuries, whether or not any of the other signs and symptoms listed below are present.

Hematuria

The presence of hematuria confirms the diagnosis of urinary tract injury, but neither the site nor the severity of the injury is proportional to the degree and intensity of hematuria.

Urethral Bleeding

Urethral bleeding is diagnostic of an injury below the vesical neck. The patient should not be asked to void, and a urethrogram should be made prior to attempts at catheterization.

Extravasation in the Perineum

Either blood or urine may extravasate within the perineum, along the lines of attachment of Buck's or Colles' fascia. This is an indication of disruption of urinary tract continuity below the urogenital diaphragm and is similarly an indication for an early retrograde urethrogram.

Rectal Examination

A rectal examination may reveal the prostate to be displaced from its usual location or replaced by a soft pelvic hematoma. Either finding is clinical evidence of transection of the urethra above the perineal diaphragm. This also is an indication for retrograde urethrogram.

Evidence of Severe Occult Bleeding

Injuries of the kidney and the renal vascular pedicle are suggested by increasingly refractory shock, increasing abdominal girth, and ecchymosis in the flank.

Pain

Pain, abdominal guarding and splinting are unreliable signs of urinary tract injury and more often reflect the severity of trauma to overlying bones or muscles.

SPECIAL TECHNIQUES FOR UROLOGIC EVALUATION

In almost all cases of injury there is ample time for

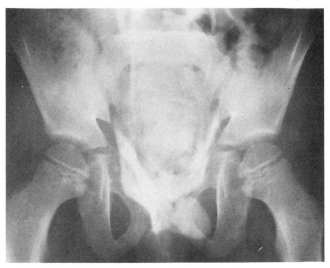

Fig. 8-2. A retrograde urethrogram showing extravasation from the supramembranous urethra. Note also fractures of the pelvis.

careful and complete evaluation of the urinary system.[2] An intravenous urogram is indicated in all cases where genitourinary injury is suspect, not only to help delineate the injury, but also to determine the structure and function of the contralateral renal unit. Prompt function and normal configuration on an intravenous urogram are sufficient criteria to indicate that a particular renal unit is capable of sustaining life. Bilateral nonfunction usually is due to poor renal perfusion secondary to hypovolemia. (Rarely it may be due to unilateral

TRAUMA TO THE KIDNEY

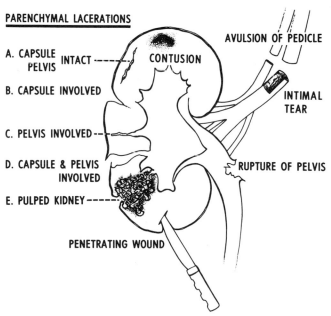

Fig. 8-3. Schematic representation of types of renal trauma.

Table 8-1. Classification of Renal Injuries Correlated with Clinical and Radiographic Findings

Injury	Clinical Findings	Radiographic Findings
Contusion	Hematuria, gross or microscopic	Normal Slight delayed function
Laceration Subcapsular	Hematuria	Distention of renal outline Delayed function

Through capsule	Hematuria, flank tenderness,
	  ± mass, signs of intraperitoneal
	  hemorrhage
		Loss of renal outline and
		  psoas shadow
		Retroperitoneal mass,
		  minimal dye extravasation
		  nephrogram phase present

Intrapelvic	May be all of above	As above plus more marked dye extravasation

Shattered Kidney
  (total or polar)
	All of above
	Shock
		As above
		Nephrogram phase may be
		  absent

Avulsion of Ureter	Hematuria, often expanding
	  flank mass
		Massive extravasation
		  prompt function

Pedicle Injuries
  Transection
	Rapid death, severe shock
	Late posttraumatic collapse
		No nephrogram
		  (if live)

Intimal tears	Flank pain Asymptomatic loss of kidney	No nephrogram

injury with contralateral absence or bilateral severe injury.) The urogram should be done when the patient's circulatory status has stabilized. The high dose infusion urogram will accurately delineate the severity of injury in 80 percent of cases.[4] The immediate "flush phase" may also indicate injury to solid viscera, such as liver and spleen.

While you await the delayed films, cystourethrograms may be done. If there is blood at the meatus, rectal or perineal hematoma or extravasation, or if a catheter cannot be passed, a retrograde urethrogram is mandatory. Figure 8-2 is a retrograde urethrogram of a 9-year-old boy who sustained an anterior compression injury to his pelvis. Blood was present at his urethral meatus, and rectal examination revealed a dislodged prostate. Retrograde urethrogram demonstrates extravasation at the supramembranous urethra and indicates disruption at this level. Special studies such as angiography and retrograde pyelography may be indicated.

SPECIFIC INJURIES OF THE UPPER TRACT

The classification and radiological signs of injury to the upper tract are summarized in Figure 8-3 and Table 8-1. Most patients will respond to conservative management with bed rest. Monitor the physical signs, urinalyses, and urographic changes carefully and frequently.

Indications for Surgical Management

1. Massive unrelenting hematuria
2. Continuous hematuria
3. Increasing extravasation of urine (Fig. 8-4)
4. Fever
5. Expanding abdominal mass
6. Severe intraabdominal hemorrhage
7. Retroperitoneal hemorrhage
8. Absent nephrogram with vascular occlusion confirmed by angiogram.

Whenever surgery is carried out for renal injury the status of the contralateral kidney must be known, if necessary by intraoperative urography. If during the course of laparotomy a retroperitoneal hematoma is found, it should be left undisturbed, provided it is stable and not enlarging. Surgical treatment may consist of nephrectomy or renal salvaging procedures, such as suture and drainage, partial nephrectomy, or renovascular reconstruction. The late complications of renal injury are hypertension, hematuria, loss of renal function, chyluria, urinoma, obstruction, cyst formation, and calcification.

URETERAL INJURIES

Injury to the ureter almost never occurs as a result of blunt trauma. Penetrating injuries and surgical procedures are the usual causes. Urinary extravasation confirmed by retrograde pyelography confirms the presence of this injury. Treatment is surgical reconstruction with adequate local and urinary drainage.

VESICAL AND URETHRAL INJURY

Injury to the urethra and bladder are the commonest urological sequelae to blunt abdominal trauma. Vesical contusion is common and is of academic significance only. When a child sustains an injury severe enough to fracture his pelvis, then there is a high probability of a surgically significant vesical injury.[7]

The cystourethrogram will reveal the nature of the injury. Two-thirds of vesical disruptions are retroperitoneal; only one-third are intraperitoneal.

All injuries of the bladder accompanied by radiologically proven extravasation must be managed surgically. The peritoneal cavity is opened and explored. If the rupture has been intraperitoneal the rent in the bladder should be repaired using two layers of absorbable sutures. If extraperitoneal, the laceration need be repaired only if easily accessible. In either instance the bladder should be drained suprapubically, and an adequate drain should be placed in the space of Retzius.

Disruption of the supramembranous urethra is the most serious urinary injury in this group. The high incidence of stricture (50 percent) and impotence (40 percent) have made its management controversial. At one extreme, some surgeons advocate complete mobilization and visualization of the affected area transpubically or perincally with direct suture repair and suprapubic urinary diversion. At the other extreme is an ultraconservative approach that avoids any surgical manipulation of the injured site and provides suprapubic drainage only.[6] This latter group of patients will for the most part later require two surgical procedures to treat their strictures. We recommend that urethral alignment be secured as atraumatically as possible, with a Foley urethral catheter under slight traction. Adequate suprapubic drainage should be provided to the bladder and space of Retzius.

The diagnosis and treatment of lower urethral injuries follows the same principles. Surgical intervention is always necessary when there is radiological confirmation of extravasation.

Suprapubic diversion, direct suture repair, and adequate local drainage remain the mainstays of treatment. Late sequelae of lower tract injury include

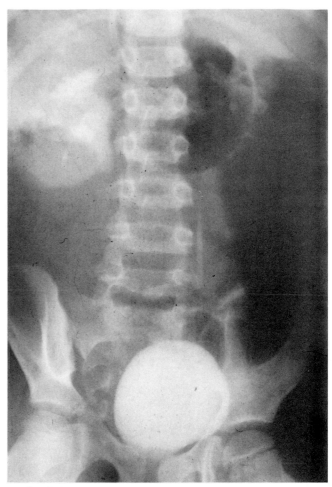

Fig. 8-4. Intravenous urogram of 8-year-old boy after blunt injury to right flank. Note extensive extravasation obscuring right renal outline.

stricture, infection, impotence, vesical dysfunction, incontinence, stone formation, abscess, and diverticula.

REFERENCES

1. Currie, D. J.: Early management of the critically injured. Canadian Med. Ass. J., *95:* 862, 1966
2. Guerrier, K., Albert, D. J., Mahoney, S. A., Igant, R. J., Jr., and Persky, L.: Delayed nephrectomy after trauma. J. Trauma, *9:* 465, 1967
3. Kaufman, J. J., and Brossman, S. A.: Blunt injuries of the genito-urinary tract. Surg. Clin. N. Amer., *52:* 747, 1972
4. Lucy, D. T., Smith, J. J. V., and Koontz, W. W., Jr.: A plea for conservative treatment of renal injuries. J. Trauma, *11:* 306, 1971.
5. Mertz, J. H., Wishard, W. N. Jr., Nourse, M. H., and Mertz, H. O.: Injury of the kidney in children. J.A.M.A., *183:* 730, 1963
6. Morehouse, D. D., and McKinnon, K. J.: Urological injuries associated with pelvic fractures. J. Trauma, *9:* 479, 1969
7. Quinby, W. C.: Fractures of the pelvis and associated injuries in children. J. Ped. Surg., *1:* 353, 1966

9

Craniocerebral Injury

E. Bruce Hendrick, M.D., B.Sc. (Med), F.R.C.S.(C)

The early diagnosis and possible complications of craniocerebral injury have been surrounded for many years with an aura of mysticism which, unfortunately, has led to an unnecessary and irrational anxiety on the part of many physicians faced with the treatment of these injuries. Because many children with limb fractures have head injuries, orthopaedic surgeons should know something about craniocerebral injuries in particular, about first aid, assessment, the indications for referral to a neurosurgical center, and the influence of a head injury on the treatment of a fractured limb.

EXAMINATION

The approach to a craniocerebral injury should be systematic and careful. Begin with a history, then go on to a general assessment and examination of the cranium and the central nervous system.

History

A careful history obtained from relatives or witnesses to the accident will do much to determine the type of injury: when it occurred? how it occurred? what was the patient's immediate level of consciousness following the injury? Did the level of consciousness decrease? Was there a lucid interval?

General State

In the initial examination the general state of the patient is much more important than any evidence of local intracranial damage.

The six "B" priorities—breathing, bleeding, brain, bowel, bladder, and bone—indicate the order in which attention must be paid to multi-system injuries. Airway patency and normal intergaseous exchange in the pulmonary system have a profound effect on cerebral blood flow, metabolism, and intracranial pressure. An obstructed airway not only carries with it the secondary pulmonary complications of atelectasis and infection, but it produces a gross abnormality in gaseous exchange so that the cerebral vascular system is perfused by arterial blood of high carbon dioxide content. This, in turn, increases cerebral blood flow and causes cerebral edema and intracranial hypertension. In addition, the struggle against an obstructed airway raises intrathoracic pressure and, eventually, intracranial venous pressure.

The patient should be carefully examined for signs of tension pneumothorax, hemothorax and aspiration. If bronchial toilet is required, bronchoscopy and endotracheal intubation should be carried out immediately in the Emergency Department.

Positioning of the patient can make the difference between life and death (Fig. 9-1). For transportation from the site of injury to the hospital, from the Emergency Department to the X-ray Department, and on the ward, the child should be in a semiprone position so that nasopharyngeal secretions may drain out rather than be aspirated.

If there can be one statement that should be repeated over and over again to a physician in charge of an Emergency Room or to people concerned with first aid, it should be the simple statement that "hypotensive shock is never due to a head injury alone." The presence of shock indicates injury elsewhere: therefore be scrupulous in examining the abdomen, chest, and extremities. Only in the head-injured patient with failing vital centers, or extensive scalp lacerations, are the classic signs of shock detected. Occult hemorrhage within the chest, abdomen, or pelvis may cause profound hypovolemic shock, which is more lethal than a head injury and certainly exacerbates the effects of the head injury.

Replacement of lost fluid by the intravenous route is mandatory. Because whole blood is more effective it should be used if it is available and can be obtained in the necessary time. There is no truth in the rumor that fluid replacement is contraindicated in craniocerebral injury.

Cranial Examination

Only after the general examination has been carried out and first aid is instituted to improve airway, restore blood pressure, and stop hemorrhage, should detailed examination of the head be undertaken. Obvious fractures of the skull with laceration of brain and extrusion of brain content on the surface need no comment. In

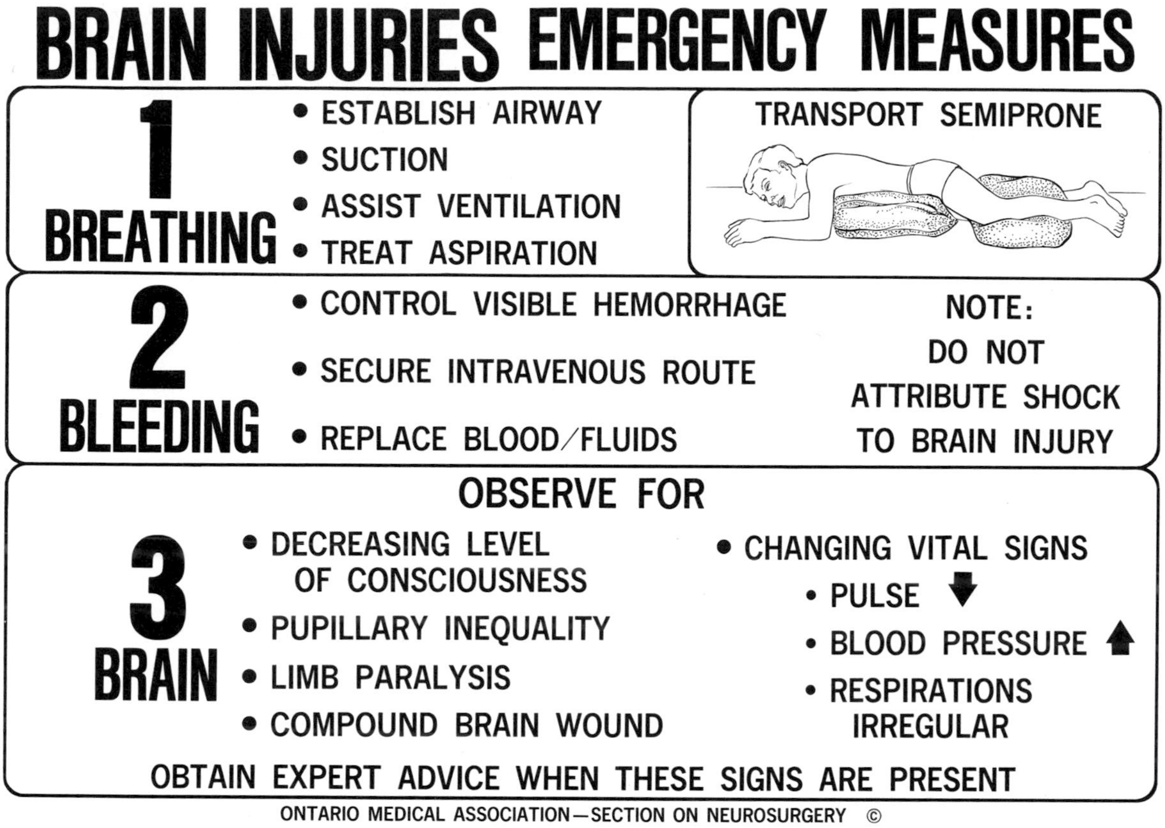

BRAIN INJURIES EMERGENCY MEASURES

1 BREATHING
- ESTABLISH AIRWAY
- SUCTION
- ASSIST VENTILATION
- TREAT ASPIRATION

TRANSPORT SEMIPRONE

2 BLEEDING
- CONTROL VISIBLE HEMORRHAGE
- SECURE INTRAVENOUS ROUTE
- REPLACE BLOOD/FLUIDS

NOTE:
DO NOT
ATTRIBUTE SHOCK
TO BRAIN INJURY

3 BRAIN

OBSERVE FOR
- DECREASING LEVEL OF CONSCIOUSNESS
- PUPILLARY INEQUALITY
- LIMB PARALYSIS
- COMPOUND BRAIN WOUND
- CHANGING VITAL SIGNS
  - PULSE ⬇
  - BLOOD PRESSURE ⬆
  - RESPIRATIONS IRREGULAR

OBTAIN EXPERT ADVICE WHEN THESE SIGNS ARE PRESENT

ONTARIO MEDICAL ASSOCIATION—SECTION ON NEUROSURGERY ©

Fig. 9-1. All emergency rooms should have a chart such as this.

patients with large masses of scalp hair, lacerations and depressions may go unnoticed unless careful palpation and examination of the whole head is carried out. Blood or spinal fluid draining from the nose or external auditory canal should be noted and taken as presumptive evidence of a fracture of the base of the skull in the anterior or middle fossa. To prevent the possibility of contamination of the intracranial content by bacteria from outside, a broad-spectrum antibiotic should be administered, in the same dosage used for meningitis, immediately upon admission to hospital.

Examination of the Central Nervous System

The importance of the first examination of the central nervous system cannot be overemphasized, because this examination assists in diagnosis and forms a base for judging subsequent progress. Much of the anxiety that often attends the treatment of a head injury in the acute stage stems from the fact that at the outset no accurate assessment was made of the patient's level of consciousness and the presence of neurological abnormalities was not noted. There are usually two reasons for this: the patient may be quite uncooperative and may not allow an ordinary neurological examination, or the presence of other injuries may make examination difficult. Yet there are few cases in which it is not possible to record accurately the level of the patient's consciousness, the size and reaction of the pupils, the tone and power of the limbs on command or stimulation, the presence or absence of reflexes, and the state of the plantar responses.

A "mini-neurological" examination will form the basis for decisions later by a team of doctors and nurses who were not present in the Emergency Room. Therefore technical language should be avoided in describing the conscious level of the patient and his reactions to the examination. A simple sentence on the patient's record stating that he is responding verbally to his name or simple commands, or indeed, responds briskly to pinprick in all four extremities by withdrawing, is of inestimable value to all who will subsequently participate in treatment. Such phrases as comatose, semicomatose, or semi-conscious should be used only by poets. This cannot be overemphasized: *The most important single factor to be observed on repeated examination and noted accurately on the chart is the patient's level of consciousness.* The return to normalcy is a sign of recovery. But if the patient recovered completely from the initial concussion and then lapsed into unconsciousness, it is obvious that some major complication has developed. A grave prognostic sign that calls for action is a decreasing level of consciousness on successive reports. Because it is difficult to estimate the progress of a patient who has been unconscious throughout, careful recording of other vital signs is invaluable. The patient's temperature, pulse, blood pressure, respiration, and pupillary reactions should be charted at regular, stated intervals. Slowing of the pulse, elevation of the blood pressure, and loss of pupillary reflexes may be the only signs of deterioration.

Deterioration of the patient's condition immediately suggests that the intracranial problem is becoming more serious. On the other hand, one should not overlook the possibility of chest complications causing cerebral hypoxia, cerebral fat embolism, metabolic disorders, and shock from other injuries. The restless agitated state seen in many patients with head trauma is often related to a full bladder, a tight encircling bandage or cast, or cerebral hypoxia. Unless these factors are taken into account, the cause of deterioration may be erroneously interpreted as intercerebral, and fruitless intracranial procedures may be instituted.

Investigations

Usually the first thought of those called to see a head injury is that a radiographic examination of the skull must be carried out. This procedure has been greatly abused and, indeed, if the patient is showing signs of rapidly increased intracranial pressure or intracranial localization, radiographs will be of little value, will delay treatment, and will adversely influence the outcome to a significant degree. Depressed fractures of the skull do require radiography to allow the surgeon to determine the extent of the fracture and the depth to which the fractured fragments have penetrated. However, in subdural or extradural hematoma, or in acute cerebral edema, radiographs should be delayed until the primary problems have been dealt with.

In the brain-injured patient, special diagnostic aids are of great help. Cerebral arteriography will help distinguish between an extradural clot and an intracerebral clot and will help with localization. If a patient who has been improving develops a delay or a levelling off in his recovery, angiography may show the presence of a chronic subdural hematoma. We do not use diagnostic ultrasound in children because it seems unreliable.

Brain scanning has been of great value in predicting the improvement of the patient with cerebral edema or cerebral infarct or damage following a localized trauma.

The simplest diagnostic procedure which comes to the mind of many doctors is a lumbar puncture. *Lumbar puncture should never be carried out in the presence of an acute head injury.* The rapid removal of fluid from the lumbar sac may produce a change in intracranial pressure relationships and subsequent coning or herniation of the cerebellar tonsils or the cerebral peduncles; either may be fatal. Lumbar punctures should be considered only when the patient develops an unexplained fever after a period of 2 or 3 days; that is when meningi-tis is a possibility. The presence of blood in the spinal fluid is of no significance except as an indication that there has been bleeding into the subarachnoid or ventricular areas.

DIAGNOSIS

A few more words might be said at this point about the differentiation of extradural hemorrhage, subdural hemorrhage, and cerebral edema. In a review of several thousand head injuries it was my intention to differentiate these three. At the end of the review it was found they could not be differentiated by their presenting features or by signs or symptoms.

The classic form of the extradural hemorrhage is consistent with a space-occupying lesion in the middle cranial fossa. The picture of an initial period of unconsciousness following injury with a subsequent lucid interval and then increasing stupor and coma is well known. The triad of an ipsilateral dilated pupil, contralateral hemiparesis, and a linear fracture in the temporal parietal area would alert most physicians to impending disaster. Review of a large series of extradural hematomas showed that the classical picture occurs in less than 10 percent. The commonest features are deepening unconsciousness and a dilated pupil, not necessarily on the side of the hematoma. *In the series, a skull fracture was present in less than 15 percent of patients.* The use of x-rays therefore, is clearly contraindicated in a deteriorating patient.

Posterior fossa extradural or subdural hematomas are rare. They present with changes in blood pressure, respiratory rate, or pulse rate. They do not tend to show lateralizing neurological deficits. They do not progress as quickly as supratentorial clots. Radiographs usually reveal a fracture crossing the transverse sinus and extending down to the foramen magnum.

Spinal Injuries

A word of warning about spinal injuries associated with head injuries: They are not common but they do occur. One should be alert to meningismus and to local tenderness in the neck or spine. Flaccid paralysis of both lower extremities in a patient with a head injury should suggest a spinal cord injury. Urinary retention may be a primary indication of injury to the spinal cord itself. These problems are easily missed because neurological deficits are attributed to brain injury, but one should be always alert to a second neurological problem. A sensory deficit to pinprick or absence of sweating below the level of a spinal cord lesion may be of some help in diagnosis.

TREATMENT

Treatment is determined by the urgency of the problem and the facilities available. *For example, a patient with obvious extradural hemorrhage cannot be transported. Minutes count.* If a neurosurgeon is not immediately available, the surgeon on call should make bur holes. Children with severe head injuries who show no signs of deterioration can be transported to the regional neurosurgical unit. Be sure that they are transported semiprone with a good airway and are not suffering hypovolemic shock due to visceral injury. If the patient is to be transferred, it should be done quickly and without delay.

If there is no evidence of increased intracranial pressure, an open depressed fracture, or progressive deterioration requiring urgent operative treatment, the patient should be admitted to hospital and placed under close observation. Head-injury patients should be nursed in the semiprone position. While unconscious, they should be turned from side to side at 2-hour intervals. They should not be placed head down in traction for a lower limb injury. Some other method of treatment should be used for the lower limb. Rectal temperatures should be recorded regularly, and pyrexia should be controlled by simple measures such as alcohol sponging and, if necessary, hypothermic blankets. Sedatives are given only if there is evidence of epileptic activity.

In head injuries cerebral edema is the problem of greatest concern. The use of hyperosmolar 20-percent mannitol simply buys time. It is not recommended, unless prior neurosurgical consultation has been obtained. If necessary, mannitol may be administered intravenously in doses of 1.5 to 2.0 g./kg. over a period of 30 to 45 minutes. *Be sure that cardiopulmonary function is adequate and kidney function intact.* The use of mannitol commits the surgeon to another course of action, whether it is the transfer of the patient from a primary care facility to a specialized unit or the preparation of the patient for immediate surgery.

Intravenous dexamethasone (14 mg. initially and 4 mg. every 6 hours intravenously or intramuscularly) is said to have some effect on cerebral edema, but the results are not dramatic.

Operative Treatment

There are only two indications for immediate surgical intervention in head injuries: (1) an open penetrating wound and (2) bur hole exploration for extradural or subdural clot in patients who have clearly displayed severe and rapid deterioration of neurological function. This deterioration is usually manifest by a decreasing level of consciousness, a dilating pupil (usually on the side of the suspected clot), and progressive paralysis of the limbs on the opposite side. A bur hole will confirm the diagnosis and permit removal of surface hematoma from the extradural and subdural space. The first bur hole is made in the temporal region on the side of the enlarged pupil. The skin incision runs upward for 2 inches from the zygoma, a finger's breadth in front of the ear and will bring one on to the fleshy belly of the temporalis muscle. The temporal artery itself will be either seen or divided. After temporal artery bleeding is controlled, the temporalis muscle is incised vertically in the same direction as the skin wound, and the muscle fibers are removed from the surface of the skull. With a perforator and bur, a hole is made in the center of the exposure and enlarged by means of rongeurs. If an epidural clot is present, it will be immediately apparent. The skull defect may be enlarged, the clot removed, and the bleeding point identified and coagulated. Do not worry about blood loss; the major concern is death from brain compression. Always make the initial bur hole in the temporal fossa, because the commonest source of bleeding in an extradural hematoma is the middle meningeal artery. Although hematoma derived from large venous sinuses have been reported and have been seen by this author, the middle meningeal artery or its branches have been responsible in 80 percent of cases.

When no extradural hemorrhage is found, the dura should be incised in a cruciate fashion and the subdural space opened to exclude subdural hematoma. If the temporal bur hole reveals no evidence of subdural hematoma, then two more bur holes should be made, one in the posterior frontal area just one half to 2 inches lateral to the midline and the other 2 inches lateral to the midline in the posterior parietal area. The dura should be opened again to exclude subdural hematoma. Bur holes must be placed bilaterally, because subdural hematomas occur on both sides in more than 50 percent of head injury patients. Simple evacuation of the subdural hematoma by suction and irrigation with warm normal saline solution produces significant improvement.

Treatment of closed depressed fractures of the skull which are not producing a gross neurological deficit can be safely delayed. An extensive open fracture should be treated by debridement and closure of the scalp wound followed by transfer of the patient to a neurosurgical facility. Removal of the bone fragments and closure of the scalp is all that is necessary as immediate treatment. Definitive repair of the dura and repair of the skull with cranioplasty can be carried out later.

OTHER PROBLEMS

Unconscious patients require a great deal of care; an experienced team is needed to stay ahead of problems.

Fluid and Electrolyte Problems

Many patients with severe head injury present nutritional and metabolic problems. Use intravenous replacement therapy (in the form of a solution of two thirds dextrose and one third normal saline) for the first 24 to 36 hours after admission to hospital. Then begin feeding through a nasogastric tube using a gastric one diet and an antacid to reduce the real risk of acute gastric hemorrhage. Vitamin supplements are necessary. A fatty diet may cause diarrhea; the problem can usually be relieved by substituting a more dilute solution containing Kaopectate administered by gastric tube.

Daily determinations of serum proteins, blood glucose, and electrolytes are invaluable in judging what is required to correct the various metabolic disorders as they arise. One of the commonest disturbances, water deprivation, usually occurs because of the doctor's reluctance to begin artificial feeding in the unconscious patient. He hopes that the patient will soon regain consciousness and be able to swallow spontaneously. Water deprivation can also be due to increased fluid loss, hyperpyrexia, and unrecognized diabetes insipidus in severe midbrain injury, although this is a very rare phenomenon. Routine dehydration for head injuries, recommended in many early texts, has proven to be an unnecessary and potentially dangerous procedure. It may lead to worsening of the patient's condition and deterioration of his level of consciousness.

Diabetes insipidus can follow hypothalamic damage. The common time of onset appears to be about the tenth day, because there is usually sufficient antidiuretic hormone to prevent the syndrome from appearing earlier. The condition can be detected from the urinary output and specific gravity. In most individuals, the diabetes is mild and can be treated by increased fluid intake. In the more severe cases injections of pitressin may be necessary. Diabetes mellitus is rarely due to head injury, but patients with head trauma often show transient glycosuria. In recent years disorders to chloride metabolism have been recognized: (1) inability to secrete chloride results in hyperchloremia and hypochloruria and (2) excessive loss of chloride produces hyperchloruria. A high mortality attends these disorders if the imbalance is not corrected; adequate laboratory investigation and appropriate replacement therapy should eliminate these problems.

Chest Problems

Problems may arise from chest injuries, such as pulmonary fat embolism, atelectasis, and penumonia.

Pulmonary fat embolism is particularly likely in a patient with associated limb fractures and accounts for a proportion of cases diagnosed as hypostatic bronchopneumonia following head trauma. Acute pulmonary edema may be produced as the result of a brain stem compression.

Bronchopneumonia in the unconscious patient is al-

ways a problem, but it can be treated with endotracheal bronchial toilet and antibiotics. Tracheostomy may be a life-saving procedure, particularly in the patient who has suffered damage to the thoracic cage or who has a repiratory infection. Tracheostomy should be considered for three groups of patients: (1) those in whom it is quickly apparent that unconsciousness is profound and will last for more than 48 hours, (2) patients with other injuries affecting the airway, such as jaw or chest fractures, (3) patients who cannot lie semiprone because of spinal injuries.

Limb Fractures

Patients with cerebral injury should not be placed head down. This will aggravate cerebral edema and bleeding and should be avoided if at all possible. Fractures of the femur can be left flat in a Thomas splint for a day or two if a rapid recovery can be expected. Alternatively 90-90 traction should be used. Fractures of the shaft of the humerus frequently require traction. When the child is very restless and seems likely to continue so, internal fixation of fractures of long bones may be advisable.

PROGNOSIS

Orthopaedic surgeons should not give laissez-faire treatment to deeply unconscious children. The prognosis for survival and function is much better in children than in adults. The same standards of fracture care should be observed as in children who have no head injury.

Summary

Treatment of closed head injuries may be summarized under four main headings:

Maintain a clear airway at all times in unconscious patients. Patients who are unconscious should be placed in a semiprone position. In the presence of excessive nasopharyngeal secretions a nasal airway is necessary with suction available at all times. With prolonged coma tracheostomy should be considered.

Chart pulse, respirations and blood pressure at 15 and 30 minute intervals after admission to the Emergency Room. Intervals for charting the vital signs may be lengthened as soon as the patient remains stable for 6 to 12 hours providing the depth of consciousness has not deteriorated.

Regularly observe
1. State of consciousness
2. Size and reactivity of pupils
3. Activity of deep tendon reflexes
4. Character of respirations

Watch for these signs which carry grave prognostic significance
1. Temperature over 39.4°C (101°F)
2. Irregular periodic respirations
3. Pupillary abnormalities
4. Paralysis of the extremities
5. Decreasing level of consciousness

At times it is dificult to decide who should be admitted to hospital and who should not. As a standard rule, all individuals with a history of head trauma who have had an episode of unconsciousness or who are unconscious should be admitted. Individuals who have altered personality or who show neurological deficit on examination should be admitted for observation.

The treatment of a head injury is similar to that of any other injury or acute illness. Proper examination, observation and correlation of the changing factors or signs and proper application of treatment in response to the dynamic changes provide the essentials of care. The treatment of the patient with head injury and multiple trauma may call for compromise, but, with the exception of hemorrhage, the head injury should be treated first, because it may be fatal. However, one should not unnecessarily delay treating other injuries on the grounds that the patient has sustained a head trauma. Treatment of the head injury becomes as time passes, more and more of a team effort involving not only the orthopaedic surgeon and neurosurgeon but the specialist in pulmonary physiology and the intensive care staffs.

RECOMMENDED READING

Alexander, E.: Medical management of closed head injuries. Clin. Neurosurg., *19:* 240, 1972.

Evans, J. P.: Advances in the understanding and treatment of head injury. Canad. Med. Assn. J., *95:* 1337, 1966.

Hagan, P. J., and Cole, J. M.: Medical management of injuries to the temporal bone and its contents. Med. Clin. N. Amer., *48:* 1605, 1964.

Harwood-Nash, D. C.: Cranio-cerebral trauma in children. Curr. Prob. Radiol. *3:* 3, 1973.

Harwood-Nash, D. C., Hendrick, E. B., and Hudson, A. R.: The significance of skull fractures in children; a study of 1187 Patients. Radiology, *101:* 151, 1971.

Hendrick, E. B., and Harris, L.: Post-traumatic epilepsy in children. J. Trauma, *8:* 547, 1968.

Hendrick, E. B., Harwood-Nash, D. C., and Hudson, A. R.: Head injuries in children. Clin. Neurosurg., *11:* 46, 1965.

Hooper, R.: Observations on extradural hemorrhage. Brit. J. Surg., *47:* 71, 1959.

Horwitz, N. H., and Rizzoli, H. V.: Postoperative Complications in Neurosurgical Practice. Baltimore, Williams & Wilkins, 1967.

Jackson, F. E.: The pathophysiology of head injuries. CIBA Clinical Symposia, *20:* 4, 1968.

Jamieson, K. G.: Extradural and subdural hematomas. Changing patterns and requirements of treatment in Australia. J. Neurosurg., *33:* 632, 1970.

Jamieson, K. G., and Yelland, J. D. N.: Extradural hematoma. Report of 167 cases. J. Neurosurg., *29:* 13, 1968.

————: Surgically treated traumatic subdural hematomas. J. Neurosurg., *37:* 137, 1972.

Jeffreys, W. H., and Hood, H.: The supportive management of acute closed head injuries. Med. Clin. N. Amer. *48:* 1599, 1964.

Jennett, W. B.: Head injuries in children. Dev. Med. Child. Neurol., *14:* 137, 1972.

Johnston, I. H., Johnston, J. A., and Jennett, W. B.: Intracranial pressure changes following head injury. Lancet, *2:* 433, 1970.

Lewin, W.: The management of head injuries. London, Balliere, Tindall & Cassell, 1966.

Lindenberg, R., and Freytag, E.: The mechanism of cerebral contusions. A pathologic-anatomic study. Arch. Pathol., *69:* 1960.

Meirowsky, A. M. (ed.): Neurological Surgery of Trauma. Washington, D.C., Office of the Surgeon General, Department of the Army, 1965.

Mullan, S.: Essential don'ts in the treatment of craniocerebral injuries. Surg. Clin. N. Amer., *43:* 115, 1958.

Peerless, S. J., and Rewcastle, N. B.: Shear injuries of the brain. Canad. Med. Assn. J., *96:* 577, 1967.

Plum, F., and Posner, J. B.: Diagnosis of Stupor and Coma. ed. 20 Philadelphia, F. A. Davis, 1972.

Potter, J. M.: Emergency management of head injuries. Brit. Med. J., *2:* 1477, 1965.

————: Head injuries. *In* Gillingham, F. J. (ed.): Clinical Surgery. Neurosurgery. London, Butterworth, 1970.

Rowbotham, G. F. Acute Injuries of the Head: Their Diagnosis, Treatment, Complications and Sequelae. London, E. & S. Livingstone, 1964.

Strich, S. J.: Shearing of nerve fibres as a cause of brain damage due to head injury. Lancet, *1:* 443, 1961.

Symonds, Sir Charles: Concussion and its sequelae. Lancet, *1:* 702, 1962.

Tindall, G. T., Meyer, G. A., and Iwata, K.: Current methods of monitoring patients with head injury. Clin. Neurosurg., *19:* 98, 1972.

White, R. J., et al.: Programmed management of severe closed head injuries. J. Trauma, *8:* 203, 1968.

Youmans, J. R. (ed.): Neurological Surgery. Philadelphia, W. B. Saunders, 1973. (See vol. 1, chap. 40–56)

10

Clavicle

Sir Robert Peel, Prime Minister of Britain in 1834, would have been amongst the first to agree that the clavicle is a badly designed bone. In 1850, he died after falling from his horse on Constitution Hill, having sustained a fracture of the clavicle which probably penetrated the subclavian vessels. The double curve of the clavicle is a poor mechanical shape, adequate perhaps in arboreal animals and quadrupeds, but definitely a point of weakness in the young male biped. The double curve can produce a very good imitation of a clavicular fracture on some radiographic projections. About half the fractures of the clavicle occur in children under the age of 10 years. In children, the clavicle is the most frequently broken bone. Injuries may occur at three sites.

SHAFT FRACTURES

Fractures of the shaft (usually the mid-shaft) are commonest, being greenstick or complete fractures (Figs. 10-1, 10-2). Fractures unite quickly, though almost invariably with malunion. Remodelling in the course of the year is complete. Despite the proximity of pleura, skin, brachial plexus, and brachial vessels, complications are almost unknown, unless open reduction is attempted. The only complication recorded in children is subclavian vein compression due to greenstick fracture with an inferior bow. The veins of the

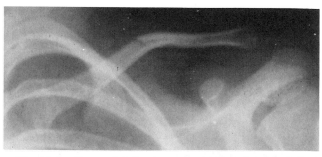

Fig. 10-1. Greenstick fractures are easily missed in infants who present because they do not move the arm. There may be no physical signs to focus the doctor's attention on the clavicle. In this girl, aged 3 years, the diagnosis was missed at first when the displacement was less than it is here.

arm become congested, and edema forms. Put the child to bed to reduce compression. Alternatively, reduce the fracture, and apply a shoulder spica when this complication is present.

As in most simple injuries, half the treatment consists of programming parents in what to expect and half consists of treating the child. A figure-of-eight bandage works well. Stuff a length of stockinette with a rolled-up length of Gamgee or *ABD* pad. Have the child sit down and hold the arms in the position of surrender (Fig. 10-3). Tie it tightly in this position, and have mother tighten the bandage occasionally over the next few days. Do not have it so tight that axillary sores are produced; there is no sense in striving for anatomical reduction. The bandage is intended to provide comfort and prevent further displacement, not to reduce the fracture. The parents should be instructed not to pull the child's arm and to lift him without yanking the shoulder. To put on a undershirt, the injured arm should be threaded through first, followed by the head and then the good arm. Three weeks' of bandaging, followed by 3 weeks' abstention from contact sports seem to be sufficient treatment. I never take a follow-up radiograph because it just confuses me and does not help with making a decision. The bandage is for comfort, not for union. Prepare the parents to expect a large lump at the site of the fracture for about a year. If you tell them it is healing bone, rather like a plumber's joint, they will be happy.

Internal fixation has no place in this injury. It will only produce a bad scar, interfere with union, and provide a point of entry for infection. The only pseudarthroses of the clavicle that I have encountered are the result of internal fixation or are congenital in origin (Fig. 10-4).

MEDIAL END

The medial end of the clavicle has an epiphysis that forms a center of ossification about the age of 18 and fuses at 25. Epiphyseal separation, usually regarded as a child's injury, can occur here in adults. Though rare, this injury mimics a sternoclavicular dislocation which occurs only in the skeletally mature. Separation of the

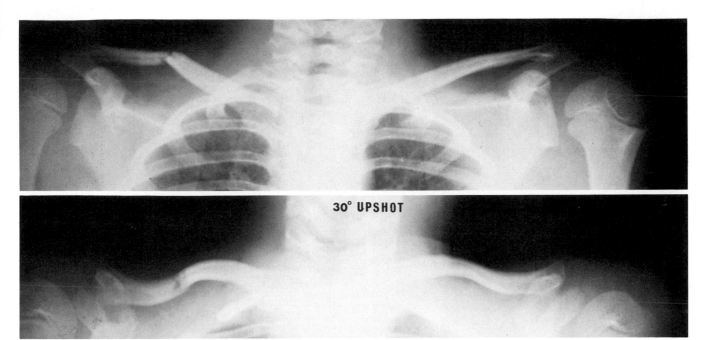

Fig. 10-2. Incomplete fractures may require two or three views to establish the diagnosis.

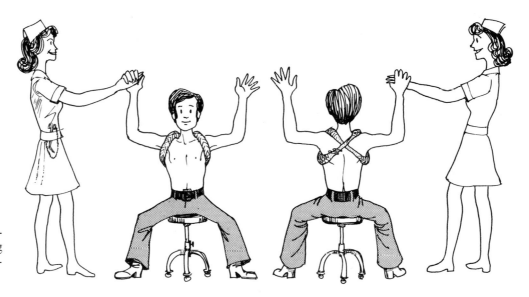

Fig. 10-3. Perhaps the easiest way to apply a snug figure-of-eight bandage without tears.

medial end of the clavicle is difficult to diagnose. Pain and swelling in the region of the sternoclavicular joint is obvious to all, but many are put off the diagnosis by a normal anteroposterior radiograph of the clavicle. Tomograms alone will demonstrate a displacement: however, the unossified epiphysis of the child will not show. The diagnosis will not leave you in doubt if you remember that epiphyseal separations are invariably the cause before the age of 18, and dislocations are invariably the cause after the age of 25.

Anterior Displacement. There is forward prominence of the clavicle.

Posterior Displacement. Compression of the trachea may produce dyspnea.

Although it is said that closed reduction can be ob-

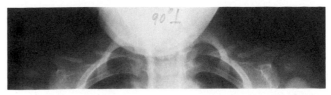

Fig. 10-4. Cleidocranial dysostosis, not strictly speaking, a pseudarthrosis.

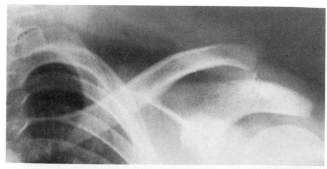

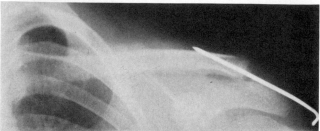

Fig. 10-5. Fracture of the lateral end of the clavicle.

tained by traction, in my experience the reduction cannot be maintained. Internal fixation is required. At operation, the joint and its meniscus are intact, but the periosteum over the medial end of the clavicle is torn. Simurda drills a hole in the medial end of the clavicular shaft and sutures the epiphysis in place with a strong suture. The periosteum is repaired, and the sternomastoid is sutured over the repair. I have used a transarticular Kirschner wire (with a hook on one end to prevent migration) to fortify the periosteal suture. The results in terms of reduction are satisfactory, but the scar is ugly.

OUTER END

Dislocations of the acromioclavicular joints are rare in children. Children sustain a little-recognized fracture of the distal quarter inch of the clavicle. The coracoclavicular ligaments remain intact, so that there is no depression of the shoulder tip. Marked anteroposterior instability is present suggesting that the injury is due to a backward blow on the shoulder (Fig. 10-5).

As at the medial end, maintenance of reduction may be a problem. Anteroposterior alignment may be most difficult to maintain. In one case I have treated, a percutaneous Kirschner wire was inserted to hold the position for 3 or 4 weeks. This may be overtreatment, but in another case left untreated, an ugly lump remained which did not remodel. The shaft of the clavicle moved forward leaving a periosteal tube posteriorly which formed a second clavicle. Unfortunately, the two did not unite.

BIBLIOGRAPHY

Brooks, A. L. and Henning, G. D.: Injury to the proximal clavicular epiphysis. J. Bone Joint Surg., *54A:* 1347, 1972

The death of Robert Peel. [Editorial] Lancet, *2:* 19; 55, 1850

Howard, F. M. and Shafer, S. J.: Injuries to the clavicle with neurovascular complications. J. Bone Joint Surg., *47A:* 1335, 1965

Kital, M. A. and Aufranc, O. E.: Venous occlusion following greenstick fracture of the clavicle. J.A.M.A., *206:* 1301, 1968

Simurda, M. A.: Retrosternal dislocation of the clavicle: a report of 4 cases and a method of repair. Can. J. Surg., *11:* 487, 1968

11

Injuries of the Shoulder and Humeral Shaft

Shoulder and humeral shaft injuries are easy to treat and produce excellent results. The temptation to operate should be strongly suppressed.

FRACTURES OF THE SCAPULA

Great violence occasionally fractures the scapula, and usually there are other injuries. Muscle pull may avulse the apophysis of the coracoid. A sling is sufficient treatment (Fig. 11-1).

DISLOCATION OF THE SHOULDER

Tramatic dislocation is only seen in older adolescents after the epiphyses have closed. This is an adult-type of injury, and will not be considered further.

SEPARATION OF THE PROXIMAL EPIPHYSIS

Birth injury may separate the upper epiphysis and produce a clinical picture resembling that of Erb's palsy. Callus seen on a radiograph at 10 days will make the distinction. A Type I separation is occasionally seen in a toddler (Fig. 11-2). These injuries should be managed by the methods described below.

ADOLESCENT TYPE-II INJURY

Adolescent Type II injuries are commonest in teen-aged girls who fall from a horse and sustain a hyperextension injury of the shoulder on landing (Fig. 11-3). Moore's description of 100 years ago cannot be improved upon.

The symptoms of this fracture are striking and uniform. The shaft of the humerus is so inclined as to carry the elbow a little backward and outward, while the superior end of the shaft is brought forward, so as to make a prominence less rounded than the head and lower down. This is usually found about an inch and a half below the acromion (the

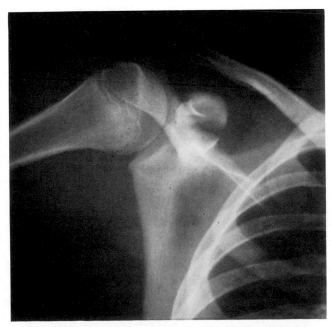

Fig. 11-1. Fracture of the coracoid process in a 13-year-old boy.

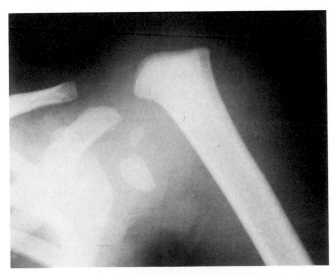

Fig. 11-2. Type I injury in a child of 2 years.

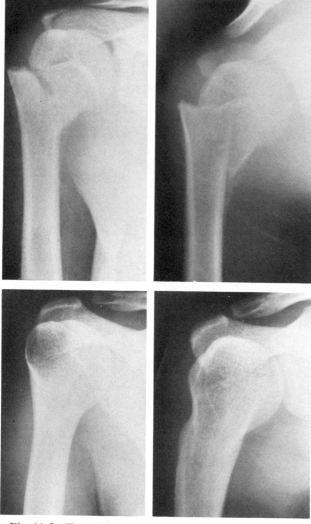

Fig. 11-3. Type II injury in a girl of 13 years. The position was accepted, and the lower films made 3 years later show excellent remodelling. Movement and appearance were normal.

distance varying a little with the size of the youth) and near the coracoid process. The curved line from the acromion down to this projection has a long sweep, instead of the small sphere of the natural head. This appearance is pathognomonic, and may be safely trusted in diagnosis without insisting upon crepitus. As in other epiphyseal fractures, this is not clear and sharp, as when the fracture is of bone, but is muffled. In addition to these striking symptoms we may add the fact of a shortening of half an inch or a little more in the length of the humerus.

At the fracture there is anterior and lateral bowing. The metaphysis buttonholes through the anterior periosteum and may tangle with the tendon of biceps. The fracture lies too far laterally to damage the neurovascular bundle.

Radiographs are often difficult to interpret. An axillary view is painful, and a shoot-through lateral is often

obscure. Two oblique radiographs taken at 45 degrees to the frontal plane are better. The relationship of the fracture to the growth plate may become apparent only after reduction.

Management

Reduction, and maintenance of reduction, can be difficult, but good results are the rule when these fractures are treated conservatively. It would seem unwise to strive officiously to reduce the fracture for the sake of a good-looking radiograph.

Neer has classified the degree of displacement into four grades:

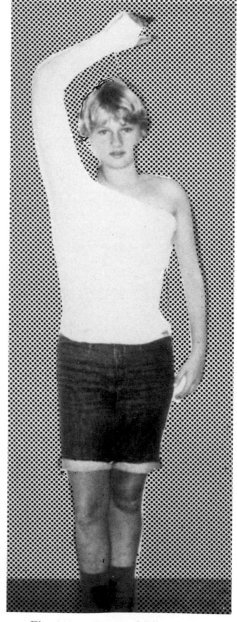

Fig. 11-4. Statue of Liberty cast.

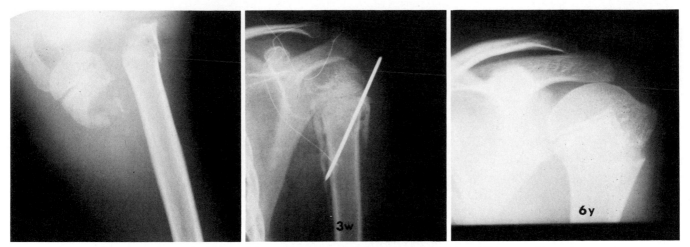

Fig. 11-5. This 5-year-old sustained a fracture of the odontoid in addition to this metaphyseal fracture. Internal fixation was required for nursing.

I. Less than 5 mm. displacement
II. One-third displacement
III. Two-thirds displacement
IV. More than two-thirds displacement

About 70 percent of patients have Grade I or II displacement and require no more than a sling. Several methods of treatment have been advocated for the more severe grades of displacement.

A Sling. This region has a great capacity for remodelling, and malunion does not limit movement. There is no cosmetic blemish, because the shoulder has thick muscle cover. Eighty percent of humeral growth occurs at the upper end, and within a year or two, all signs of angulation will disappear. Movement should be commenced at about 3 weeks.

Traction. The position can be improved by manipulation of the fracture under anesthesia, by the method described by Moore. The arm is moved forwards and upwards into a vertical line. Skin tape traction can be used to maintain the arm in this position for about 2 weeks. Not all fractures will stay, and any degree of slip must be accepted. After 2 weeks, the fracture is sticky, and the arm can be mobilized for a few days before being placed in a sling.

Cast Immobilization. After reduction by Moore's method a shoulder spica can be used to hold the arm in the Statue of Liberty position. This gives excellent control of the reduction (Fig. 11-4). At 3 weeks, the child has to be admitted to hospital for cast removal, because the arm is stiff in abduction and requires some time to come down to the side again. Bed rest is needed during this time. Never leave this cast on for more than 3 weeks if you wish to avoid prolonged stiffness.

A Statue of Liberty cast puts the child in a very inconvenient position, as he cannot get into a car. Also, my enthusiasm for this position was dampened by a case of incomplete brachial plexus palsy that developed after a few days and took a long time to recover. A colleague had a similar experience with one of his cases. Another child was unstable in this position, and reduction could only be maintained with the arm in full internal rotation and extension—in the "Napoleon position." For these reasons, I prefer traction if the fracture cannot be held in apposition with the arm at the side after reduction.

Open Reduction. Results of *laissez-faire* treatment are at least as good as those of open reduction. Open reduction leaves a large scar (an important consideration in girls). It is not an easy operation. The internal fixation may pull out and occasionally produces a growth disturbance.

At operation, the tendon of biceps may be found interposed, and this finding has been the justification for surgery in the past. The only justification for it today is in the minds of surgeons who harbor the illusion that anatomical reduction is important in this fracture. I mention it only to condemn it.

Results

All children recover full movement and a normal-looking arm. Shortening due to premature closure of the growth plate is common. Neer found 1 to 3 cm. of shortening in 10 percent of children with undisplaced fractures and in 40 percent with severely displaced fractures. Smith found shortening in 20 percent, regardless of the method of treatment used. This degree of shortening is seldom noticed by the patients.

Hippocrates wrote, "It sometimes happens that the head of the humerus is fractured at its epiphysis; and this, although it may appear to be a much more troublesome accident, is, in fact, a much milder one than the other injuries at this joint."

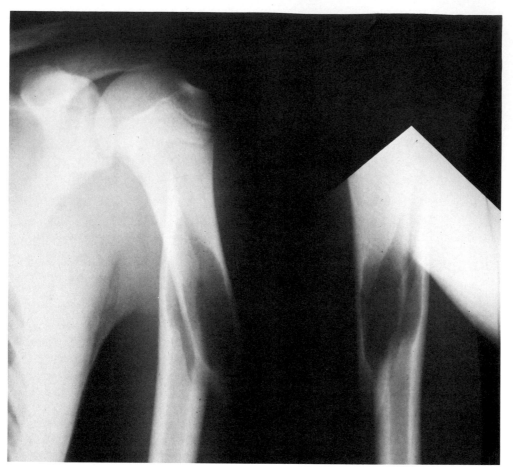

Fig. 11-6. Spiral fracture of the humerus. If a bulky pad is placed between the body and the arm, the deformity will be increased. Did you notice the bone cyst?

After reviewing a large series, Smith concluded that this was an overtreated fracture and hoped that in the future the routine treatment should border on *laissez-faire.*

FRACTURES OF THE UPPER METAPHYSIS

Greenstick fractures are common and are seldom displaced. A Velpeau bandage, smartened up with a roll of plaster so that it will last for 2 to 3 weeks, provides a comfortable solution.

Completely displaced metaphyseal fractures are more difficult than Type II injuries. The shaft penetrates the deltoid to lie subcutaneously. A short incision may be required to disengage the distal fragment and push it back into place. This is a stable reduction in a sling without internal fixation (Fig. 11-5).

FRACTURES OF THE HUMERAL SHAFT

Transverse humeral shaft fractures are the result of a direct blow. Spiral fractures are produced by a twist; even muscular violence will do this. Spiral fractures are a common injury in soldiers learning to throw hand grenades.

Fractures are easily treated because they reduce themselves under the influence of gravity (Fig. 11-6). The only important part of treatment is to maintain good public relations with the family. There are many ways of treating the fracture. A Velpeau bandage held in place with one roll of plaster or a stockinette Velpeau (Fig. 11-7) is simple for minimally displaced stable fractures. A U-slab provides better fixation. For very unstable fractures we use a thoracobrachial box, because

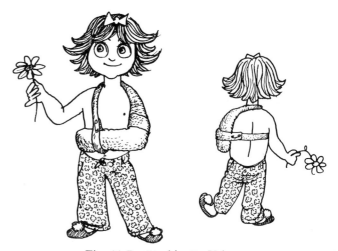

Fig. 11-7. Stockinette Velpeau.

Fig. 11-8. The upper figures show the methods of treating a fracture of the humerus in a child with a head injury. We now prefer ASIF screw traction to a transverse ulnar pin. The methods in the lower figures are suited to ambulant children.

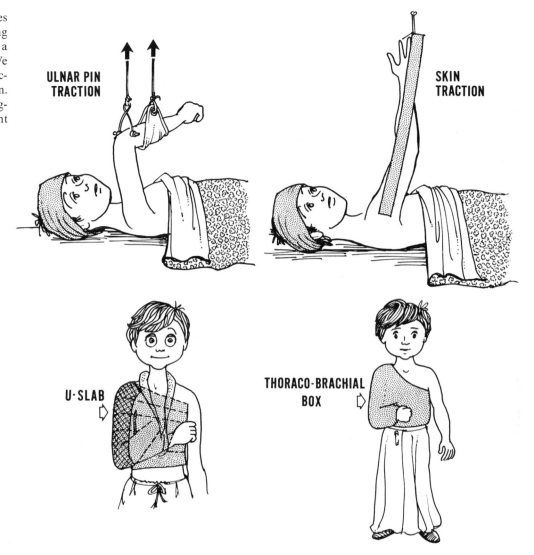

ULNAR PIN TRACTION

SKIN TRACTION

U-SLAB

THORACO-BRACHIAL BOX

it prevents crepitus, which families find very disturbing (Fig. 11-8).

For a week, an attempt should be made to prop the child up at night for sleep. Bayonet apposition is satisfactory because overgrowth of about 1 cm. can be expected. Varus angulation is common and can be kept at less than 20 degrees. At the lower end, angular malunion may show and should be corrected; this is accomplished by manipulating the cast a bit. Immobilization for 3 to 4 weeks is sufficient (Fig. 11-9).

Open fractures with bone loss at the lower end may not unite. Grafting and compression plating may be required and should be carried out before the elbow becomes stiff.

SPECIAL PROBLEMS

Multiple Injuries

The combination of a fracture of the femur, a fracture of the shaft of the humerus and a head injury is not unusual as a result of a car striking a child. It is not possible in such cases to use the dependent weight of the arm to keep it straight. Some form of overhead traction should be used. Most popular is skeletal traction through the proximal ulna. The pin is inserted about 1 inch distal to the olecranon from the medial side, and the ulnar nerve is carefully avoided. Since one boy had a temporary ulnar nerve palsy after this, I prefer to use skin traction; the arm is pulled upwards in the position of a fascist salute. When skeletal traction is required, a screw into the subcutaneous border of the ulna, as advised by the ASIF group, seems safer.

Radial Nerve Palsy

In children, a supracondylar fracture is more likely to produce a radial nerve palsy than a fracture of the shaft. Spontaneous recovery can be expected; look for this first in the brachioradialis. Radial nerve palsy is particularly likely to occur in fractures at the junction

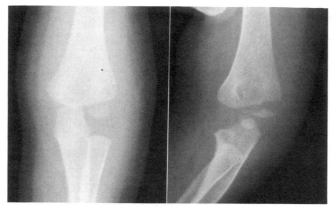

Fig. 12-2. The only way to make the diagnosis was to obtain a stress film.

however, most of these fractures were only partially reduced initially. Early radiographs from one angle may cast a rosy shadow, but subsequent radiographs, taken from a different angle, produce the truer image. However, it is customary to blame slippage within a cast on instability of the fracture, a poorly applied cast over a lot of swelling, or lack of support of the cast by a sling.

Malunion

Full extension of the elbow is usually only possible some weeks after the cast comes off. This may be the first time that everyone becomes aware that the arm is

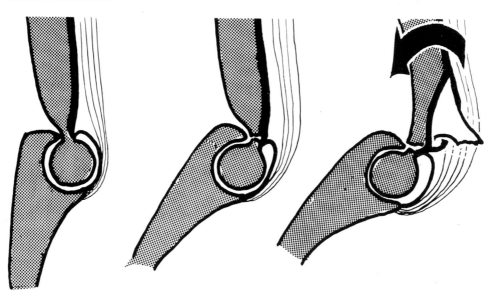

Fig. 12-3. Experimental production of an extension type of supracondylar fracture. The olecranon forms a fulcrum when the elbow is hyperextended. The periosteum remains intact until the arm is twisted. Then the sharp corner of the metaphysis tears the periosteum to allow displacement.

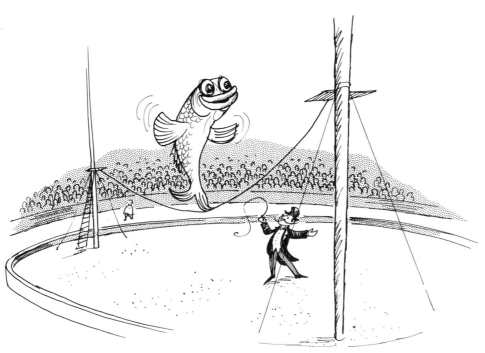

Fig. 12-4. Reduction can be a balancing act.

crooked. It is impossible to tell whether an arm is straight or crooked when it is flexed. Some blame this—unjustly—on a growth disturbance; it is always due to malunion. Properly interpreted radiographs will preserve you from this trap.

Stiffness

Never immobilize the elbow in full flexion for more than 3 weeks. Disregard radiographic signs of union or absence of union at this time. Remember that supracondylar fractures do not displace after 3 weeks (unlike radiographs, which may be misplaced at almost any time).

Armed with these general principles, we will now examine the individual injuries.

SUPRACONDYLAR FRACTURES

A supracondylar fracture of the greenstick type is produced experimentally by forcibly hyperextending the elbow to nearly 90 degrees. The level of fracture is determined by the olecranon forming a fulcrum in the supracondylar region, while the collateral ligaments of the elbow, attached to the metaphysis, prevent a dislocation. Fractures are transverse, signifying an angulatory, not a rotatory force.

In experiments, the periosteum remains intact so long as the force is pure hyperextension (Fig. 12-3). When the fracture is forcibly rotated, the sharp corner of the proximal fragment tears the periosteum, permitting gross displacement. With progressively more force, the sharp edge will first tear the brachialis and then the skin.

The rent in the periosteum is L-shaped and leaves two-thirds of the periosteum around the fracture intact

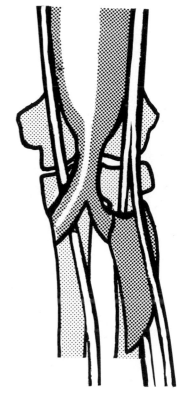

Fig. 12-6. The median and radial nerves lie anterior to the elbow and are equally liable to injury in extension fractures.

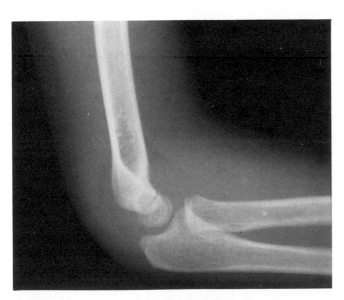

Fig. 12-5. Fat pad sign.

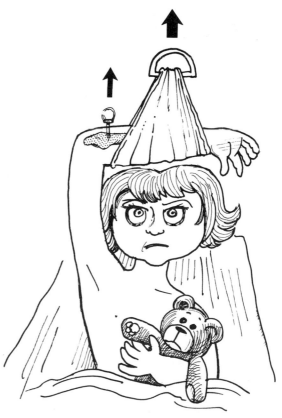

Fig. 12-7. Traction for difficult problems. An ASIF screw is preferred to a transverse pin because there is no risk to the ulnar nerve. Furthermore the problem of side-to-side slip does not arise.

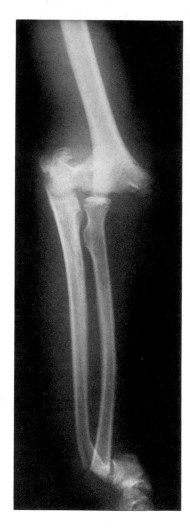

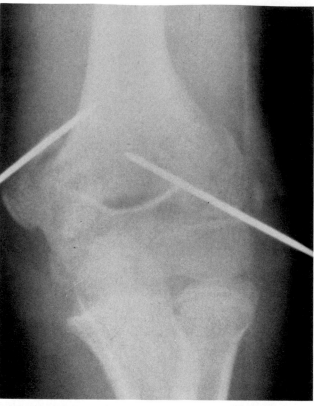

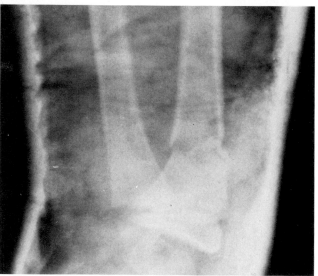

Fig. 12-8. Two fractures in the same arm were the reason for percutaneous pinning. The pins inserted with a hand drill, should have been more vertical and deeper. A power drill is essential for accurate placement. The fractures healed in anatomical position; after 3 months the boy had a full range of movement.

to form a useful hinge that aids reduction. The periosteum is stripped off the shaft for several inches depending on the degree of displacement at the time of injury. The humerus at the level of fracture is shaped like a fish tail: its sharpness produces the damage already described, and may in addition interfere with the radial nerve, the brachial artery, and the median nerve: its narrowness can turn a stable reduction into a balancing act (Fig. 12-4).

Angulated Greenstick Fractures

A small crack or a fat pad sign may be all there is

to see of this injury (Fig. 12-5). While it is probably sufficient to apply a collar-and-cuff sling for 3 weeks in order to produce union, anxious parents and children require an arm cast in order to be convinced that there is a fracture that needs protection.

If the fracture is angulated more than about 20 degrees, the child should be anesthetized, so that the elbow can be flexed above a right angle to facilitate reduction. Radiographs should be taken before the cast is applied. In our series of supracondylar fractures, cubitus varus has occurred in this group because the initial displacement was underestimated and treatment was perfunctory.

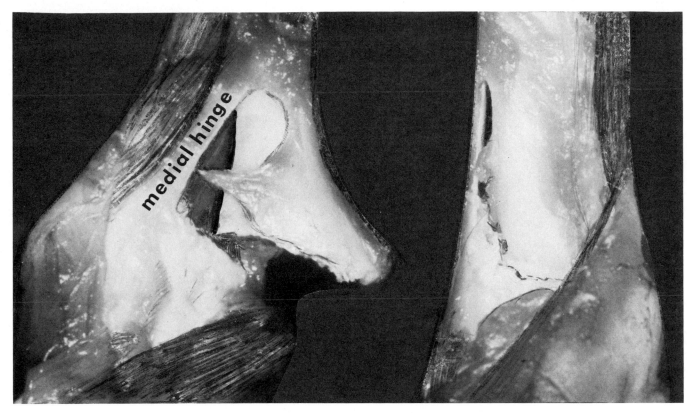

medial hinge

Fig. 12-9. An experimentally produced fracture shows the medial hinge and offers a glimpse of the posterior hinge. After reduction, the soft tissues hold the fragments in place. The better the reduction, the greater the security.

The Classical Displaced Supracondylar Fracture

INITIAL CARE

Look first for signs of ischemia and then for signs of nerve palsies. Radial and ulnar palsies are easily recognized. The median palsy (usually incomplete and often overlooked) may only result in loss of flexion of the distal interphalangeal joint of the index finger, loss of flexion of the interphalangeal joint of the thumb, and numbness of the tip of the index finger (Fig. 12-6).

As first aid, splint the fracture in extension. Flexing a displaced supracondylar fracture in a sling only compresses the artery. It is foolish to have a child waiting for radiographs with an ischemic limb. Put the splint on before the radiographs are taken to prevent the technicians from twisting the arm through the fracture.

Reduction should be undertaken as soon as a child's stomach is legally safe for anesthesia because reduction is easiest before edema is added to hematoma. At least four methods of reduction have been advocated.

REDUCTION

Traction

Skin and skeletal traction (Fig. 12-7) have the following advantages:

1. Safety. Volkmann's ischemia is less of a hazard than with closed reduction.
2. Good results. Varus and valgus deformities are very infrequent.
3. Traction is applicable to fresh fractures and fractures a few days old.
4. It is suitable for stable and unstable or irreducible fractures.

Traction should be set up after the fracture has been reduced under general anesthesia. Traction requires prolonged hospitalization and a considerable amount of attention in order to keep it in good shape. Dodge reviews his results with Dunlop traction and describes the method in detail.

Closed Reduction and Cast

This is our method of choice and is applicable for 90 percent of these fractures. The advantage is that good results can be obtained with brief hospitalization. Vascular problems have not occurred in our patients, nor has malunion been a problem. However, closed reduction is not a method for the uninitiated, for unstable fractures, nor for fractures that cannot be flexed above a right angle. When there is gross displacement accompanied by diffuse fusiform swelling of the arm,

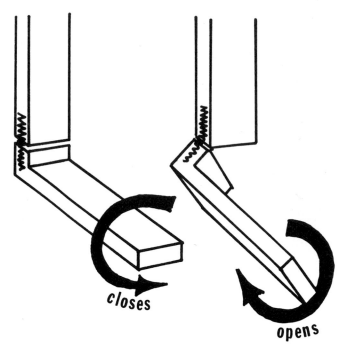

Fig. 12-10. The forearm is used to control the position of the distal fragment.

the hematoma is not contained; reduction is easy, and the elbow can be flexed without obliterating the pulse. By contrast, a circumscribed firm anterior hematoma with moderate displacement indicates that the antecubital fascia is intact. The pulse may be expected to disappear when the elbow is flexed to 90 degrees. For these problems the following method should be used.

Closed Reduction and Percutaneous Kirschner Wire Fixation

This method was introduced for all supracondylar fractures to prevent redisplacement, particularly when the elbow cannot be flexed beyond a right angle. After the fracture has been reduced by closed methods, one Kirschner wire is inserted through the medial epicondyle, and another through the lateral epicondyle (Fig. 12-8).

Open Reduction and Internal Fixation

This method has been tried and condemned by a number of surgeons because of the frequency of stiffness. For older adolescents with T-shaped fractures, open reduction with ASIF fixation may be the ideal method. The results of exposing the fracture through a short anteromedial incision (just sufficient to insert a finger) followed by percutaneous K-pinning are good.

The degree of proficiency with which any of these methods is followed is probably more important than the method used.

The Technique of Closed Reduction

There is no lack of advice about technique. In 1896 Smith evolved a method, based on his anatomical dissections, that still works well for us. The use of intact periosteal hinges to aid and maintain reduction is the key to success. Everyone knows that there is a posterior hinge of periosteum in a posteriorly displaced fracture. After the fracture is reduced the fracture gap is impacted by flexing the elbow strongly.

Similar collateral hinges are present to permit control of valgus and varus, though they are less well known. When there is medial displacement, a medial periosteal hinge is always present (Fig. 12-9). When the fracture is reduced this hinge can be tightened to impact the lateral part of the fracture. If the fracture remains open laterally, a varus deformity due to malunion will be evident. But how can this medial hinge be tightened? Smith originally pointed out (and others have confirmed) that pronation of the forearm tightens the medial periosteal hinge. Figures 12-10 and 12-11 elucidate the mechanics of this maneuver.

The few fractures that have lateral displacement have a lateral hinge. These fractures are best held in supination.

With the child under general anesthesia, go through these steps (Fig. 12-12):

1. Palpate the bony landmarks. Check the direction of displacement.

2. Apply traction with the arm flexed to about 10 degrees. The proximal fragments will be returned into the periosteal tube. Correct any lateral displacement.

3. Push the olecranon anteriorly to correct the posterior displacement. Flex the elbow to about 40 degrees.

4. Externally rotate both arms to correct the usual internal rotation deformity. Both arms should rotate an equal amount.

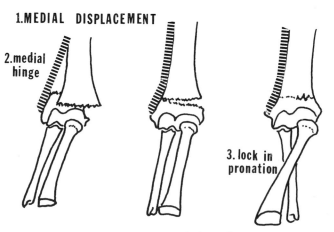

Fig. 12-11. When the bone ends have been brought into contact (and not before) rotation of the forearm will close the fracture using the medial hinge. If the fracture remains open laterally cubitus varus is the result.

5. Continue to flex the elbow above a right angle while maintaining pressure on the olecranon. Be sure that the posterior displacement is reduced *before* this is done, otherwise the brachial artery will be crushed in the fracture. In order to use the posterior hinge to close the fracture completely the elbow should be flexed until the olecranon lies anterior to the epicondyle (Fig. 12-13).

6. If the displacement was initially medial, pronate the forearm to lock the fracture. About 10 percent of supracondylar fractures are laterally displaced; these should be set in supination.

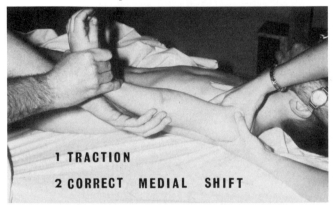

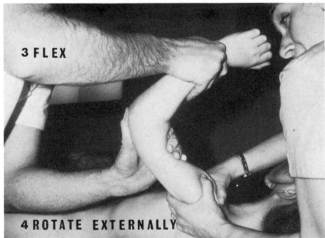

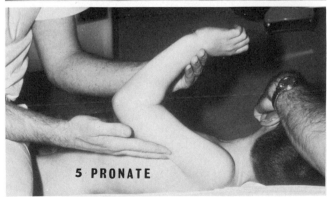

Fig. 12-12. The steps in reduction of a supracondylar fracture. At the final stage the elbow should be flexed more acutely.

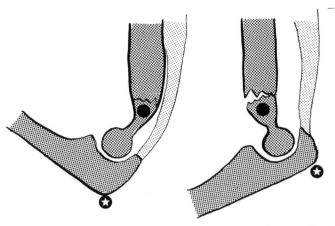

Fig. 12-13. Flex the elbow until the olecranon lies anterior to the epicondyles in order to lock your reduction.

7. Put a gauze square in the elbow crease to prevent blistering and intertrigo. Apply an Ashurst bandage to avoid compression of the front of the elbow (Fig. 12-14).

8. Radiograph the elbow as shown in Figure 12-15. Do not obtain a lateral by twisting the arm. You may lose reduction.

9. If the radiograph is satisfactory apply a very light shell of plaster and a collar-and-cuff sling. The sling takes the weight of the cast off the fracture and prevents rotation of the limb.

10. Admit the child for 48 hours, and order observation of the circulation, sensation, and movement of the hand. Do not give analgesics. They might mask Volkmann's ischemia. Check active and passive extension of the fingers. Pain on passive extension of the fingers is the early sign of Volkmann's ischemia.

Decisions to Be Made During Reduction

How Much Flexion? About 120 degrees of flexion is necessary to ensure stability (Fig. 12-16). The radial pulse may disappear for a few minutes after reduction. Ignore this if the fingers are pink, but if the fingers are white, reduce the degree of flexion. If flexion to a right angle is not possible without circulatory impairment, see that the posterior displacement is corrected. If the fracture is anatomical, three options are open:

1. Fix with two percutaneous Kirschner wires.
2. Cast in this position, and increase flexion when the swelling is less, on the third to seventh day.
3. Put in traction.

What Do the Radiographs Show? The radiographs are difficult to interpret in the heat of the moment. Oblique films sometimes help. Figure 12-17 shows the various possible appearances and may help you to recognize faults.

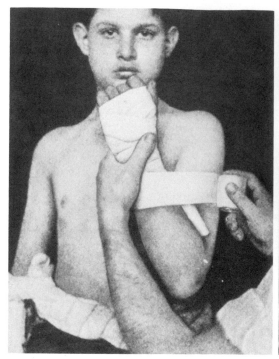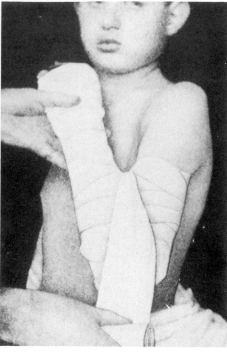

Fig. 12-14. Hold the reduction with a flannel bandage. (Ashurst, A. P. C.: Fractures of the Elbow. Philadelphia, Lea & Febiger, 1910)

Follow-up

Repeat radiographs should be taken before the child goes home. Radiograph the fracture again a week after injury. If the position is unsatisfactory, a further attempt at reduction should be made, or the child should be placed in traction. (This is almost never necessary.)

Remove the cast at 3 weeks and radiograph again. Do not leave the cast on for longer than 3 weeks. Warn the parents that it may take at least 3 months for the elbows to regain full movement, and perhaps longer. A small proportion of children have permanent limitation of elbow movement.

PROBLEMS AND VARIANTS

In a review of 200 consecutive patients with supracondylar fractures requiring reduction, the following features emerged. After closed reduction two-thirds of the patients had no problems, whereas one-third of the patients had early problems: nerve palsy, poor position, instability, two fractures in the same limb, or fracture variants.

Soft-Tissue Problems

Nerve Injuries, 14 percent. Half of these were noted before reduction and half, after. Perhaps some were missed initially, but others developed progressively. The radial nerve and median nerve each accounted for 6.5 percent, while the ulnar nerve was injured in 3.5

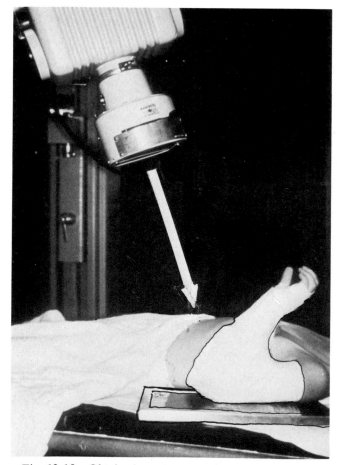

Fig. 12-15. Obtain the anteroposterior radiograph before the cast is applied.

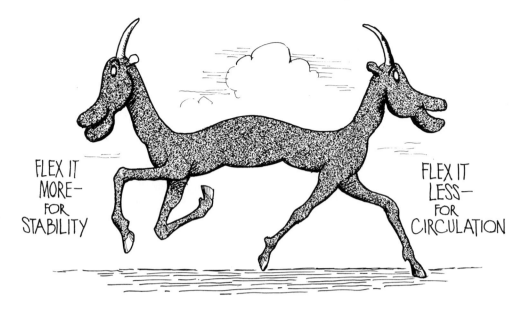

Fig. 12-16. Dr. Dolittle's analysis of the problem in supracondylar fractures of the elbow. (Adapted from Lofting, H.: The Story of Doctor Dolittle. Philadelphia, J. B. Lippincott, 1920. Copyright 1920 by Hugh Lofting. Copyright 1948 by Josephine Lofting)

FLEX IT MORE— FOR STABILITY

FLEX IT LESS— FOR CIRCULATION

percent. The majority recovered completely within a few months. This has been the experience of most authors. An occasional case does not recover. I have seen one radial nerve disappear into the bone at the time of supracondylar osteotomy (in a child with a complete radial palsy and malunion). This was 4 years after injury. Another child with a partial median palsy had no recovery after a year.

Vessels. In this series of 200 cases, only one case of Volkmann's contracture occurred, and that was referred into hospital with the condition already established. If Volkmann's contracture is a common problem at your hospital it would suggest that the treatment of this fracture should be improved. Volkmann's contracture is largely a preventable condition. When it does occur, radical, urgent fasciotomy and exploration of the vessels is required (as described in Chap. 5). Absence of a radial pulse is not an indication for exploration if the finger are pink and can be painlessly extended.

Skin, 1 percent. The occasional open fracture requires surgical toilet and may then be managed in the same fashion as a closed fracture. We have had no problems of infection.

Bone Problems

Comminution of the medial column occurred in a few fractures and rendered the reduction less stable. Closed treatment is still usually possible.

A flexion injury produced anterior displacement in 2 percent; these injuries were treated in extension (Fig. 12-18). In children of 15 and 16, fractures of the adult type occurred. Comminuted Y- and T fractures present problems with reduction. In some, a good reduction can be obtained by wrapping an Esmarch bandage around the arm for a few minutes and then using skeletal traction for 3 weeks (Fig. 12-19). Others can be treated by open reduction and internal fixation using ASIF equipment (Fig. 12-20).

At the other end of the scale are epiphyseal separations in the first year of life. Since they mimic dislocations clinically, they are hard to recognize. None were encountered in the series of 200.

Two fractures in the same limb were seen in 4 percent,

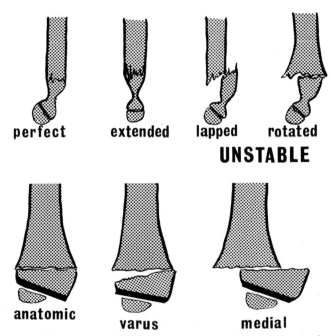

perfect   **extended**   **lapped**   **rotated**
UNSTABLE

anatomic   **varus**   **medial**

Fig. 12-17. Possible appearances in the anteroposterior and lateral radiographs. In the anteroposterior film, look at Baumann's angle; the thick black line should be at 70 degrees to the humeral shaft.

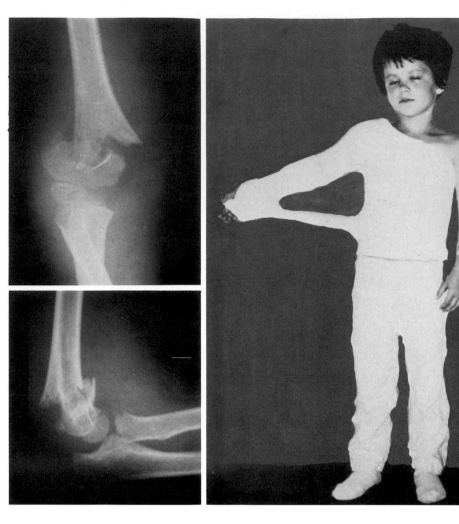

Fig. 12-18. The flexion type of supracondylar fracture.

mostly involving the distal forearm, but occasionally through the shaft of the humerus. Diagnosis was easily missed. At least one radiograph should include the entire humeral shaft and the forearm bones. The forearm fractures were held satisfactorily in a supracondylar-type cast. Those fractures involving the humerus required skeletal traction.

PROBLEMS WITH REDUCTION

Closed reduction was the initial treatment of 95 percent. The remainder were treated either by traction or Kirschner wire fixation, largely depending on personal-preference. For skeletal traction, a 3-mm. Steinmann-pin is introduced from the medial side of the ulna as

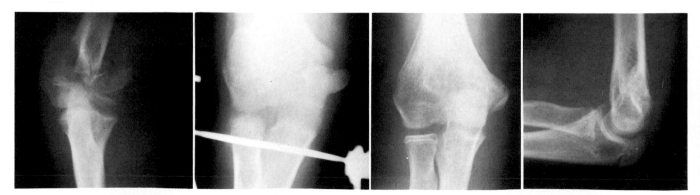

Fig. 12-19. This comminuted **T** fracture in a 13-year-old boy was treated in traction. Follow-up films, taken 6 months later, show anatomical union. He had a full range of movement.

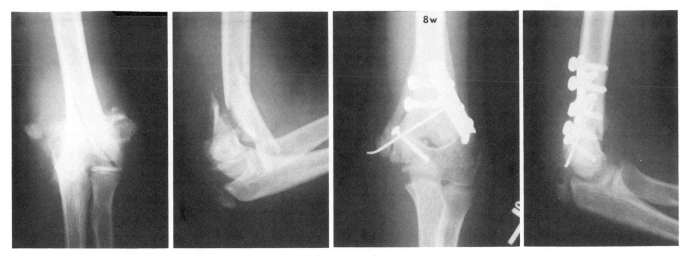

Fig. 12-20. Even through a posterior approach this was a tedious operation, and the patient, a 12-year-old boy, lost the last 20 degrees of extension.

the thumb pushes the ulnar nerve away. The pin is inserted 1½ inches distal to the olecranon, so that when the arm is hanging over the head, it balances well. Although this has been the standard method for several years we now use a winged ulnar screw for traction, because the risk of nerve damage is avoided and because valgus and varus can be controlled easily. After 3 weeks the device is removed, and active movement may begin.

Nine percent of fractures treated by closed means required further "alterations." (A tailor introduced me to this useful term.) A few of the unsatisfactory reductions were corrected by traction. In others—those in which insufficient flexion was obtained initially—the arm was flexed further at about 5 days. Most of those thought to have slipped had, in fact, either a poor initial reduction, which was not appreciated, or a poor cast. Do not expect to reduce this fracture after a week.

The chief causes of stiffness are immobilization beyond 3 weeks and forced movement thereafter.

VARUS AND VALGUS DEFORMITY

The techniques of management described are very effective in preventing malunion (Fig. 12-21). The only patient of ours who required treatment for malunion was wrongly thought to have no displacement initially, and the fracture went unreduced.

The deformity is only recognized when the arm is fully mobile again. It is due to malunion and not to a growth disturbance. A gunstock deformity consists of varus, medial rotation, and extension deformity (Fig. 12-22). It should be corrected only after the elbow has regained full mobility. Though corrective supracondylar osteotomy is frequently dismissed as an easy operation, our results in 28 cases suggest that the problems

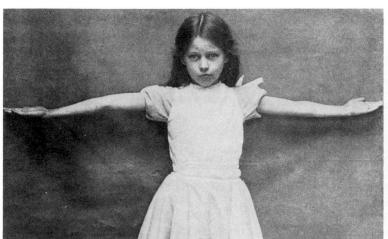
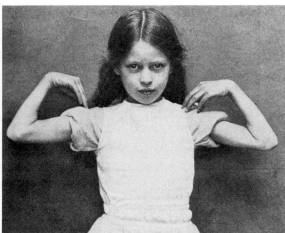

Fig. 12-21. Minor degrees of malrotation do not matter. Hey Groves' (1916) illustration shows the frequent result of a right supracondylar fracture. Slight hyperextension, slight loss of flexion, and slight external rotation are present.

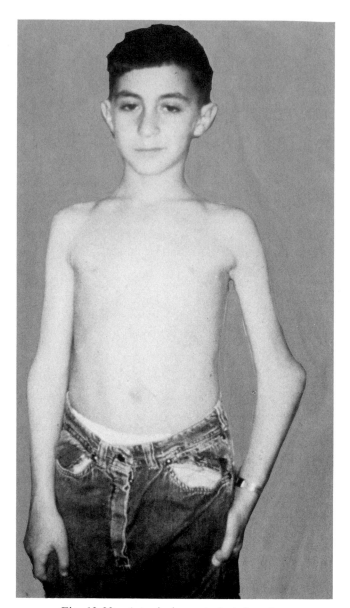

Fig. 12-22. A typical gunstock deformity.

ALIGNMENT AFTER SUPRACONDYLAR OSTEOTOMY

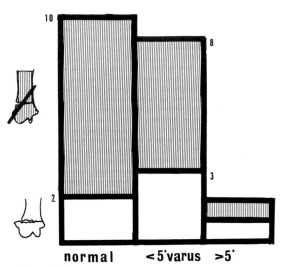

normal   <5˚varus   >5˚

Fig. 12-23. The results of supracondylar osteotomy in 25 patients. The osteotomy was held by a Kirschner wire in the shaded columns; in the white column a cast provided the only fixation. The carrying angle was restored in only half the patients.

similar injury to the artery, and had nerve palsies and skin loss as a result. Another developed infection of the bone. The overall results are shown in Figure 12-23 and Table 12-1.

Other methods of fixation have been advocated. Langenskiold used a 4-hole plate, but found two out of 11 osteotomies required further correction. French advocated a wire loop wound around two screws, as illustrated in Campbell's *Operative Orthopaedics*. No results have been published. Other surgeons have used the staple, and some have immobilized the arm in full extension for 3 weeks. Tachdjian advocates external pin fixation with Roger Anderson apparatus.

have been underestimated. For a varus deformity, a lateral incision should be made over the supracondylar region, and the periosteum lifted. A lateral wedge is removed leaving a medial hinge intact. The medial hinge should be cracked to obtain the desired position. The problem comes in holding the position. We have tried fixation in a cast with the elbow flexed and the forearm fully pronated and found that the position was lost in three out of eight patients while in the cast, and required further correction.

In 20 patients the osteotomy was held by a single Kirschner wire. Seventeen of the 20 were satisfactory, but several dangerous complications ensued. One patient developed an aneurysm of the brachial artery because the Kirschner wire penetrated the artery. Another developed gross swelling of the arm suggesting a

Table 12-1. Supracondylar Osteotomy

14 complications in 25 patients	
General	
poor scar	3
stiffness	2
No Internal Fixation	
displaced	3/7
neuropraxia	1/7
Internal Fixation	
displaced	2/18
pin problems*	3/18
	14/25

*Aneurysm, pin-track infection, hematoma, skin loss, and neuropraxia

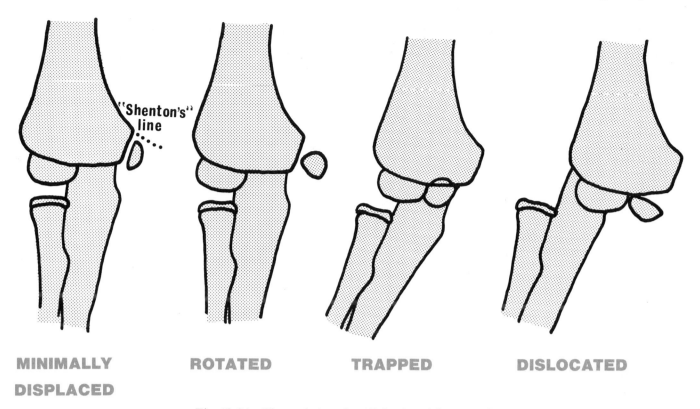

"Shenton's" line

MINIMALLY DISPLACED   **ROTATED**   **TRAPPED**   **DISLOCATED**

Fig. 12-24. The varieties of medial epicondyle separation.

Malunion is obviously more difficult to correct than to prevent. A foolproof method of correction has yet to be established.

MEDIAL EPICONDYLE

Valgus strain applied to the elbow of a cadaver fractures the radial neck. A medial epicondyle seems likely to be avulsed, either by the contraction of the flexor muscles at a time when the valgus strain is applied or by a dislocation.

In children between the ages of 5 and 15, the clinical signs of a medial hematoma may be more obvious than the radiographic ones. A film of the normal elbow will eliminate doubts.

The degree of displacement should be assessed (Fig. 12-24) and the presence of other injuries noted, such as fracture of the radial neck and injury of the ulnar nerve, which lies close by.

Diagnostic traps exist; the unossified apophysis in a child less than 5 years old casts no shadow, and avulsion is a matter of conjecture (Fig. 12-25). Until the age of 11 or 12 years, separation of the medial *condyle* may masquerade as an epicondylar separation and be-

Fig. 12-25. This child had an open dislocation of the elbow joint. Air is in the joint. Though there is no sign of injury to the medial epicondyle it was found to be separated during joint toilet.

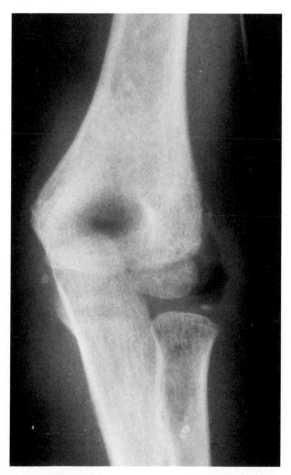

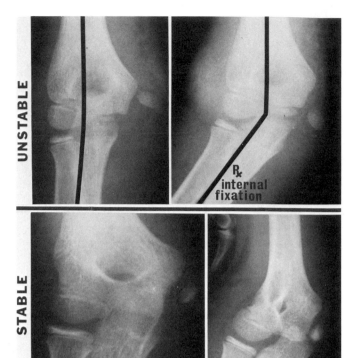

Fig. 12-26. Assess the stability of the medial epicondyle under anesthesia.

cause the ossific nucleus of the medial condyle does not appear until this age the diagnosis may be overlooked. A neglected fracture of the medial condyle is as bad as a neglected fracture of the lateral condyle. It may be possible to avoid this trap in children under the age of 5 who have soft-tissue swelling on the medial aspect of the joint by examining the elbow under anesthesia. Instability should be treated by exploration.

Treatment

There are no published reports of long-followed cases, and the choice of treatment is somewhat empiric. Prior to 1950 the majority of patients at this hospital were treated by closed reduction under anesthesia. The elbow was held at 90 degrees in full pronation, with the wrist flexed to relax the flexor muscles; local pressure applied over the medial epicondyle helped to secure reduction. Fibrous union was common. It is my understanding that elbow movement returned more slowly than with open reduction. Some required late excision of the fragment because of discomfort. But instability was not a problem. Since 1950 open reduction has been the most popular. Our current practice is as follows:

Minimal displacement and soft tissue swelling. Apply a cast to protect the fracture.

Definite displacement. Under anesthesia test the stability of the medial side of the elbow. If the injury is the result of a valgus strain, the elbow is unstable, and an open reduction is carried out. Separation due to a posterior subluxation tears the anterior attachments of the medial epicondyle but not the superior attachments. The elbow is stable after the dislocation is reduced and may be casted. This variety was found in only two out of 100 cases (Fig. 12-26).

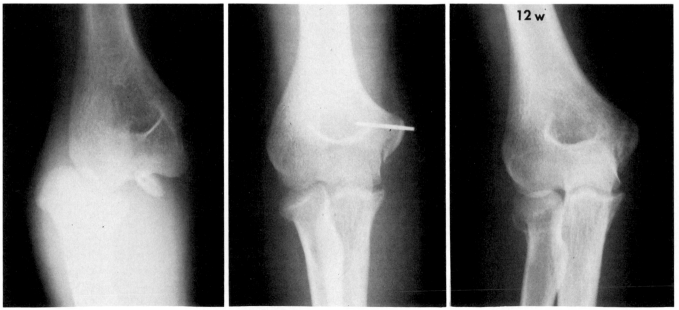

Fig. 12-27. Separation of the medial epicondyle accompanied by dislocation and by a fracture of the radial neck. The fragment is pinned back. Three months later the growth plate is closing.

Displacement and dislocation. Quickly reduce the dislocation under demerol in order to assist the circulation and relieve pain. Perform open reduction as soon as the child is fit for anesthesia.

Trapped fragment. The fragment can be extricated by applying a valgus strain or by supinating the forearm but it will seldom return to its bed. Perform open reduction.

Open Reduction. If you operate with the child lying on his back you will be wrestling; either you cannot see the fracture, or you will be engaged in a tug-of-war to hold the fragment in position. Have the child prone with the arm in the half-Nelson position (in other words, behind the back) with a tourniquet in place. A transverse incision leaves a better scar, but a longitudinal incision, (slightly posterior so that the child cannot see the scar) has tradition behind it. Divide the skin and subcutaneous fat and then you will find fracture hematoma. The tissues will be so stained with blood that identification of important structures is difficult. Wash everything clean and milk the blood out of the joint. The fragment then comes into sight. Hold it with a towel clip and pull distally in order to find the ulnar nerve. The nerve can and must be found by looking through the tear in the posterior periosteum. Often stained red, the nerve is easily recognized by the nutrient artery on its surface. Do not dissect the nerve free or put tapes around it. About 5 percent of our cases have had a transient postoperative ulnar nerve palsy that was associated with overelaborate displays of the nerve.

The fragment will usually fall back into position. The fracture surfaces are easily recognized, and the rotation can be checked by lining up the flexor muscle fibers with the line of the forearm. Hold the fragment in place with a superficially placed towel clip while it is secured with a Kirschner wire (Fig. 12-27). A few absorbable sutures around the periosteum will complete the fixation. I prefer a Kirschner wire because I do not completely trust absorbable sutures, but some surgeons are content with sutures alone. An above-elbow cast is applied with the elbow flexed to 90 degrees, the forearm pronated (to relax pronator teres) and the wrist slightly flexed. At 3 weeks the cast is removed. The pin has often worked through the skin by this time, because there is so little subcutaneous fat over the condyle to hide it after the swelling has receded. The pin is removed. If it is still subcutaneous, remove the pin at 4 to 5 weeks under local anesthesia.

Problems. A review of the charts of about 150 patients (and a search of my conscience) brought very few problems to light.

Movement. Full extension is often slow to return and may never be achieved. A word of warning to the

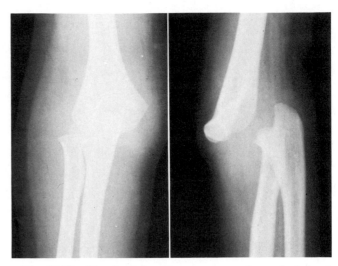

Fig. 12-28. Simple dislocations are rare; always look hard for a fracture as well.

parents in advance is better than a thousand words of explanation afterwards.

Complications after closed reduction. One child had been immobilized for 6 weeks and had persistent stiffness treated by 2 manipulations under anesthesia with some benefit. No elbow should be immobilized this long.

Another child had a posterior dislocation with avulsion of the epicondyle treated by closed reduction. About 3 months after injury the elbow was still very stiff, and signs of median nerve impairment were noted. The nails of the index and middle fingers developed clubbing and the girl began to bite her nails. Nearly a year later, the median nerve was explored because the signs were unchanged and the elbow had only 40 degrees of movement. The nerve was found to pass into the humerus at the fracture site and through a bony tunnel into the elbow joint before resuming its normal course. The nerve was freed and restored to its anatomical position.

We encountered only one un-united medial epicondyle producing pain and requiring late excision of the sesamoid-like bony nodule.

A problem encountered at open reduction. A child presented with an acute dislocation of the elbow and a widely displaced epicondyle. The dislocation was reduced with difficulty. Attempts to carry out an open reduction of the medial epicondyle met with even more difficulty until it was realized that this child had a fresh dislocation and an old un-united separation of the medial epicondyle. The fragment was excised and the soft tissues repaired.

In conclusion, medial epicondylar fractures seem to have good prognoses. We favor open reduction if the elbow is unstable under anesthesia.

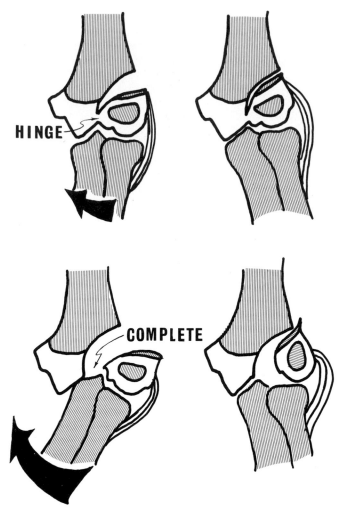

Fig. 12-29. The experimental production of a fracture of the lateral condyle in a cadaver. (*Top*) A varus force avulses the later condyle but leaves a hinge of cartilage intact. When the elbow is released the fracture reduces. (*Bottom*) When the force is greater the hinge tears and the elbow dislocates. When the elbow is released the fragment rotates and does not reduce. (Courtesy Dr. Roland Jakob).

DISLOCATION OF THE ELBOW

Dislocation, unaccompanied by fracture, is rare in children. Always look for a fracture. Figure 12-28 is an example of a simple dislocation, but, even here, we suspected an occult separation of the medial epicondyle.

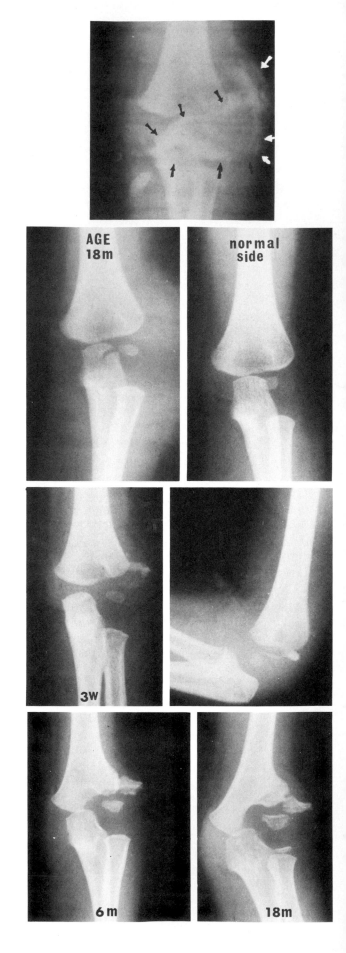

Fig. 12-30. This child, aged 18 months, was admitted with the diagnosis of a fracture of the lateral condyle. At rounds, the surgeon was persuaded to carry out an arthrogram to confirm the diagnosis, and this was wrongly interpreted as normal. The elbow was placed in a cast. Later the child revealed all the problems of an un-united displaced fracture of the lateral condyle. The varus fracture of the olecranon seen in the initial film is a clue to a fracture of the lateral condyle.

FRACTURES OF THE LATERAL EPICONDYLE

An ossification center appears at the age of 12 and fuses with the lateral condyle at the age of 14. The center for the lateral epicondyle is often irregular and beginners often confuse it with a fracture. We have encountered only one patient with separation of this epiphysis. It was explored because it looked so like a fracture of the lateral condyle.

FRACTURES OF THE LATERAL CONDYLE

Fracture of the lateral condyle has an evil reputation. However, most of the children we treat do not come back to the clinic more than once following cast removal. For most orthopaedic surgeons, this is a solved fracture.

The mechanism of the fracture is controversial. Dr. Roland Jakob has produced the fracture experimentally in a cadaver by applying a varus strain to the extended elbow at this hospital. The trochlear ridge on the ulna behaves as a fulcrum for avulsion of the lateral condyle by the lateral ligament (Fig. 12-29). The bone separates, but the articular cartilage remains intact as a hinge. The fracture reduces when varus angulation is corrected. But if, instead, the angulation is increased, the cartilage hinge tears, the fracture displaces, and the elbow may dislocate. The fragment displaces through 90 degrees in two planes.

The child with a fracture of the lateral condyle has a swollen tender area over the lateral part of the elbow. Circulatory and neurological complications were unknown in our series of 100 displaced lateral condyles.

Grossly displaced fractures are obvious on radiographs, but hairline fractures can be missed easily (Fig. 12-1). When there is clinical evidence of a fracture but no radiographic signs you should take further views until the fracture shows up. Stress films are a last resort. In a very young child, the center of ossification may be so small that the nature of the injury may be misunderstood (Fig. 12-30). The only problems we have encountered in recent years were in children in whom the diagnosis was overlooked.

Lateral condylar fractures are Type IV injuries. The majority, however, pass through the cartilaginous epiphysis and are unlikely to affect growth for the reasons explained on page 10. About 5 percent pass through the ossific nucleus of the capitellum, and the risk of growth arrest is theoretically higher in these.

The complications an orthopaedic surgeon should keep in his mind are malunion resulting in stiffness and cubitus valgus, and nonunion, the commonest problem when treatment is inadequate. There are several rea-

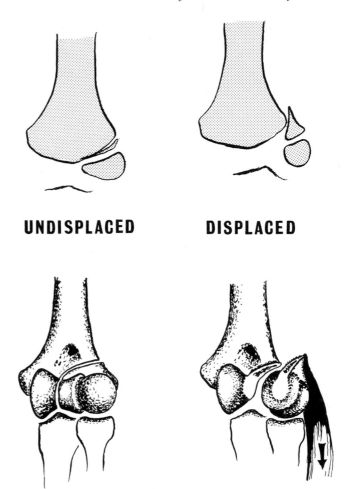

UNDISPLACED   **DISPLACED**

Fig. 12-31. Undisplaced and displaced fractures. Because the apex of the fracture is the trochlear notch, displaced fractures are often accompanied by lateral subluxation of the ulna.

sons for nonunion; lack of immobilization, synovial fluid bathing the fracture, and soft-tissue interposition. The elbow looks ugly, and there is marked cubitus valgus, which inevitably leads to a tardy ulnar nerve palsy. Smith recently reported an 80-year followup study of a patient with nonunion. The functional disability was minimal, but the ulnar nerve palsy was complete!

Classification

From the practical point of view fractures of the lateral condyle are displaced or undisplaced (Fig. 12-31). The undisplaced fractures appear horizontal and are moderately stable, the cartilage hinge is intact. The displaced fractures appear oblique and are widely displaced (Fig. 12-32).

Treatment

Undisplaced fractures may be immobilized in an above-elbow cast with the elbow at 90 degrees. Further

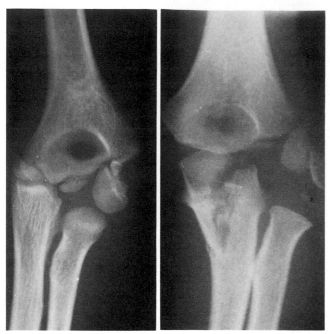

Fig. 12-32. Associated injuries are common in all fractures of the elbow. The 8-year-old (*left*) has a medial dislocation. The 5-year-old (*right*) has a varus type of olecranon fracture associated with a lateral condylar fracture.

flexion tends to displace the fragment. Radiographs should be obtained every 3 to 4 days for the first 2 weeks, because displacement is not unknown.

Three, or at most 4, weeks in a cast is sufficient to achieve union and to avoid stiffness.

Displaced Fractures. Twenty years ago closed reduction had its advocates, who based their view on adequate results in about two-thirds of children. McLearie and Merson noted that reduction was possible if the elbow was first dislocated again. Then the fragment was pushed into place, and the dislocation was reduced. If nonunion and redisplacement occur, however, they are difficult to correct.

For this reason, all these fractures must be treated by immediate open reduction and internal fixation. The results are consistently better.

Technique. With the patient supine and a tourniquet inflated, an incision is made directly over the lateral condyle. As soon as the subcutaneous layer is incised fracture hematoma will flow out. Mop this up and milk clots out of the elbow joint. Irrigate the joint to obtain a clear view. The fragment requires no dissection (which carries the risk of avascular necrosis), but it will be found rotated through 180 degrees. Slip a long-bladed retractor into the joint anteriorly, in order to visualize the head of the radius and the fracture bed. Now try to set the fragment back in place. The periosteum of the humeral shaft may need to be lifted in order to define the bed. It is easy enough to get the lateral margin replaced, but it is very difficult to see that

the joint surface is repositioned. It may be helpful to divide a little synovium to get a better view. If the joint surface is not perfect, stiffness and delayed union are more likely to be a problem. Hold the fragment in place with one or two towel clips while it is transfixed with two parallel Kirschner wires. Engage the opposite cortex.

At this stage, take radiographs to be sure that reduction is anatomical. While everything is exposed you will be prepared to strive for perfection; when the dressing is in place you will be content with anything short of disaster.

Suture the periosteum. Cut the pins below skin level, and apply a cast with the arm at 90 degrees.

Three weeks in a cast is sufficient. Leave the wires in place until they penetrate the skin, but not over 6 weeks (Fig. 12-33).

Results of Treatment

Hardacre et al. have demonstrated clearly that open reduction and internal fixation yield much better results in displaced fractures than traction or closed reduction. Wadsworth has observed, however, that premature growth plate closure is not uncommon even in undisplaced fractures.

I wrote to 100 patients who had had immediate open reductions for displaced fractures. Twenty-seven were examined and radiographed. The commonest age for this injury was between 4 and 8 years. The average length of follow-up was 6 years (2 to 12 years).

Range of Movement. Perfect in 24 of 27; the remainder had lost no more than 10 degrees.

Carrying Angle. Normal in 26 of 27; one had slight varus that had not been noticed.

Lump. The lateral condyle was larger in 15 of 27. This area is subcutaneous, and several patients had noticed the lump.

Scars. All acceptable; the most posterior scars were the narrowest.

Method of Fixation. Suture, 1 pin, or 2 pins were used in equal numbers and made no difference to the outcome. Obviously an absorbable suture inserted through a drill hole in the metaphysis and then through the extensor mass circumvented the need to pull out pins.

Radiographs. In only five patients was it impossible to judge which elbow had been fractured. All the remainder had telltale signs. In children aged 10 to 11 at time of follow-up, premature fusion of the growth plate was seen (Fig. 12-34). In all nine skeletally mature patients the trochlear notch was deepened (Fig. 12-35 and 12-36). This was due to a failure of growth of the epiphysis at the site of the fracture line. Crushing at the time of injury is a possible cause. Delayed union

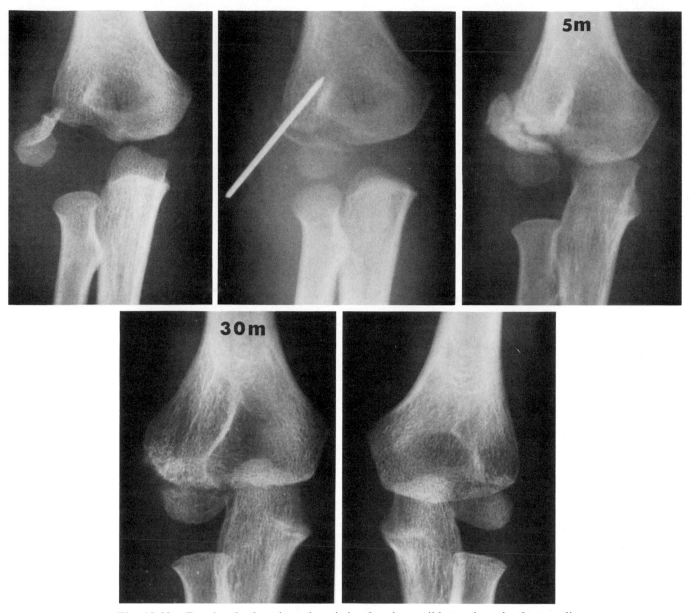

Fig. 12-33. Despite the best intentions it is often impossible to close the fracture line completely. Union was delayed in this 5-year-old child. When seen 3 years after fracture, he had a full range of movement and no deformity.

had occurred in at least two patients and did not seem to affect the result.

The Late Case

Occasionally a child presents after several weeks with a displaced fracture of the lateral condyle. Should this be accepted or corrected? The results of late surgery are not good because of stiffness and avascular necrosis. It is probably wiser to accept some lateral displacement. Figures 12-37 and 12-38 provide some evidence for this point of view. Old un-united fractures are not surgically rewarding, either. Instability is replaced by some limitation of movement. Which would you pre-fer? After reviewing the results of operation in displaced fractures more than 4 weeks old and comparing them with similar fractures that had gone untreated I would favor a "hands-off" policy.

Conclusion

Undisplaced fractures (about half the total) heal well with cast immobilization.

There is no place for a trial of conservative treatment in displaced fractures. Immediate open reduction and internal fixation is mandatory and provides excellent results.

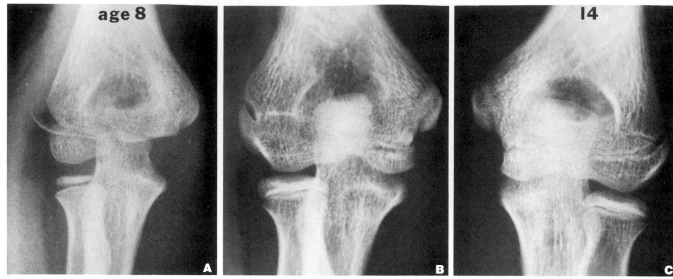

Fig. 12-34. (*A*) Displaced fracture of the lateral condyle which was replaced and held with two pins. (*B*) The same elbow 6 years later. It was perfect clinically, but there is premature closure of the growth plate. (*C*) A view of the normal elbow for comparison.

FRACTURES OF THE MEDIAL CONDYLE

Fractures of the medial condyle are rare (Fig. 12-39). They usually occur in older children and may be overlooked if only two views of the elbow are accepted. Fractures of the medial condyle produce the same problems as fractures of the lateral condyle (Fig. 12-40) and deserve the same treatment.

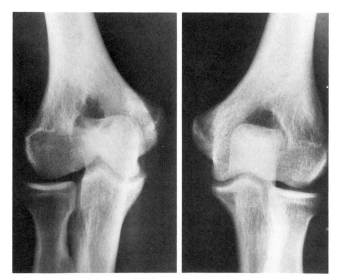

Fig. 12-35. John, aged 19, sustained a fracture of the lateral condyle at the age of 7 and the fragment was sutured in place. He now has a full range of movement and no symptoms. The lateral condyle is prominent. The radiograph (*left*) shows deepening of the trochlear notch—almost a universal finding some years after this fracture. Compare the normal elbow (*right*).

FRACTURES OF THE PROXIMAL RADIUS

Adults sustain radial head fractures; children injure the radial neck. The majority are due to a valgus injury; some are a sequel to posterior dislocation (Jeffrey); and the remainder are accompanied by fractures of the ulnar shaft reminiscent of a Monteggia fracture.

Other fractures around the elbow are present in nearly half the children with displaced radial neck fractures, and they influence management.

Mechanism of Injury

Valgus Radial Neck Fractures. The normal carrying angle of the elbow makes valgus injury likely in any

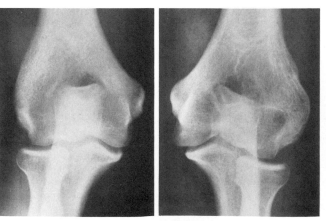

Fig. 12-36. (*Left*) The normal elbow. (*Right*) Ten years after pinning there is a slight lateral subluxation. Clinically the elbow is perfect.

fall on the outstretched arm. Anatomically, it can be demonstrated that the position of the elbow determines whether the ulna will be fractured too. In full extension the elbow is close packed: the ligaments around the elbow are tight, and the olecranon keys into the olecranon fossa so that valgus and varus movements are prevented. In this position a pure valgus force fractures the radial neck, and the olecranon sustains an oblique fracture (Fig. 12-41). In a little flexion, the olecranon is no longer held within the olecranon fossa and is free to rotate slightly: a solitary fracture of the radial neck results from valgus force. If great displacement is produced, the ulna may fracture anywhere.

Posteriorly Displaced Fractures. If a child sustains a simple posterior dislocation of the elbow and then falls down, landing on the same elbow, a posteriorly displaced fracture of the radial neck is produced. Open reduction is usually necessary, because it is almost impossible to reduce by manipulation (Fig. 12-42). Wood has demonstrated that manipulation carries the risk of replacement upside down. This is probably the cause of nonunion, which Bohler illustrates as a complication of radial neck fractures.

Other Features of Fractures of the Radial Neck

Displacement. The annular ligament hugs the radial metaphysis to the shaft of the ulna. The displaced radial head is not merely angulated but is also shifted laterally.

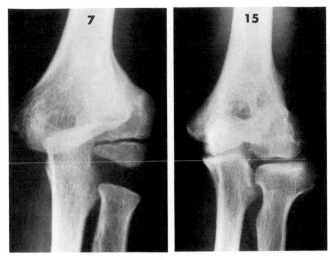

Fig. 12-37. Radiograph of an 8-week-old fracture previously treated by closed reduction. Because there is malunion an open reduction and pinning were carried out, and postoperatively a transient ulnar nerve palsy was noted. Eight years later, the elbow is pain-free but lacks 35 degree extension and 30 degree pronation, and the radial head shows posterior subluxation. The enlarged radial head and capitellum are due to prolonged hyperemia.

Assessment of displacement. Very often radiographs of the flexed elbow are compromise views of the upper forearm and the distal humerus. Well centered anteroposterior and lateral views of the radial neck should be obtained. The exact degree of tilting and shift can only

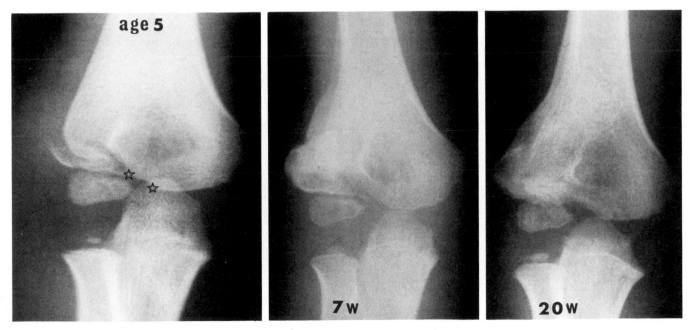

Fig. 12-38. This displaced fracture was first treated 2 weeks after injury. Manipulation did not alter the position, and the position was accepted. One year later the elbow is clinically normal.

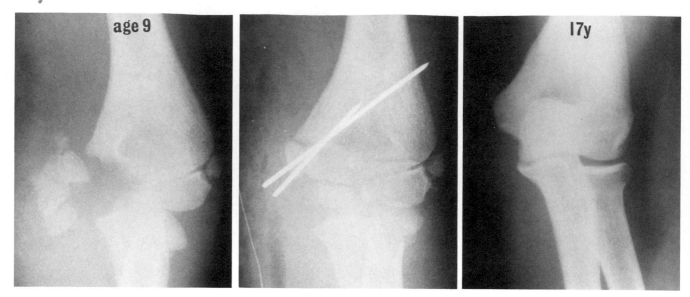

Fig. 12-39.   Though rare, fractures of the medial condyle require internal fixation.   Did you notice the fracture of the radial neck?

be measured on films taken at right angles to the plane of angulation.

The Site of Fracture.   The cartilaginous head of the radius fits the metaphysis like a bottlecap.   For this reason, the majority of fractures are metaphyseal, and only a few are epiphyseal separations.   The lateral part of the metaphysis is crushed (Fig. 12-43).

Blood Supply.   The epiphysis of the radial head is completely cartilage covered so that the blood supply may be damaged by epiphyseal separation.   However, the usual level of injury through the metaphysis is distal to the entry of the vessels, and for this reason avascular necrosis is seldom seen.   Even when the head is completely separated, avascular necrosis is not necessarily

a major problem, because revascularization of such a small volume of tissues is quickly accomplished, and because this is not a weight-bearing joint.

Associated Injuries.   In a group of 48 radial neck fractures requiring reduction that we followed, exactly half had associated injuries: olecranon, 15; ulnar shaft, 3; medial epicondyle, 2; and one example each of a posterior dislocation, and intercondylar, supracondylar, and medial condylar fractures.

Treatment

Treatment depends on the degree of displacement and the presence of other injuries.   The aim of treatment

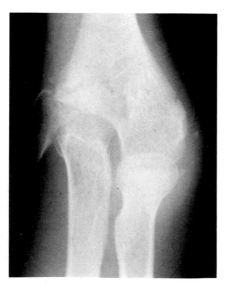

Fig. 12-40.   Nonunion of a neglected fracture of the medial condyle.

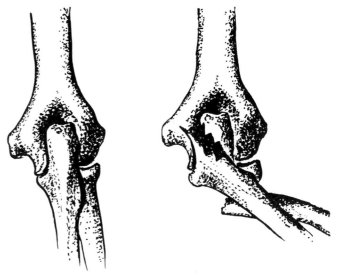

Fig. 12-41.   In full extension the olecranon keys into the olecranon fossa.   Valgus injury produces a characteristic oblique fracture of the olecranon and a radial neck fracture.

is to restore a normal range of forearm rotation. Twenty or 30 degrees of tilting of the radial head is compatible with a normal range of motion.

Minimally Displaced Fractures (up to 20 degrees). The majority fall into this category. Reduction is not necessary because the fracture will remodel (Fig. 12-44). It is customary to protect the arm in an above-elbow cast for 3 weeks. Function rapidly becomes perfect.

Moderately Displaced Fractures (more than 30 degrees). Reduce these fractures under general anesthetic with facilities available for open reduction. Put a varus force on the elbow, and rotate the forearm back and forth until the maximal prominence of the radial head is felt. Push hard with the thumb on the radial head whilst rotating the forearm gently. Often there is no sense of reduction. If reduction is unsuccessful, it is useful to take anteroposterior radiographs with the forearm in various degrees of rotation. In this way the best position can be determined for application of a reducing force. Sometimes winding an Esmarch bandage around the arm during preparation for open reduction accomplishes something that was not possible with thumb alone.

When an epiphysis cannot be reduced to within 30 degrees of the normal position, open reduction should be carried out. The sooner it is done after the injury, the easier it is. Make an incision beginning just above the lateral condyle, aiming for a point 1½ inches distal to the tip of the olecranon. Enter the elbow joint between the extensor carpi ulnaris and anconeus. Do not venture distal to the annular ligament, and keep the forearm fully pronated to avoid damaging the posterior interosseus nerve. Open the synovium; wash out the joint with saline to clear the view. Visualize the radial head and lever it into position with a small periosteal elevator, rotating the forearm to aid this. Once the fracture is reduced, it is usually stable. However, there is a small incidence of redisplacement if no form of fixation, other than a cast, is used. Several methods

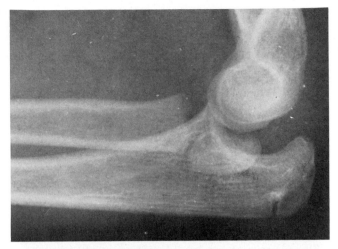

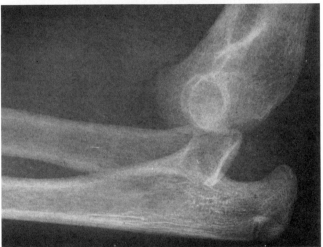

Fig. 12-42. Posterior displacement of the radial neck in a girl of 11 years. (*Top*) A dislocation with partial separation of the radial head. (*Bottom*) When the elbow is reduced the radial head is pushed completely off. The articular surface faces inferiorly. Open reduction is required.

of fixation are available for fractures that are unstable because of comminution.

1. Sutures are difficult (because there is no proximal periosteum) but possible.

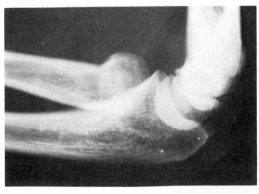
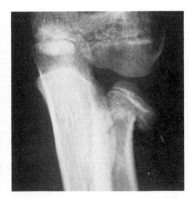
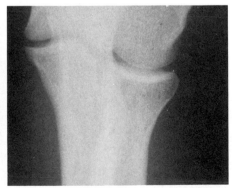

Fig. 12-43. The typical metaphyseal fracture of the radial neck in a 13-year-old boy. Seven years after closed reduction there is no sign of a previous injury.

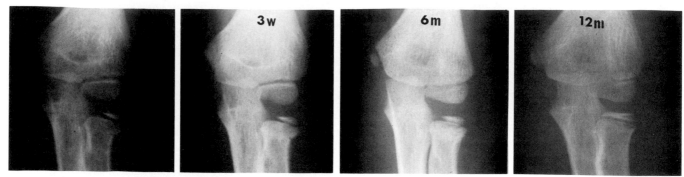

Fig. 12-44.   Remodelling will take care of minor degrees of angulation.

2. Kirschner wire through the capitellum is secure but carries the risk of infection tracking into the elbow joint as well as fracture of the wire at the joint line (which makes removal almost impossible).   This method is not recommended.

3. An oblique Kirschner wire avoiding the humerus is the method I favor.   When the wire is removed at 3 weeks, movement may be commenced.

The radius of a growing child should never be decapitated.   Although it may be completely separated, revascularization is the rule.

Concomitant Injuries.   The presence of other injuries, which may themselves require open reduction, does not mean that the radial head will require open reduction.

The commonest combination is a fracture of the radial neck and an oblique fracture of the olecranon.   The

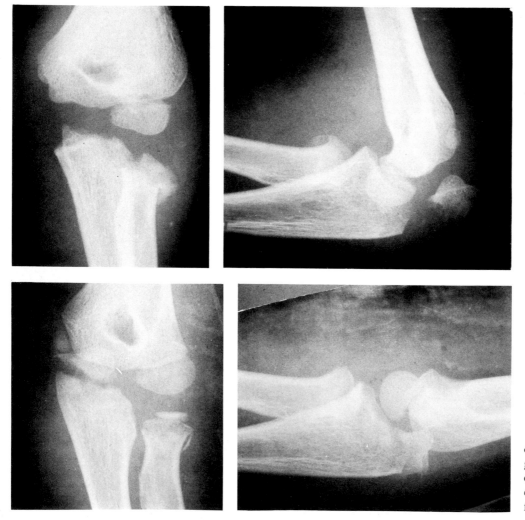

Fig. 12-45.   Fracture of the olecranon and radial neck in a girl, aged 8 years.   Treated by closed reduction and casted in extension, the elbow was perfect 10 years later.

Fig. 12-46. A similar fracture to that in the previous figure, this in a 9-year-old girl. Open reduction has been followed by radioulnar synostosis. Do not open these fractures unnecessarily.

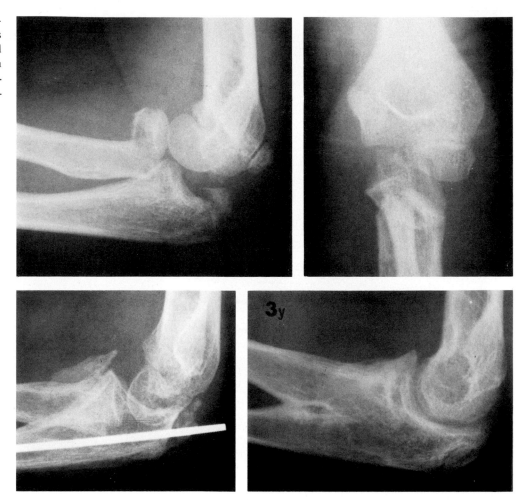

obliquity of the olecranon fracture and the intact periosteum over it make closed reduction possible (in about half the children) when the elbow is extended. A quarter of the children required open reduction of both the radial head and the olecranon (Fig. 12-45 and 12-46).

Results

Following fracture, return of full rotation of the forearm may take several months. Very little permanent disability is seen after this injury. Full flexion and extension of the elbow can be expected, but forearm rotation may be limited in some.

In our series of 48 patients requiring reduction, 28 had clinically normal elbows, and 7 had lost 45 degrees or more of forearm rotation. Thirteen had minor sequelae.

The imperfect results were much more common in the operated cases (13 of 20) than in conservatively treated cases (7 of 28). There was a higher correlation with the method of treatment than with the severity of the injury. Henrikson, in a conservatively treated series, found that 15 percent of patients had a degree of restriction whereas Reidy had 45 percent of patients with this degree of limitation in an operatively treated group. The lesson to be learned is that you should not give up closed reduction until you have tried every trick you know.

Synostosis. Though rare, synostosis is a hazard of even closed reduction. The clearance between the proximal radius and ulna is very small. Not only does synostosis block rotation, but it may result in cubitus varus (Fig. 12-47).

Heterotopic Ossification. A flake of bone may form and lie parallel to the radial shaft in the vicinity of the biceps tendon. Rotation is reduced; it was only seen after open reduction (Fig. 12-48).

Avascular Necrosis. Avascular necrosis of the whole head is rare, even when the head is completely displaced (Fig. 12-49). Necrosis of part of the head is more frequent (Fig. 12-50).

Irregularity of the head and premature closure of the growth plate are common. The carrying angle is increased in about 30 percent of children due to premature closure of the growth plate (Fig. 12-51). Irregularity of the head contributes to slight loss of rotation.

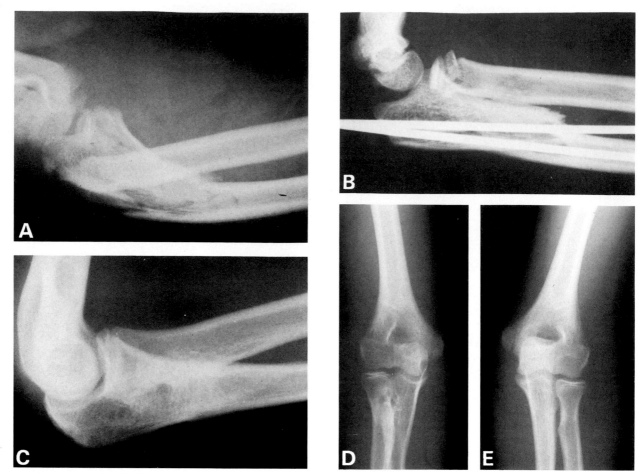

Fig. 12-47. (*A, B*) This 10-year-old had his arm out of a bus window. He sustained a degloving injury, and fractures of the radial neck and ulnar shaft. (*C*) A synostosis formed and recurred after excision. (*D*) At the age of 13 the carrying angle is reduced, because growth in the radial head has continued. Compare the normal elbow (*E*).

Nonunion. We have not seen nonunion, but Bohler and Reidy have illustrated examples. It may be due to the head having been replaced back-to-front.

In our experience, the poor results are in cases that require open reduction, a fact that leads me to wonder whether it would be wiser to leave fractures in a displaced position rather than operate on them. Jeffrey is of the opinion that the degree of initial displacement determines the quality of the result. In a child of 7 or 8, it may be wiser to accept 30 degrees of angulation after closed reduction than to carry out an open reduction. Henrikson has shown this amount of malunion will disappear during the remodelling process.

FRACTURES OF THE OLECRANON

The structure of a child's olecranon is different from that of an adult. The bone appears more spongy so that the fracture line may be more difficult to identify. The layer of articular cartilage is thick and permits osteochondral fractures. An epiphysis forms poste-

riorly. It is often irregular and, though rarely separated, it frequently looks injured.

While solitary fractures of the olecranon are seen, the majority are associated with fractures of the radial neck. When the fracture is displaced there may be angulation or separation. Angulation—valgus, varus, or extension—can usually be corrected by manipulation. When the periosteum is torn, the fragments may separate. If the fracture is not reduced by extending the elbow, some form of internal fixation is required. We have found that the ASIF technique (two Kirschner wires and a figure-of-eight tension wire) is excellent (Fig. 12-53).

DISLOCATIONS OF THE ELBOW JOINT

In children elbow dislocations without fracture are decidedly unusual. Whenever you see a dislocation of the elbow, assume that there is an occult bony fragment

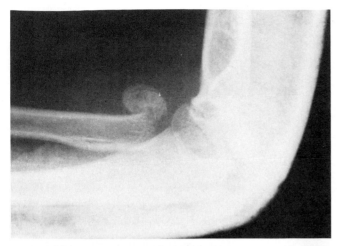

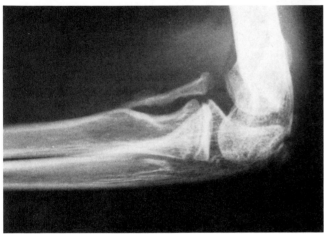

Fig. 12-48. Heterotopic ossification after open reduction. Six years after injury she had a full range of flexion and extension. Rotation was reduced by 10 degrees.

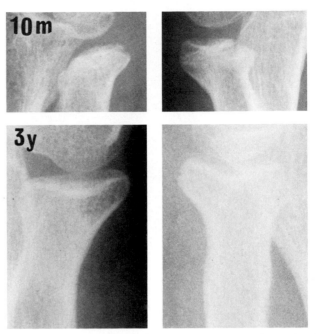

Fig. 12-50. Partial avascular necrosis. This girl sustained fractures of the radial neck and proximal ulna at 10 years. Open reduction was carried out. Ten months later growth arrest and head irregularity is evident. Three years later the growth plate on the normal side was still open, but the injured plate had closed. Movement was full except for loss of 10 degrees of supination. The carrying angle was slightly increased.

that may become trapped in the joint after reduction or may prevent reduction.

Dislocations with Occult Fragments

Medial Epicondyle. The avulsed medial epicondyle is usually overshadowed by the humerus. The best sign that it has been avulsed is that you cannot see the epicondyle in its proper position. Radiograph the opposite elbow to confirm this. This ossification center is usually present at age 7.

The dislocation should be reduced soon to relieve pain and improve circulation. If the child has a full stomach, administer intravenous demerol and place the child face down to reduce dislocation. The arm should rest on the stretcher with the elbow flexed over the edge so that the forearm hangs vertically downwards. When the child relaxes, a little pressure over the olecranon with correction of any sideways displacement usually reduces the dislocation. Most of the pain will disappear. Radiograph the elbow again, and anticipate replacing the medial epicondyle operatively at a convenient time.

If the stomach is legally empty the whole procedure can be carried out under general anesthesia.

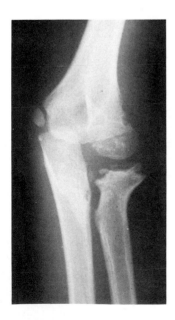

Fig. 12-49. Avascular necrosis after open reduction of a totally separated epiphysis.

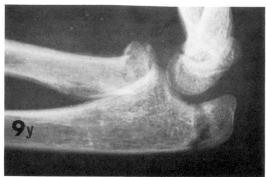

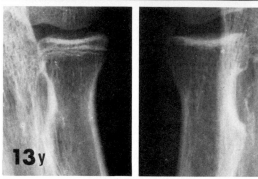

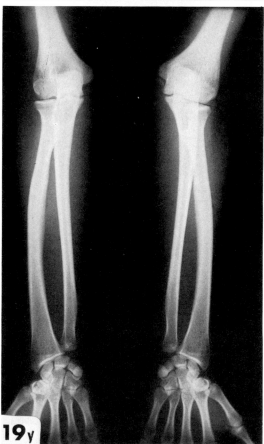

Fig. 12-51. At age 9 years this patient had fractures of the radial neck and olecranon reduced by manipulation. Premature closure of the plate occurred by the age of 13 years leaving the radius 5 mm. short. At 19 the carrying angle was increased.

Articular Surface of Ulna. Dr. Robert Gillespie drew my attention to this injury. A flap of articular cartilage and subchondral bone is lifted up from the articular surface of the ulna. The osteochondral fragment is barely perceptible on initial radiographs. After reduction there is crepitus and a restricted range of movement. Arthrotomy is required to push down the flap or excise it in order to secure concentric reduction.

Dislocations with Obvious Fractures

Fractures of the lateral condyle, olecranon, and radial neck are commonly seen with dislocation and present no traps in management.

True Dislocations

These are less common than in adults and can usually be reduced easily, either by the method described above or under general anesthesia. It is our custom to protect the elbow in a cast for 3 weeks afterwards to avoid the slight risk of recurrent dislocation.

DISLOCATION OF THE RADIAL HEAD

This is a rare injury in children because they rarely tear ligaments. Two varieties are seen, both accompanied by ulnar fractures.

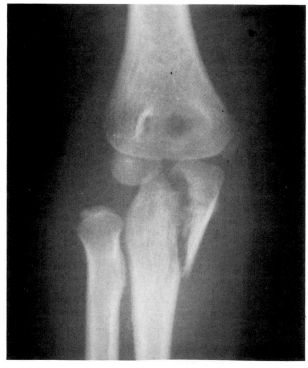

Fig. 12-52. Fracture of the olecranon is commonly accompanied by dislocation or fracture of the proximal radius. Girl aged 6 years.

1. The Monteggia injury is characterized by damage to the annular ligament producing *radioulnar* dislocation (Fig. 13-29).
2. Radiohumeral dislocation: fracture through the olecranon or coronoid allows the radial head to dislocate, leaving the radioulnar joint and the annular ligament undisturbed (Fig. 12-53).

Both varieties of dislocation are reduced when the ulnar fracture is replaced. This subject is discussed in Chapter 13.

Solitary

Solitary dislocation of the radial head has been described but the published radiographs show a bent ulna, suggesting that some of these cases are really Monteggia injuries (Fig. 13-27).

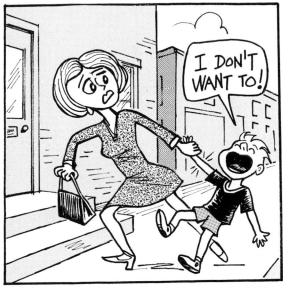

Fig. 12-54. Pulled elbow is very common in children.

Long-Standing

Confusion may arise when a child with a congenital or pathological dislocation falls on the elbow. The ensuing radiographs may mimic an acute injury. Examine and radiograph both elbows (Fig. 13-26). The diagnosis of a long-standing dislocation can be made (1) when the condition is bilateral or (2) if unilateral, when the affected radius is longer, the head misshapen, and ossification more advanced than on the opposite side.

PULLED ELBOW

The commonest elbow injury has been left until last. We see about two patients a week with pulled elbow.

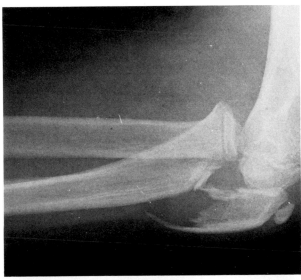

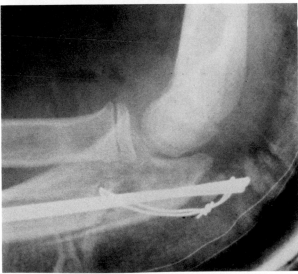

Fig. 12-53. Fracture of the olecranon with radiohumeral dislocation treated by ASIF fixation.

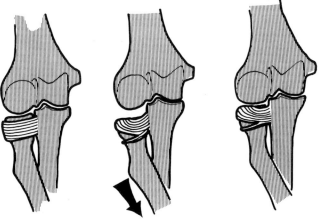

Fig. 12-55. The pathology of pulled elbow. The annular ligament is torn when the arm is pulled. The radial head moves distally and when traction is discontinued the ligament is carried into the joint.

The clinical picture is characteristic. A child between 1 and 4 years suddenly refuses to move an arm and holds it slightly flexed and pronated. Often parents think the arm is paralyzed or that the child has a fractured clavicle. They seldom mention that the problem began as the child was being pulled along by the wrist—the usual cause (Fig. 12-54).

Pathology

Salter and Zaltz found that when longitudinal traction is applied to the arm (with the forearm in pronation), the annular ligament tears at its attachment to the radius. The head of the radius moves distally. When traction is released, the ligament is carried up and becomes impacted between the radius and capitellum (Fig. 12-55). Because the shape of the radial head is not completely regular, the ligament can be replaced by slight flexion and supination. Usually reduction is carried out by the radiographers as they supinate the arm to obtain a true anteroposterior radiograph of the elbow.

Treatment

Reduction is easy: supinate the slightly flexed elbow, and often you will hear a click. The child stops crying and starts to move the arm again. Warn the parents not to pull the arm again. Recurrence and irreducibility are both unusual. It is remarkable that not all children experience a pulled elbow.

BIBLIOGRAPHY

Supracondylar Fractures

Ashurst, A. P. C.: Fractures of the Elbow. Philadelphia, Lea & Febiger, 1910

Carcassone, M., Bergoin, M., and Hornung, H.: Results of operative treatment of severe supracondylar fractures of the elbow in children. J. Pediatr. Surg., *7:* 676, 1972

d'Ambrosia, R. D.: Supracondylar fractures of humerus—prevention of cubitus varus. J. Bone Joint Surg., *54A:* 60, 1972

Dodge, H. S.: Displaced supracondylar fractures of the humerus in children—treatment by Dunlop's traction. J. Bone Joint Surg., *54A:* 1408, 1972

French, P. R.: Varus deformity of the elbow following supracondylar fractures of the humerus in children. Lancet, *2:* 439, 1959

Haddad, R. J., Saer, J. K., and Riordan, D. C.: Percutaneous pinning of displaced supracondylar fractures of the elbow in children. Clin. Orthop., *71:* 112, 1970

Hagen, R.: Skin traction treatment of supracondylar fractures of the humerus in children. Acta. Orthop. Scand., *35:* 138, 1964

Henriksen, B.: Supracondylar fractures of the humerus in children. Acta. Chir. Scand., [*Supp*] *369:* 1, 1966

Hordegan, K. M.: Neurologische Komplikationen bei kindlichen suprakondylären Humerusfrakturen. Arch. Orthop. Unfall Chir., *68:* 294, 1970

Jones, K. G.: Percutaneous pin fixation of fractures of the lower end of the humerus. J. Bone Joint Surg., *50:* 53, 1967

Kaplan, S. S. and Reckling, F. W.: Fracture separation of the lower humeral epiphysis with medial displacement. J. Bone Joint Surg., *53A:* 1105, 1971

Langenskiold, A. and Kivilaakso, R.: Varus and valgus deformity of the elbow following supracondylar fracture of the humerus. Acta. Orthop. Scand., *38:* 313, 1967

Macafee, A. L.: Infantile supracondylar fracture. J. Bone Joint Surg., *49B:* 768, 1967

Mann, T. S.: Prognosis in supracondylar fractures. J. Bone Joint Surg., *45B:* 516, 1963

Ramsey, R. H. and Griz, J.: Immediate open reduction and internal fixation of severely displaced supracondylar fractures of the humerus in children. Clin. Orthop., *90:* 130, 1973

Siffert, R. S.: Displacement of the distal humeral epiphysis in the new born infant. J. Bone Joint Surg., *45A:* 165, 1963

Smith, H. C.: Position in the treatment of elbow joint fractures: an experimental study. Boston Med. Surg. J., *131:* 386; 411, 1894

Wainwright, D.: *In* Modern Trends in Orthopaedics, Clarke, J. M. P. (ed.). London. Butterworth, 1962

Lateral Condyle

Crabbe, W. A.: The treatment of fracture-separation of the capitular epiphysis. J. Bone Joint Surg., *45B:* 722, 1963

Flynn, J. C. and Richards, J. F.: Non-union of minimally displaced fractures of the lateral condyle of the humerus in children. J. Bone Joint Surg., *53A:* 1096, 1971

Hardacre, J. A., Nahigian, S. H., Froimson, A. I., and Brown, J. E.: Fractures of the lateral condyle of the humerus in children. J. Bone Joint Surg., *53A:* 1083, 1971

McLearie, M., and Merson, R. D.: Injuries to the lateral condyle epiphysis of the humerus in children. J. Bone Joint Surg., *36B:* 84, 1954

Smith, F. M.: An eighty-four-year follow-up on a patient with ununited fracture of the lateral condyle of the humerus. J. Bone Joint Surg., *55A:* 379, 1973

Wadsworth, T. G.: Injuries of the capitular (lateral humeral condylar) epiphysis. Clin. Orthop., *85:* 127, 1972

Medial Epicondyle

Fahey, J. J., and O'Brien, E. T.: Fracture-separation of the medial humeral condyle in a child confused with fracture of the medial epicondyle. J. Bone Joint Surg., *53A:* 1102, 1971

Kilfoyle, R. M.: Fractures of the medial condyle and epicondyle of the elbow in children. Clin. Orthop., *41:* 43, 1965

Radial Neck

Bohler, L.: The treatment of fractures. New York, Grune & Stratton, 1958

Dougall, A. J.: Severe fractures of the neck of the radius in children. J. Roy. Coll. Surg. Edinb., *14:* 220, 1969

Fielding, J. W.: Radio-ulnar union following displacement of the proximal radial epiphysis. J. Bone Joint Surg., *46A:* 1277, 1964

Henrikson, B.: Isolated fractures of the proximal end of the radius in children. Acta Ortho. Scand., *40:* 246, 1969

Jeffrey, C. C.: Fractures of the head of the radius in children. J. Bone Joint Surg., *32B:* 314, 1950

Jones, E. R. W., and Esah, M.: Displaced fractures of the neck of the radius in children. J. Bone Joint Surg., *53B:* 429, 1971

O'Brien, P. I.: Injuries involving the proximal radial epiphysis. Clin. Orthop., *41:* 51, 1965

Patterson, R. F.: Treatment of displaced transverse fractures of the neck of the radius in children. J. Bone Joint Surg., *16:* 695, 1934

Reidy, J. A., and Van Gorder, G. W.: Treatment of displacement of the proximal radial epiphysis. J. Bone Joint Surg., *45A:* 1355, 1963

Schwartz, R. P., and Young, F.: Treatment of fractures of the head and neck of the radius and slipped radial epiphysis in children. Surg. Gynec. Obstet., *57:* 528, 1933

Strachan, J. C. H. and Ellis, B. W.: Vulnerability of the posterior interosseous nerve during radial head resection. J. Bone Joint Surg., *53B:* 320, 1971

Vastal, O.: Fractures of the neck of the radius in children. Acta Chir et Traumat. Cechoslov., *37:* 294, 1970

Wood, S. K.: Reversal of the radial head during reduction of fracture of the neck of the radius in children. J. Bone Joint Surg., *51B:* 707, 1969

Wright, P. R.: Greenstick fracture of the upper end of the ulna with dislocation of the radio-humeral joint or displacement of the superior radial epiphysis. J. Bone Joint Surg., *45B:* 727, 1963

Pulled Elbow

Salter, R. B. and Zaltz, C.: Anatomic investigations of the mechanism of injury and pathologic anatomy of "pulled elbow" in young children. Clin. Orthop., *77:* 141, 1971

Tachdjian, M. O.: Pediatric Orthopedics. Philadelphia, W. B. Saunders, 1972

Crenshaw, A. H. (ed.): Campbell's Operative Orthopaedics. St. Louis, C. V. Mosby, 1971

13

Radius and Ulna

Fractures of the radius and ulna are common in children and somewhat different from those of adults. For example, shattering injuries of the articular surfaces of each end of the radius do not occur, and fractures are seen that have no adult equivalent. Union is certain. Treatment is different; fractures of the shafts of both bones of the forearm can usually be managed closed and represent a challenge that adult forearm fractures do not.

THE MECHANISM OF INJURY

When a child puts out the palm of the hand to break a fall, he may sustain a greenstick fracture. As he falls all the muscles holding the forearm in pronation are tensed; landing on the thenar eminence first, a sudden supinational force is applied. This displacement of the fracture appears on radiographs to be anterior angulation, but the displacement is usually rotational. Test this for yourself with a strip of paper as shown in Figure 13-1. If the tyro accepts the angulation at face value and corrects it, the rotational deformity will remain uncorrected. The fracture should be reduced by applying a pronational force to the hand.

The radiographic appearance of greenstick fractures of the forearm can be very confusing until it is realized that the only fractures with true anterior or posterior angulation are produced by children doing cartwheels

with an arm trapped in a drainpipe. All the rest owe this appearance to rotatory deformity.

If the violence is sustained a complete fracture of both bones may be produced—an entirely different situation. The distal fragment may be in any position, but the proximal fragments take up a position dictated by the pull of muscles and other soft tissues.

The aim of treatment is to discover what this position is, so that the distal part of the limb may be lined up accurately: an old principle of fracture care. There is no other way to secure a reduction. It is useful to look at a few anatomical points to realize the importance of accurate reduction.

ANATOMY AND PATHOLOGY

The forearm bones are subcutaneous in the lower half of the forearm. The quality of reduction can be reasonably easily appreciated, not only by the surgeon, but also by the patient when the cast comes off.

Forearm rotation has a range of 180 degrees, perhaps the greatest range of rotation of any joint in the body. Although a decrease of motion by 50 percent may go unnoticed, fractures should be reduced well to avoid loss of motion. Fractures were produced in cadavers and plated with various types of malunion to determine the effects of each:

1. Ten degrees of malrotation limits rotation by 10 degrees (Fig. 13-2).

2. Ten degrees of angulation limits rotation by 20 degrees, because it produces widening and narrowing of the interosseous membrane during rotatory movements (Fig. 13-3).

3. Bayonet apposition does not limit rotation.

4. Pure narrowing of the interosseous distance is important in proximal fractures. Narrowing impedes rotation by causing the bicipital tuberosity to impinge on the ulna. Malalignment of fractures of the ulnar metaphysis increases the tension on the articular disc so that the head of the ulna is not free to rotate (Fig. 13-4).

Loss of rotation is a common problem after forearm fractures. Knight and Purvis found residual rotational deformity of between 20 and 60 degrees in 60 percent.

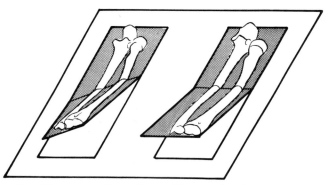

Fig. 13-1. Angulation is usually associated with rotation. Use a strip of paper to prove this yourself.

Evans found malrotation *deformity* of more than 30 degrees in 56 percent. The distal fragment was pronated so that supination was lost. Let us see how this can be prevented.

Recognition of Rotational Deformity

Clinical Examination

Look at the forearm in the position of displacement. You will be able to tell from the shape of the arm how the distal fragment lies in relation to the proximal part (Fig. 13-5). It sometimes helps if first the part of the arm below the fracture is blocked off from vision with a hand, and then the part above. If the upper part of

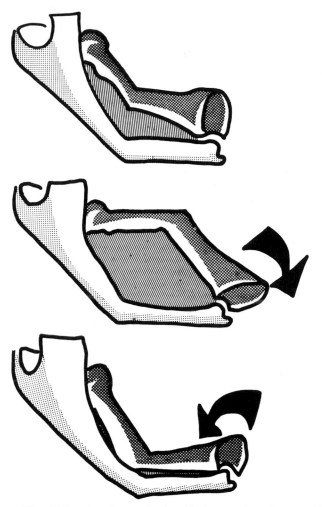

Fig. 13-3. Angular malunion limits rotation, because the interosseous membrane cannot widen and narrow.

the arm lies in supination, and the distal part looks as if it is pronated, all you should do to reduce the fracture is supinate the distal fragment. The first person who sees the child has a great advantage, because he is the only one who can see the limb as it lies.

Testing the Range of Movement. Occasionally, with a stable reduction, the range of movement can be tested before the cast is applied. A full range of movement indicates accurate reduction.

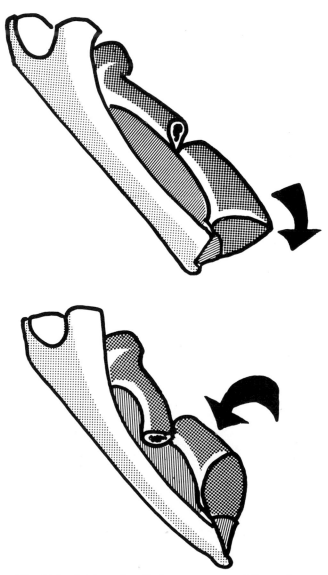

Fig. 13-2. Malrotation limits movement. Ninety degrees of pronation deformity, as shown here, limits pronation to the mid-position, because the proximal radioulnar joint has reached the limit.

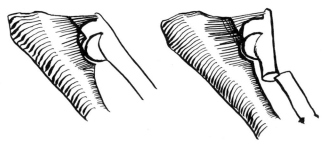

Fig. 13-4. Angulation of the distal ulna prevents the radius rotating around the head of the ulna.

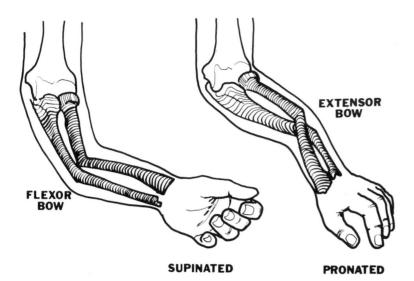

FLEXOR BOW

EXTENSOR BOW

SUPINATED   PRONATED

Fig. 13-5. Flexor bow indicates supinational deformity. Extensor bow indicates pronational deformity.

Radiographic Aids

The Radius is a curved bone that is pear-shaped in cross section. Malrotation of the radius is recognized by a break in the smooth curve of the bone and a sudden change in the width of the cortex (Fig. 13-6).

Angulation. Angulation of the bones that produces a volar prominence is conventionally described as volar angulation or bowing. The distal fragment is said to be dorsally deviated. This is worth stating clearly because telephone conversations about fractures are frequently bedevilled by semantic ambiguities. In greenstick fractures of the forearm volar or flexor bowing is the outward and visible sign of a pronational deformity. Dorsal or extensor bowing signifies supinational deformity.

The Position of the Bicipital Tuberosity. Mervyn Evans, whose classic paper on forearm fractures is essential reading, drew attention to this radiographic sign. The tuberosity normally lies medially when the arm is fully supinated; it lies posteriorly in the mid-position, and laterally in full pronation (Fig. 13-7). Intervening positions can be judged to 30 degrees by reference to a carefully positioned radiograph of the normal elbow or by reference to the figure.

In complete fractures the rotational position of the proximal fragment can be identified by this method, and reduction becomes a scientific exercise. The distal fragment is lined up in the same degree of rotation as the proximal fragment, which always returns to its own position. This takes the guesswork out of reduction—and the need for silent communications with the spirit of Nicholas Andry.

Prior to the discovery of x-rays, surgeons had to guess the position of the proximal fragment and some surgeons still do, using the traditional argument that muscle pull determines the position of the proximal frag-

ments. "In the case of fractures above the insertion of pronator teres, the proximal fragment is invariably pulled into supination by supinator. The fracture should be immobilized in supination. Fractures below the insertion of pronator teres are invariably pulled into pronation by this muscle and should therefore be immobilized in this position." Though this theory is often repeated and has a certain logic, it is usually not true. Do not work by rote, cerebrate. Use Mervyn Evans' method.

Remodelling

Remodelling will correct 30 to 40 degrees of displacement of an epiphysis in a child with growth ahead (Fig. 13-8). But remodelling does little more than round off the ends of malunited fractures of the diaphysis. Any loss of motion is permanent (Fig. 13-9).

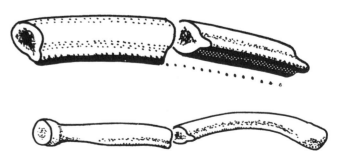

RADIAL MALROTATION

Fig. 13-6. A change in the diameter of the radius, the width of the cortex, and the smooth curve of the radius indicate malrotation.

supination · neutral · pronation

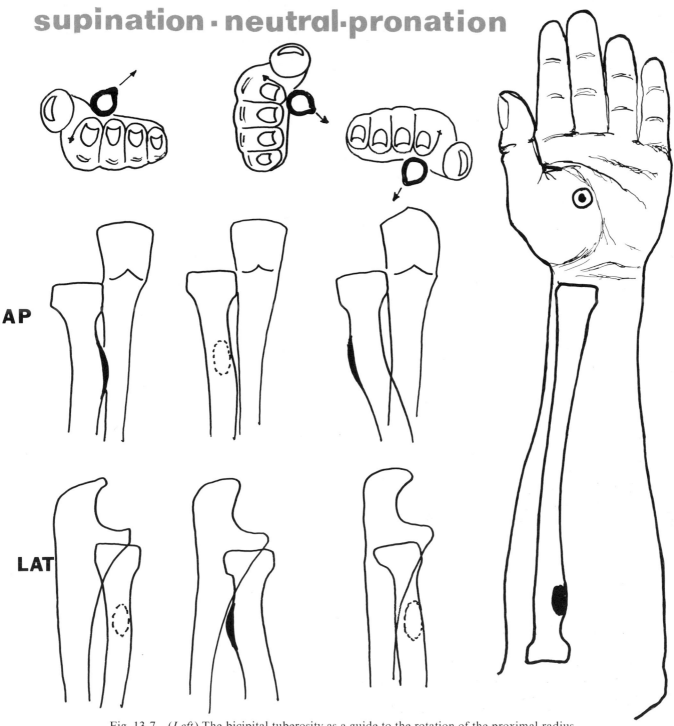

AP

LAT

Fig. 13-7. (*Left*) The bicipital tuberosity as a guide to the rotation of the proximal radius. (*Right*) If you cannot remember where the bicipital tuberosity should be put an ink mark on your palm at the site indicated. The prominence of the tuberosity always points in this direction.

Other Effects of Injury

Nerves and Vessels

Nerves and vessels are seldom injured primarily in forearm fractures. The median nerve is protected from the radius by an intervening layer of muscles. The ulnar nerve is close to bone and may occasionally be damaged, especially in open fractures near the lower end. Despite the presence of closed fascial spaces in the forearm, the risk of ischemic contracture is low if well padded casts are used.

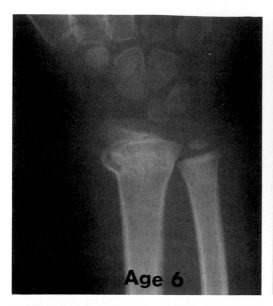

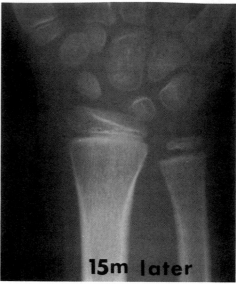

Fig. 13-8. Remodelling is effective at the ends of bones in young children.

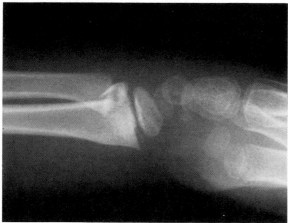

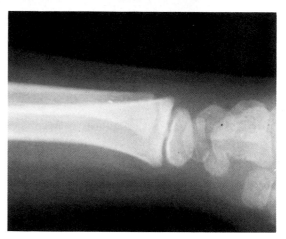

Growth

The distal end of the radius is a classical site for growth disturbance due to crushing of the plate. At first it masquerades as a sprain, and there is no great radiological evidence of injury. It is only later, when Madelung's deformity begins to appear, that the true nature of the injury is appreciated (Fig. 13-10).

At the upper end of the radius, complete separation of the head may cause avascular necrosis when the periosteum carrying all the blood vessels to the epiphysis is torn. Growth stops, and cubitus valgus is the result.

INDIVIDUAL FRACTURES

Greenstick Fractures

Displaced greenstick fractures should be slightly overcorrected by slow manipulation to take the spring out of the fracture. You will hear a crack as the bony hinge yields. If this is not done the deformity often reappears in the succeeding weeks.

A greenstick fracture of the radius at the junction of the metaphysis and diaphysis with supinational deformity is common and has an evil reputation because angulation tends to recur after reduction (Fig. 13-11). It has always been our custom to hold the fracture in full pronation in an above-elbow cast. The intact periosteum locks the fracture in place, and full pronation stops a supinational deformity from developing. Pollen advances an entirely new and different approach: he considers brachioradialis the deforming force. In pronation, brachioradialis displaces the fragment, whereas in supination the pull of brachioradialis holds the reduction. Perhaps we should enliven the care of this fracture by running a controlled trial. Certainly anything less than full pronation and full supination should be avoided, because this is a troublesome injury. The fracture should be radiographed every week for 3 weeks, and the slightest suggestion of deformity should be corrected. The cast can be removed at 6 weeks. For some reason, refracture is common at this site.

Angulated greenstick fractures of the midshaft require slight overcorrection. The periosteal tube is intact, and

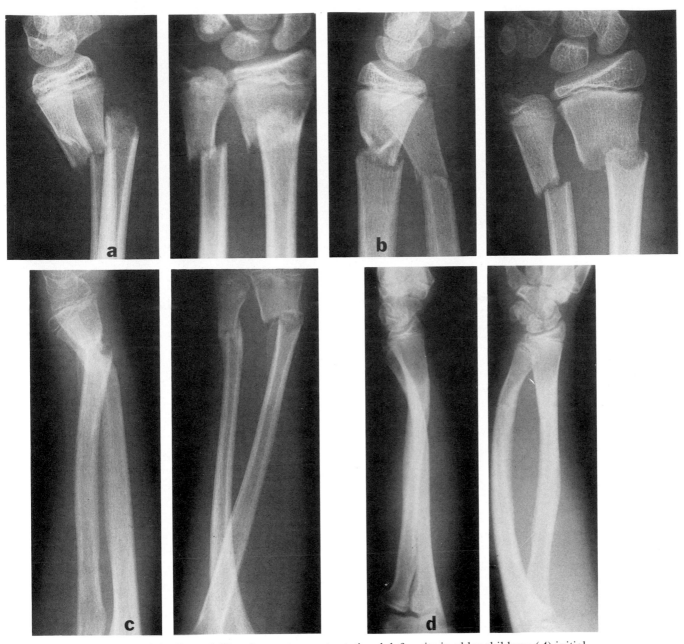

Fig. 13-9. Remodelling does not correct rotational deformity in older children: (*A*) initial injury in a 14-year-old boy. (*B*) After manipulation the distal fragment of the radius has been rotated through 90 degrees. Note the difference in the width of the bone. (*C*) When the cast is removed the fracture has angulated. (*D*) Two years later he has only a jog of rotation. The combination of 90 degrees of deformity and angulation has prevented movement, but the ends have rounded off. Look at the position of the bicipital tuberosity; what is the position of the proximal fragment?

reduction is easy. Supination injuries are pronated and then given a push to get rid of the anterior angulation, at which time a crack is heard. The cast should be well molded. Greenstick fractures are very much easier to manage than complete fractures (Fig. 13-12).

Minimally displaced fractures are very common. The deformity may be corrected with pressure while the cast is setting.

Complete Fractures of Both Bones

Complete fractures of the radius and ulna can be very

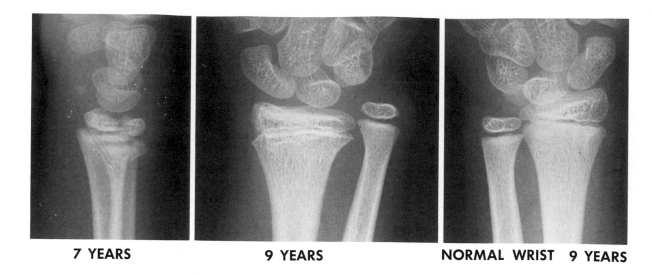

7 YEARS   **9 YEARS**   **NORMAL WRIST 9 YEARS**

Fig. 13-10. Growth arrest due to a type IV injury. If this had been accurately repositioned by open reduction this complication may have been prevented. (Courtesy Mr. Lipmann Kessel, to whom this girl was referred at the age of 9).

challenging to manage. Reduction may be difficult and unstable, particularly in older children, in high fractures, and in those that are comminuted or oblique. There are several general rules to guide you:

1. Good reductions last better than poor reductions, particularly in a well-molded cast.

2. Cortex-to-cortex apposition is adequate if rotation is correct, if the interosseous space is preserved, and if there is no angulation.

3. Immobilize the fracture in the position—any position—in which the alignment is correct and the reduction feels stable.

4. Minor improvements can be made at 3 weeks when the fracture is sticky.

5. Be prepared to carry out open reduction and internal fixation, particularly in children over the age of 10, rather than accept a poor position. Overlap of both bones in the forearm of a child under the age of 10 is probably acceptable so long as there is no malrotation or angulation. In children over 10, permanent loss of motion is the price to be paid. Skin traction is a neglected method of controlling longitudinal instability in younger children.

6. Always warn the parents before you reduce the fracture that remanipulation is often necessary later and that there will be a bump when the cast comes off.

Technique of Reduction

Examine the radiograph to determine the position of the proximal fragment. If necessary, take tuberosity views of the normal elbow in varying degrees of rotation to be sure. Reduction is best carried out by retracing the events of the fracture. Increase the deformity until the overlapping bones can be hitched together by thumb pressure. Do one at a time, then correct the deformity, and set the arm in the desired degree of rotation. Test longitudinal stability by attempting to telescope the arm. (Increasing the deformity looks repugnant to some. I can well remember trying to catch a fainting nurse and hold a reduction at the same time.)

It is always difficult to hold the limb while the cast is being applied. Having tried many different ways, the way I like best is with the forearm parallel to the floor, with the periosteal hinge uppermost to hold the fracture (Fig. 13-13).

Mold the cast well, as shown in Figure 13-14. A good cast may leave the child's grandmother complaining that the arm looks more crooked now than it did before reduction. The cast should be pear-shaped in cross section. The ulnar border should be straight, with the elbow at a perfect right angle. Close molding just above the elbow should prevent the cast telescoping up and down the arm. If the radius is comminuted or tends to shorten, include the thumb in the cast. A bad cast looks like a loose shirt sleeve. Hold the fracture with a thin cast while radiographs are being taken. Supervise them personally in order to obtain a true lateral and AP. At this time, all should be peaceful and serene. The room should be free of distractions, such as an anesthetist struggling with a patient, a nurse hurrying you out of the plaster room, or a radiographer serving up overexposed keyhole views of the limb. Remember that the quality of reduction that is accepted

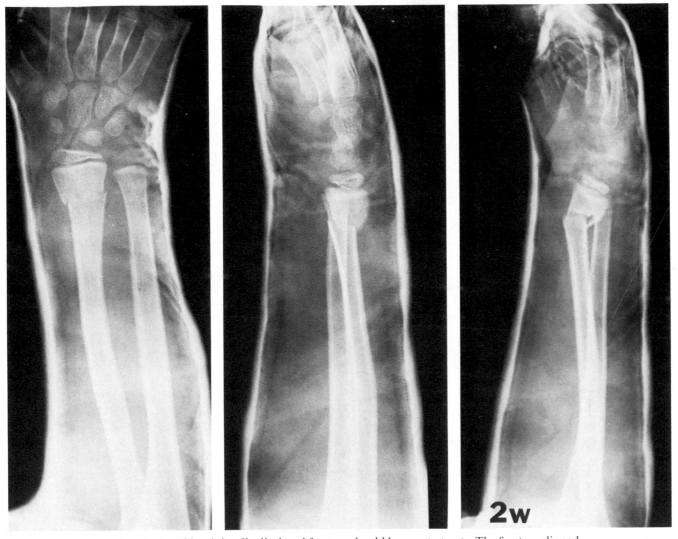

Fig. 13-11. This minimally displaced fracture should be easy to treat. The fracture slipped because of three errors. (1) The cast is round in cross section, (it should be oval); (2) there is no moulding; and (3) the arm is not in full pronation as it should be. All the errors are evident in the radiographs. The fracture was remanipulated.

is inversely proportional to the difficulties involved in changing it. If the position is not satisfactory, try again. Look at the radiographs in order to decide if the arm should be supinated further, or pronated further, or left in the midposition. An image intensifier can be useful if the reduction is very difficult. When the position is satisfactory, put on a good strong cast, because children are very destructive. Support the weight of the cast with a neck hoop, so that the weight of the cast will not act as a deforming force at the fracture site (Figs. 13-15 to 13-17). Include the thumb in the cast if the fracture is very unstable.

Many authors advocate an alternative method of reduction: traction is used to reduce and hold the limb while the cast is applied. Counter traction is provided by a padded sling around the arm. The sling is fixed

to a hook on the wall or a post on the table. An assistant pulls on the hand while the surgeon manipulates the bone ends. The cast is applied, and then the sling is pulled out. I have not liked this method because

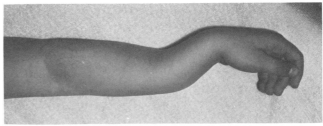

Fig. 13-12. A typical greenstick fracture in a 7-year-old boy. It is easily reduced.

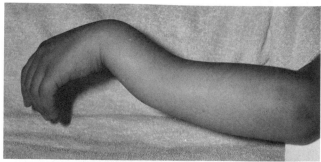

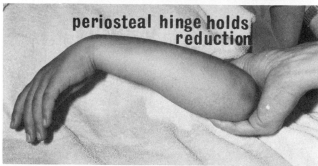
periosteal hinge holds reduction

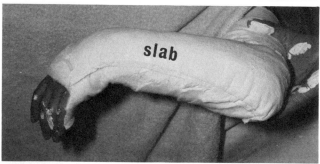
slab

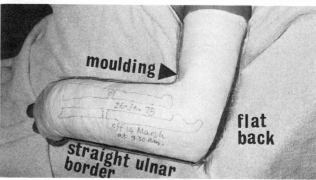
moulding ▶
flat back
straight ulnar border

Fig. 13-13. Reduction and casting. The supinational deformity is corrected, and then the fracture is held by the periosteal hinge. A slab is allowed to harden, after which the circular layers are applied and moulded. Write on the cast. It helps the radiographer provide well centered follow-up films and saves embarrassment if the written record is lost.

the intact periosteum must be stretched to allow the overlapping ends to jump into end-to-end contact. It is like trying to force a door shut when something is in the way of the hinge. Fearsome traction is required. The hand becomes white, and the sling can produce

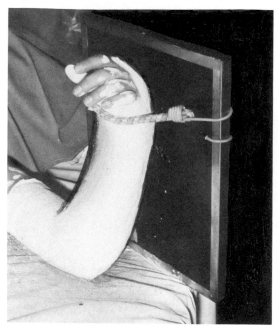

Fig. 13-14. Mold the cast well around the anterior surface of the radius. The rubber straps holds the cassette and the arm very conveniently.

nerve palsies. The sling gets in the way of cast application and leaves a depression in the cast.

Open Reduction. There is the feeling around that open reduction is *"verboten"* for children, but not all fractures of both bones can be managed by closed reduction. There are bad results! Internal fixation is preferable to malunion. The only indication is failure to achieve satisfactory alignment after one or two sessions of manipulation by an experienced surgeon.

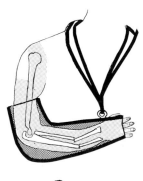
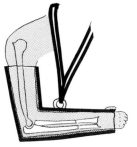
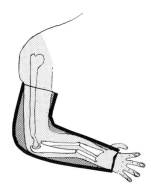

Fig. 13-15. The fracture will not support the weight of the cast. Incorporate a loop in the cast for attachment to a collar of stuffed stockinette.

Fig. 13-16. (*A, B*) The best position that could be obtained in an open fracture in an 11-year-old boy. Both bones are hitched, the rotation is correct, and there is no angulation. The cast is well molded and incorporates a collar. (*C, D*) Nine months after the injury, the arm looks normal and has a full range of motion. Bayonet apposition is perfectly acceptable but requires a good cast to maintain position.

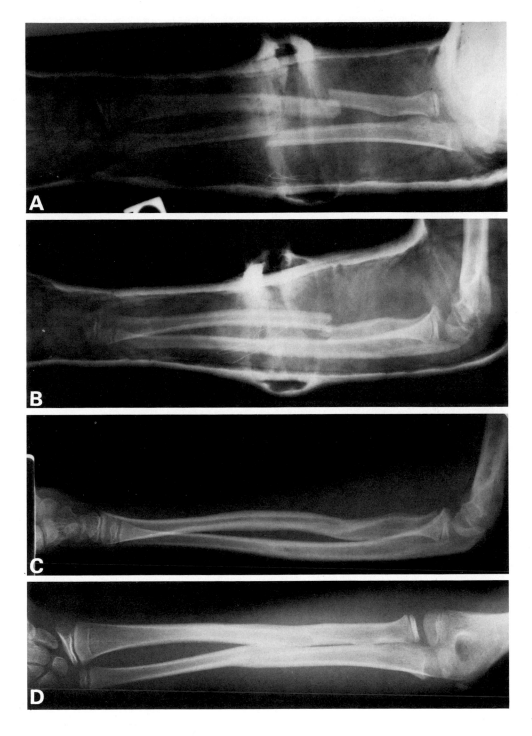

Teenagers with high oblique fractures are particularly likely to require open reduction. Open reduction without internal fixation can be disastrous. Semitubular compression plates require a large exposure in small arms. An intramedullary Kirschner wire in the radius alone or in the ulna as well provides sufficient fixation and can be inserted through an oblique hole drilled through the cortex an inch or two away from the fracture. The end is left long to allow easy removal (Fig. 13-18).

Epiphyseal Separation of the Distal Radius

Type I Injuries

Type I injuries are seen in younger children, are seldom much displaced, and are diagnosed on clinical suspicion more than by radiographic findings. Swelling and tenderness at the growth plate, despite normal radiographs, are our grounds for making this diagnosis. Protection for 3 weeks in a cast is more than enough treatment. You may think this is overdiagnosis, but the

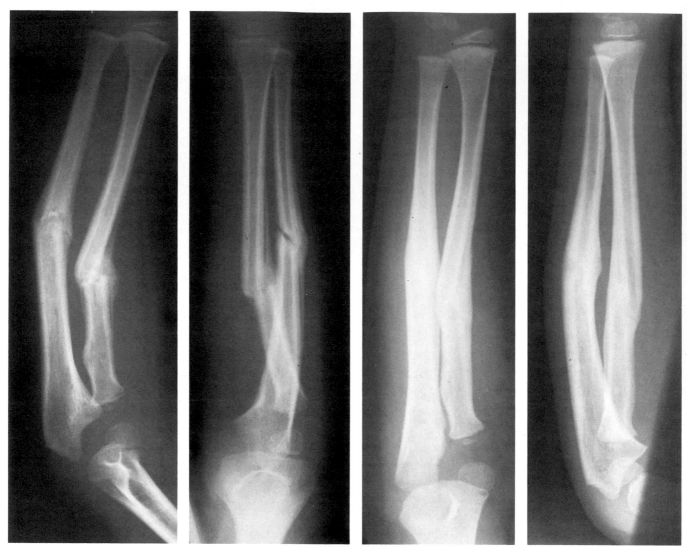

Fig. 13-17. Four weeks after the fracture was originally manipulated the bones were still end-to-end but had become angulated. The fracture was manipulated again, and the radiograph taken 6 months later shows an excellent result. The range of movement was full. Boy aged 5 years. Correction of angulation when a fracture is sticky is a useful technique.

entity is common, real and painful. A cast relieves the symptoms and stops the parents worrying and telephoning.

Type II Injuries

Type II injuries are the commonest, usually associated with posterior displacement, and frequently accompanied by a chip off the ulnar styloid. They are easily reduced by direct pressure under anesthesia. Wrist flexion does not help to hold reduction, because the wrist joint flexes easily to 80 degrees before the capsule tightens enough to exert any influence on the distal fragment. In order to achieve anything with wrist flexion more than 80 degrees of flexion will be required, and such a position is intolerable. Therefore, leave the wrist in a neutral position. Apply a below-elbow cast with scrupulous three-point molding. In 3 weeks the fracture will be united, and the cast can be removed (Fig. 13-19).

Buckle Fractures

Buckle fractures are common and usually dismissed by the family for a day or two as a sprain. The diagnosis is usually accompanied by guilty feelings on someone's part. Protect these injuries for about 3 weeks with a below-elbow cast (Fig. 13-20).

Overlapping Solitary Radial Fractures

The ulnar styloid is usually avulsed. Armed with

strong thumbs and an awareness of the periosteal hinge, you can reduce all these fractures closed, as shown in Figure 13-21. If the fragments are still in cortex-to-

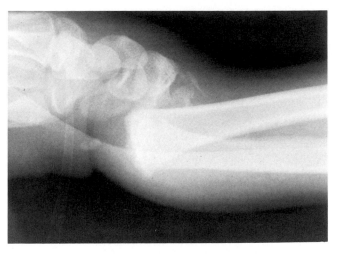

Fig. 13-19.   Type II epiphyseal separation in a boy of 15 years.   This is easily and completely reduced.

cortex apposition, repeat the maneuver with more thumb pressure. Be careful not to dislocate your own thumb in the process, as a surgeon in our group did. Set the arm in full pronation to hold the reduction.

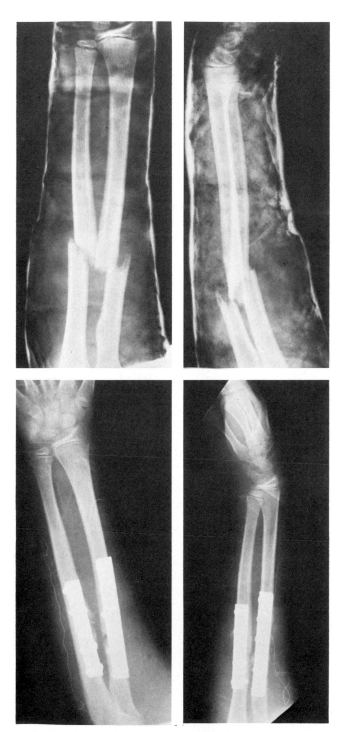

Fig. 13-18.   (*Top*) Proximal fracture in a boy of 15 years. The best position that could be achieved after several attempts was not good enough.   Open reduction produced an excellent result.   (*Bottom*) Simple Kirschner wire fixation is sometimes indicated for unstable fractures in small children.

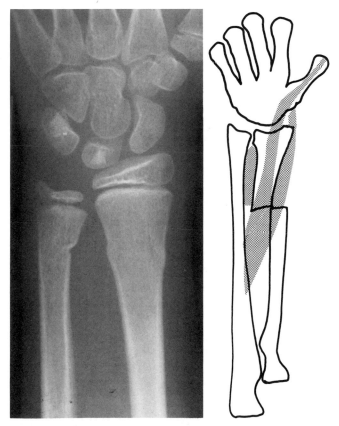

Fig. 13-20   (*Left*) A buckle fracture in a girl of 10 years. (*Right*)   Medially displaced fracture of the radius. The outcropping thenar muscles and pronator quadratus contribute to the deformity.

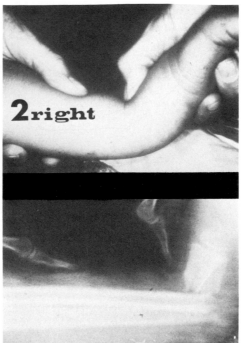

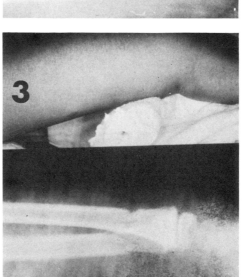

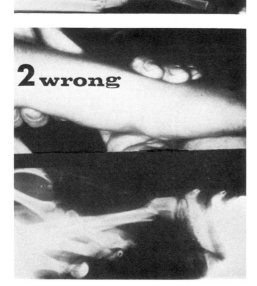

Fig. 13-21. Reduction of a forearm fracture with overlap.

Medially Displaced Solitary Radial Fractures

Outcropping thenar muscles contribute to this deformity. Reduce the fracture in supination to relax them, and include the thumb in the cast. Complete reduction is often difficult but, fortunately, slight displacement gives little or no functional disability (Fig. 13-20B).

Displaced Fractures of the Distal Radius and Ulna

If both bones are overlapping, reduce them one at a time by increasing the deformity as described above. Hold the fracture in the midposition, with firm three-point molding. If the fracture is put up in either full pronation or supination, one fragment will be angulated anteriorly, while the other is posteriorly angulated (Fig. 13-22).

Fractures of the Radial Neck and Olecranon

Fractures of the radial neck and the olecranon are discussed in Chapter 12.

FRACTURE DISLOCATIONS

Monteggia's Fracture Dislocation

For practical purposes there is no such thing as an isolated fracture of the ulna (Fig. 13-23). Giovanni

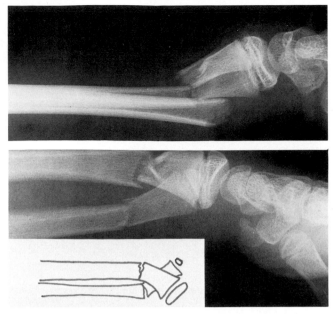

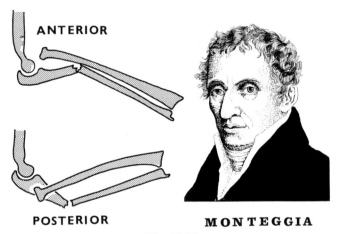

Fig. 13-22. Forced pronation of fractures at the distal end of the radius and ulna will produce angulation.

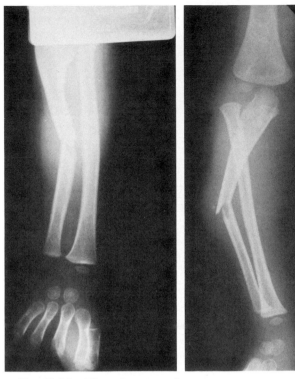

Fig. 13-24. There is a conspiracy to prevent recognition of the dislocated radial head. Either the film does not include the elbow joint or the name goes over it.

Monteggia's 1814 experience is still being repeated. Here is Monteggia's original account:

I unhappily remember the case of a girl who, after a fall, seemed to me to have sustained a fracture of the ulna in its upper third. It might have been that some commotion of the dislocated bone misled me at the beginning of treatment, or else it might have been that there really was a fracture of the ulna with a dislocation of the radius, as I undoubtedly

ANTERIOR

POSTERIOR   **MONTEGGIA**

Fig. 13-23.

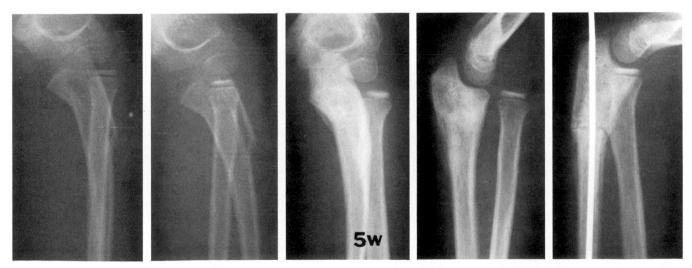

Fig. 13-25. Initial films did not include a lateral of the elbow. Anterior dislocation was missed until the cast was removed. Osteotomy of the ulna and open reduction of the radial neck was required.

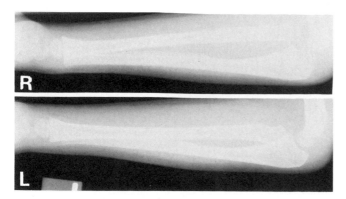

Fig. 13-26. Congenital dislocation of the radial head may be confusing when the elbow is radiographed after an acute injury. The radius is longer, and the ossific nucleus is larger.

found in another case. The fact is that at the end of the month, when the bandage was removed and all the swelling had disappeared (which, however, in simple dislocation of the radius is usually slight), I found that on extending the forearm the head of the radius jumped outwards, forming a hard ugly prominence on the anterior surface of the elbow, showing in an extremely obvious way that this was a true anterior dislocation of the head of the radius. When compressed it went back into place, but left to itself it came out again especially on extension of the forearm. I applied compresses and a new bandage to hold it in, but it would not stay in place.

Monteggia did not have radiography to help him. All radiographs of the forearm should include the wrist and elbow joints (Fig. 13-24). *A line through the long axis of the radius should pass through the capitellum in*

all views (Fig. 13-25). The radial head may be displaced anteriorly, laterally, or (occasionally) posteriorly. Closed reduction is usually possible in children (unlike adults)—perhaps because the orbicular ligament is avulsed from the ulna rather than torn.

There are two catches to this diagnosis. Congenital dislocation of the radial neck may masquerade as a new injury; however the radial head is too big, eccentric, and slightly irregular, and the radius is too long to permit serious confusion (Fig. 13-26). Acute radial dislocation may be accompanied by bending of the ulna, which may go unrecognized until the normal ulna is radiographed (Fig. 13-27). A separated radial epiphysis is another variety of the Monteggia injury seen in children (Fig. 13-28).

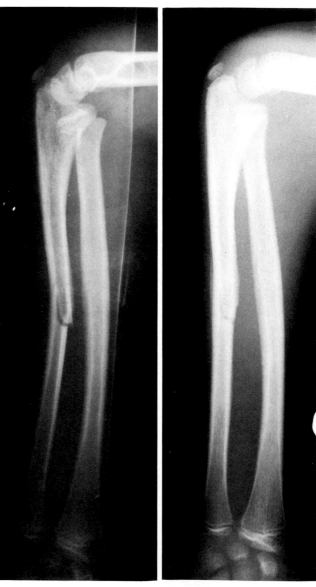

Fig. 13-28. Separation of the radial head with a fracture of the ulna in a boy of 12 years. Views before and after reduction.

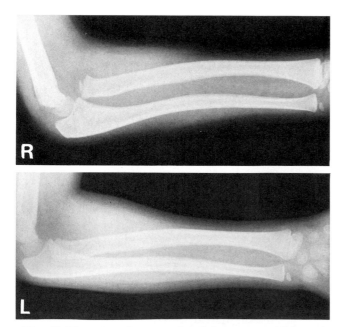

Fig. 13-27. The ulna may bend in young children in association with a dislocation of the radial head.

Fig. 13-29. Reduction of an anterior Monteggia fracture dislocation is by flexion and supination. (*Bottom left*) Insufficient flexion to reduce the radial head. (*Bottom right*) More flexion achieves reduction.

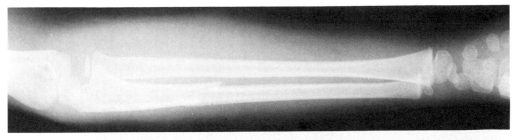

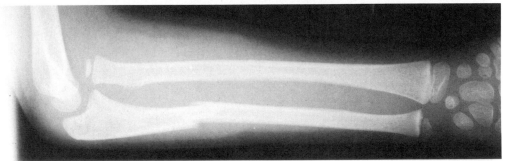

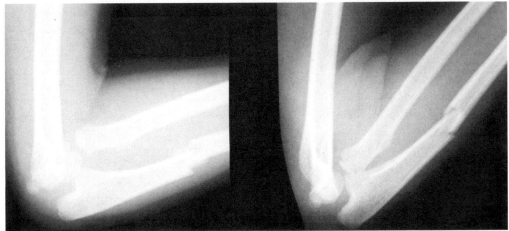

Treatment

Anterior Dislocation. Apply traction with the forearm extended and supinated. Press the radial head back into position while flexing the elbow. Immobilize the elbow in full supination with as much flexion as the circulation will tolerate (Fig. 13-29).

Lateral Dislocation. Traction in extension followed by flexion to 90 degrees and supination will reduce the radial head (Fig. 13-30).

Posterior Dislocation. Apply traction to the forearm with the elbow in as much extension as the deformity will permit. Push the radial head forward, and immobilize the elbow in extension.

Galeazzi's Fracture Dislocation

Fracture of the radius with dislocation of the inferior radioulnar joint is less common than Monteggia's injury

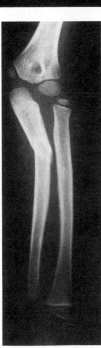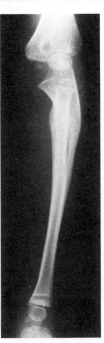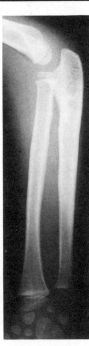

Fig. 13-30. The lateral type of Monteggia injury is difficult to reduce. The ulnar deformity has not been fully corrected. One year later pronation is restricted by 10 degrees.

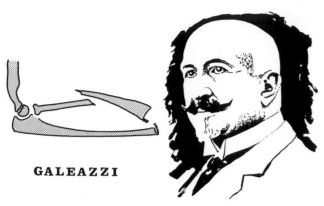

GALEAZZI

Fig. 13-31.

and less definite. It is easily managed by reduction of the displacement of the radius (Fig. 13-31).

FOLLOW-UP CARE

Apart from buckle fractures, all these injuries should be considered unstable. Many a good reduction has been lost. Gandhi et al. studied 1767 forearm fractures in children under the age of 12 and found that 2.5 percent had significant angulation when the cast came off. The causes of angular deformity in these children were:

1. Children missed follow-up radiograph at 1 week.
2. Nothing was done about tilting at 1 week.
3. Fractures of the distal one third of the forearm were immobilized in midpronation.
4. Incomplete reduction was accepted.
5. Neglected cases which presented late.

In this group Gandhi noted that angulation at the distal end corrects well if the growth plate has 5 or more years of activity. Some degree of angulation can be accepted in children under the age of 10.

In the mid-forearm angulation corrects poorly and limits rotation. Every effort should be made to maintain a reduction free of angulation or rotation.

We usually radiograph forearm fractures weekly for the first 3 weeks. The cast is removed at 6 weeks. If the fracture is very unstable, we may radiograph every week. If union is poor at 6 weeks, the cast should remain in place longer.

CONCLUSIONS

Fractures of the forearm and wrist are the commonest injuries in childhood. While the majority are easily treated, the occasional case will be underestimated or the patient will miss follow-up appointments and return with poor result. It is always difficult to know what to do with the child who presents with malunion a few weeks after the cast has been removed at Elsewhere General Hospital. Angular deformity at the lower end in a young child always improves. Rotational deformity at the lower end, midshaft deformity, and deformities in teenagers do not remodel well. It does not help to send these individuals away with reassuring words. They must either accept what they have or gamble on redressement of the fracture.

BIBLIOGRAPHY

Boyd, H. B., and Boals, J. C.: The Monteggia lesion: a review of 159 cases. Clin. Orthop., *66:* 94, 1969

Bryan, R. S.: Monteggia fracture of the forearm. J. Trauma, *11:* 992, 1971

Christensen, J. B., Cho, K. O., Adams, J. P., and Miller, L.: A study of the interosseous distance between the radius and ulna during rotation of the forearm. J. Bone Joint Surg., *46B:* 778, 1964

Cooper, R. G.: Management of common forearm fractures in children. J. Iowa Med. Soc., *54:* 689, 1964

Evans, E. M.: Fractures of the radius and ulna. J. Bone Joint Surg., *33B:* 548, 1951

Gandhi, R. K., Wilson, P., Mason Brown, J. J., and Macleod, W.: Spontaneous correction of deformity following fractures of the forearm in children. Brit. J. Surg., *50:* 5, 1962

Giberson, R. G., and Ivins, J. C.: Fractures of the distal part of the forearm in children. Correction of deformity by growth. Minnesota Medicine, *35:* 744, 1952

Knight, R. A., and Purvis, G. D.: Fractures of both bones of the forearm in adults. J. Bone Joint Surg., *31A:* 755, 1949

Monteggia, G. B.: Instituzioni Chirugiche *5:* 130, 1814. Milan: Maspero (Translated by Helen Rang)

Onne, L., and Sandblom, P.: Late results in fractures of the forearm in children. Acta. Chir. Scand., *98:* 549, 1949

Patrick, J.: A study of supination and pronation with especial reference to the treatment of forearm fractures. J. Bone Joint Surg., *28:* 737, 1946

Pollen, A. G.: Fractures and Dislocations in Children. Edinburgh, Churchill Livingstone, 1973

Stein, F., Grabias, S. L., and Deffer, P. A.: Nerve injuries complicating Monteggia injuries. J. Bone Joint Surg., *53A:* 1432, 1971

Theodorou, S. D.: Dislocation of the head of the radius associated with fracture of the upper end of the ulna in children. J. Bone Joint Surg., *51B:* 700, 1969

Tompkins, D. G.: Anterior Monteggia fracture. J. Bone Joint Surg., *53A:* 1109, 1971

Warren, J. D.: Anterior interosseous nerve palsy as a complication of forearm fractures. J. Bone Joint Surg., *45B:* 511, 1963

14

Hand

In our Emergency Department the hand is radiographed for possible fractures more often than any other part, yet interesting hand fractures are rare in children. Three-quarters of the injuries can be managed by a little strapping and reassurance that everything will be all right again in a few weeks. Carpal dislocations and multiple unstable fractures of the metacarpals are not seen, and challenging industrial hand injuries are missing. This leaves only a few varieties of phalangeal fractures to win an orthopaedic surgeon's interest.

PROBLEMS OF FINGER FRACTURES

Malrotation

Malrotation does not remodel. The fingers become entangled when flexed. Rotation should be checked in two ways: (1) ensure that all the fingernails are in the same plane (Fig. 14-1) and (2) ensure that the fingers remain adjacent when flexed, and do not converge or diverge. Malrotation does not show on a radiograph. Only by these simple clinical tests can the problem be recognized. When the fingers are immobilized in a flexed position, as they should be, this problem does not usually arise. Correction of malrotation in a fresh fracture is easy, but if it heals with malrotation, only osteotomy will correct the position.

Angulation

Angulation is usually apparent on radiographs and is easily detectable clinically. Straighten the finger and splint it to the adjacent finger using strapping or cast (Fig. 14-2). Never immobilize a solitary finger. When one finger alone is immobilized, there is a great chance that angulation will develop by the time the cast is removed.

Malarticulation

Patients are very sensitive about finger stiffness because it is so easy to make comparisons with the other finger joints. Stiffness and swelling after an injury often lasts for several months, even when the injury does not alter a joint surface. However, these problems will certainly be permanent if you do not correct irregularities in the joint surface (Fig. 14-3).

Interposition

When interposed tendon or capsule prevents closed reduction of a fracture or dislocation, an open reduction will be required.

INDIVIDUAL INJURIES

Carpal Fractures

Scaphoid fractures are very unusual in children and should be casted for 6 weeks. Nonunion is a possible complication and may require grafting.

Injuries of the Thumb Metacarpal

Impacted Fracture of the Base of the Thumb

Impacted fractures of the base of the thumb are commonly the result of fighting. There is a flexion deformity (Fig. 14-4). Up to 30 degrees of angulation can be accepted; the thumb is protected in a scaphoid cast. Warn the parents that a bump will remain for a year after the cast is removed. Angulation over 30 degrees should be corrected under anesthesia. Press on the base of the thumb and apply counter pressure on the head of the metacarpal. Apply a scaphoid cast and mold it in the same way. The common error is to hyperextend

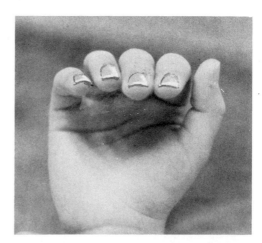

Fig. 14-1. The fingernails should be in the same plane. When there is malrotation, one finger is in a different plane.

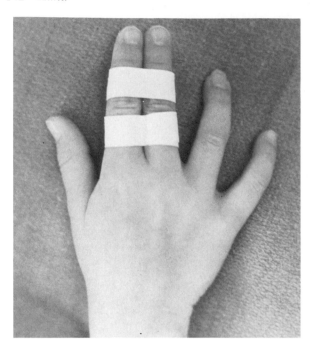

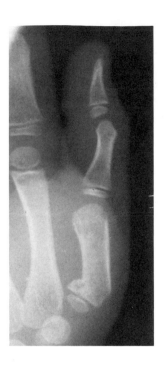

Fig. 14-4. Buckle fracture of the thumb.

Fig. 14-2. Strap two fingers together for minor injuries.

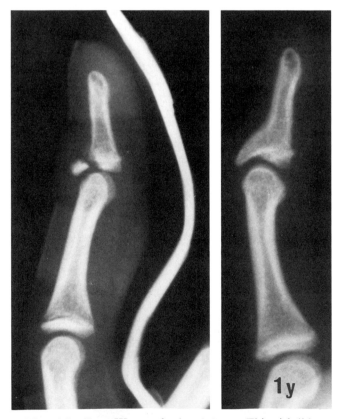

Fig. 14-3. Type III growth plate injury. This girl did not come for treatment for 3 weeks, and the position was accepted. The fracture united, but she has a marked swan-neck deformity.

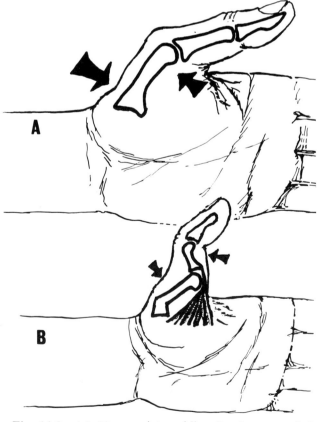

Fig. 14-5. (*A*) Three-point molding for fractures of the thumb with flexion deformity. (*B*) The common error.

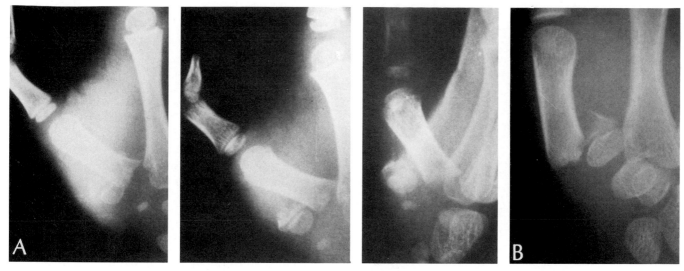

Fig. 14-6. (*A*) Ulnar displacement of a Type II fracture usually defies closed reduction. This one was left because of severe head injury. The thumb was short and bumpy, but it moved well. (*B*) Radial displacement is easily corrected by closed reduction, as indicated in the previous illustration.

the metacarpophalangeal joint by applying counter-pressure too far distally, which does nothing to correct the deformity. A well-applied cast leaves the meta-carpophalangeal joint slightly flexed (Fig. 14-5). It may be removed after 3 weeks.

Type II Injuries

Some Type II injuries are minimally displaced and require only protection. Occasionally there is complete displacement that buttonholes through the periosteum

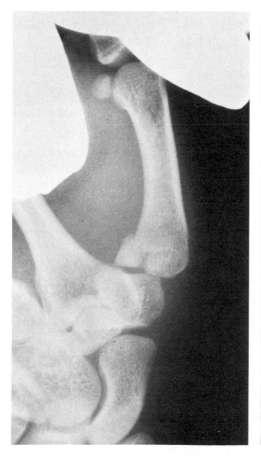
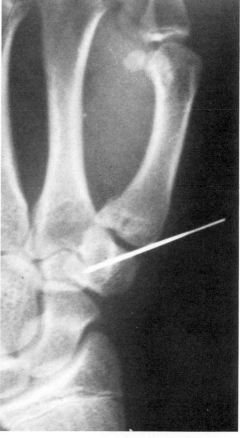

Fig. 14-7. Bennett's fracture dislocation. A pin passed percutaneously will hold the reduction. In children the fragment is too small to be held with a screw.

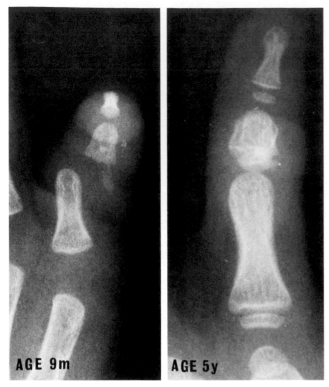

AGE 9m   AGE 5y

Fig. 14-8. An irreducible dislocation is always an indication for surgery. The proximal plate of the middle phalanx had been rotated through 180 degrees. After open reduction the finger was straighter, but growth was affected.

anteriorly. Although closed reduction is worth attempting, these injuries usually require open reduction to lever the metaphysis back into position (Fig. 14-6).

Type III Injuries

The medial part of the growth plate closes last, and adolescents may separate the medial corner of the epiphysis. This is just the same as a Bennett's fracture and requires accurate repositioning. Under anesthesia, traction usually reduces the fracture dislocation; a thin percutaneous Kirschner wire can be inserted just proximal to the base of the metacarpal into the trapezium to maintain reduction (Fig. 14-7). A scaphoid cast completes the immobilization. Three weeks is sufficient.

Injuries of the Fifth Metacarpal

Impacted fractures of the neck of the fifth metacarpal are very common after fights. There is no satisfactory method of holding the fracture reduced without hazard. Cleverly molded casts produce stiffness and sores. For this reason, I usually put a bandage around the palm for comfort, and warn the parents that the knuckle will be less prominent for a year or two. The functional results are excellent. Tell the child in the future to fight

only with a tightly clenched fist, like a real fighter. Strongly contracted muscles protect the hand from injury.

Other Metacarpal Fractures

Fractures of the metacarpal shaft are much less common in children than in adults. Marked swelling appears on the dorsum of the hand. Elevate the arm, apply a front slab of plaster, and apply a well-padded, yielding bandage around the palm and forearm. Encourage finger movements, and remove the cast after 2 to 3 weeks.

Phalangeal Fractures

Children's former friends step on fingers, bend them back, and damage them with baseballs.

Injuries of the Proximal End of the Phalanx

Type I. In the infant, the proximal epiphysis is unossified, a fact that may lead to diagnosistic difficulties. I recall an infant of 9 months whose little finger was caught in a car door. When the swelling went down after a couple of weeks, the finger was crooked at the level of the proximal interphalangeal joint. Radiographs suggested a dislocation. At operation, the proximal epiphysis was found rotated through 180 degrees. After reduction, the appearance was improved, but the joint had only half the normal range of movement and the epiphysis did not grow well (Fig. 14-8).

A more typical Type I injury produces a mallet deformity of the distal interphalangeal joint. This is easily held with a splint or strapping until union is solid at 3 weeks (Fig. 14-9).

Type II. Type II injuries are commonest in the proximal phalanges. A minor degree of displacement is usual and almost impossible to correct. The extra octave fracture of the little finger is the commonest and usually requires nothing more than strapping to the ring finger (Fig. 14-10). Greater degrees of displacement may be associated with gross swelling. Such a case

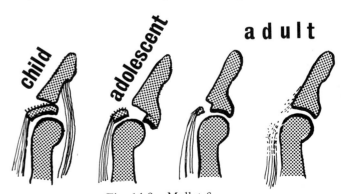

Fig. 14-9. Mallet finger.

Fig. 14-10.   The extra octave
fracture of the little finger.

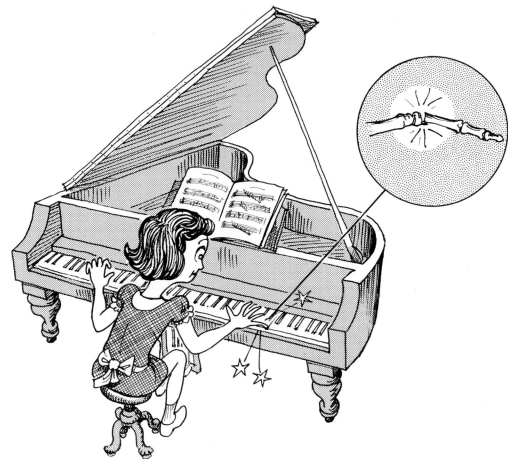

requires admission, elevation, and reduction later (Fig.
14-11).

Type III.   In the adolescent, a mallet deformity is
most commonly the result of a Type III fracture-dislocation.   It requires open reduction and fixation with two
fine Kirschner wires (Fig. 14-12).

Corner fractures of the epiphysis are the equivalent
of collateral ligament injuries in adults.   If the articular
surface is involved, these should be accurately replaced
(Fig. 14-13).

Fractures of the Shaft of the Phalanx

The majority of phalangeal shaft fractures are undisplaced injuries that require only protection.   When
displacement is minimal, strap two fingers together for
about 3 weeks.   If there is much swelling and there is
a risk of displacement, use a slab of plaster in front of
the fingers, and strap them down to it.   The fingers
should be well flexed in order to ensure that alignment
and rotation remain correct.

Injuries of the Distal End of the Phalanx

Cartilaginous Injuries.   The cartilage cap of the phalanx has no epiphysis and is occasionally separated.

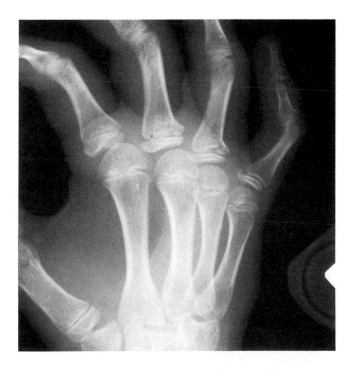

Fig. 14-11.   When skating this girl hyperextended her fingers.   Gross soft-tissue swelling is evident on radiographs, and
there are Type II injuries of the middle- and ring fingers.
The hand required elevation, but reduction was not necessary.

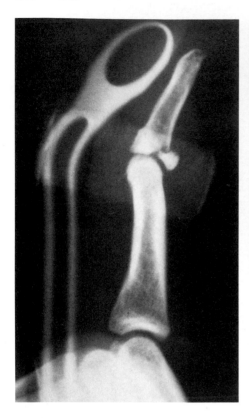
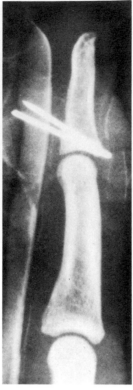
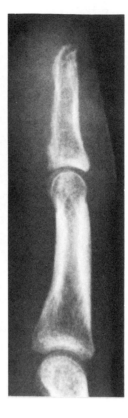

Fig. 14-12. Closed reduction did nothing for this 15-year-old. Open reduction was performed. The pins were left protruding anteriorly to facilitate skin closure. The length is easily adjusted. They are removed from the front.

This is not immediately obvious, but the passage of time reveals subperiosteal new bone formation and explains the cause of prolonged stiffness (Fig. 14-14).

Unicondylar Fractures. Undisplaced unicondylar fractures are almost unknown. Minimally displaced ones are easily overlooked (Fig. 14-15). They can be reduced by closed manipulation and held with a fine percutaneous Kirschner wire (Fig. 14-16). Grossly displaced fractures that cannot be reduced should be opened; loose fragments may have to be removed before the fracture is held reduced with two fine Kirschner

wires. The wires and the cast should be removed at 3 weeks. These injuries are *commonly undertreated* and result in angulation and stiffness in the finger.

Bicondylar Fractures. Some bicondylar fractures are little cracks, but others are widely displaced (Fig. 14-17). Dixon and Moon described fractures with 180 degrees of displacement. You might think that this degree of displacement would be obvious, but unless you look for it, it will pass unnoticed. This degree of wide displacement denotes complete periosteal severance, and open reduction is required. Leave the pins

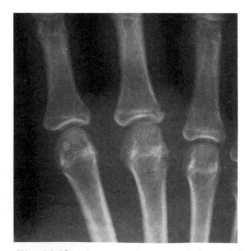
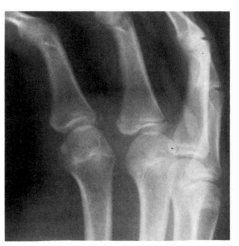

Fig. 14-13. A corner fracture of the epiphysis of the index finger and a Type III injury of the middle finger. The fingers were strapped together.

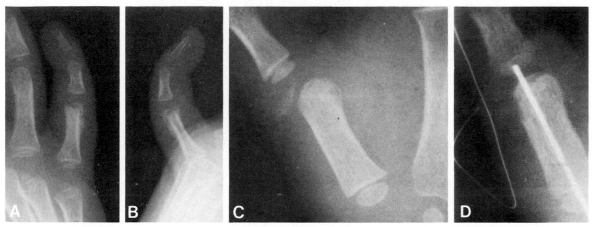

Fig. 14-14. (*A, B*) Three weeks after a crushing injury of the cartilaginous cap of a phalanx. No injury was recognized on the initial films. (*C*) A fresh osteochondral fracture of the metacarpal of the thumb. Closed reduction was impossible. At operation the fragment was found to be flipped over. (*D*) After open reduction and fixation with a fine wire.

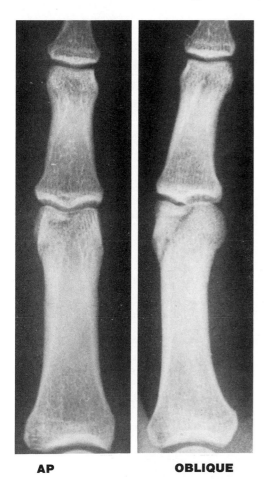

AP   OBLIQUE

Fig. 14-15. Different projections are needed to show some condylar fractures. The fracture could not be seen on antero-posterior films (*left*) but would have been visible on an oblique view (*right*). This was "held" in a cast, slipped, and the patient now has a slightly crooked finger. It should have been pinned percutaneously.

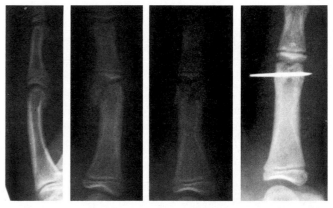

Fig. 14-16. Percutaneous pinning of a unicondylar fracture.

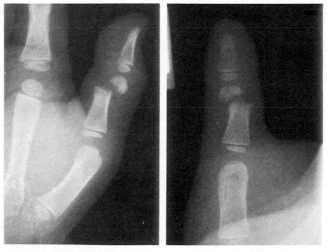

Fig. 14-17. This car door injury healed well with cast immobilization.

in place for 6 weeks, because healing may be slow. Avascular necrosis, surprisingly, has not been described.

Stiffness after an injury, which is such a nuisance in adults, is not a great problem with finger fractures in children.

Dislocations

Dislocation of the metacarpophalangeal joint of the thumb is common and can usually be reduced with traction under anesthesia. Cast immobilization with the thumb flexed is advisable for 3 to 6 weeks, to allow healing of the volar plate and prevent repeated dislocation (Fig. 14-18).

Trigger thumb may present as a dislocation, but the signs are obvious and the radiographs are normal.

Posterior dislocations of the metacarpophalangeal joint of the finger usually requires open reduction through a palmar incision. The metacarpal head may become trapped by the flexor tendons and the palmar fascia, or the capsule may become interposed.

MISCELLANEOUS INJURIES

Frostbite

The growth cartilage is much more sensitive to cold than either skin or vessels. Permanent growth arrest may result from children riding bicycles in extremely cold weather. In the months that follow this, parents realize

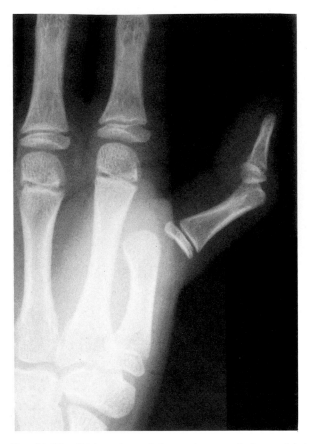

Fig. 14-18. Dislocation of the metacarpophalangeal joint of the thumb.

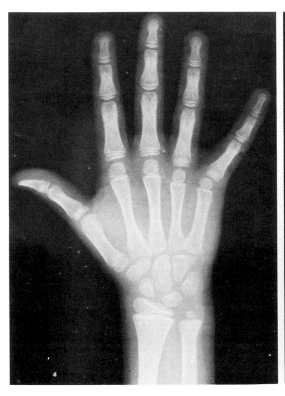 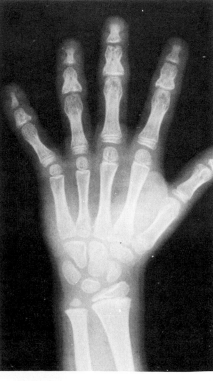

Fig. 14-19. Frostbite injury. The fingers of one hand are short.

Fig. 14-20. Growth arrest in the left hand due to an old wringer injury.

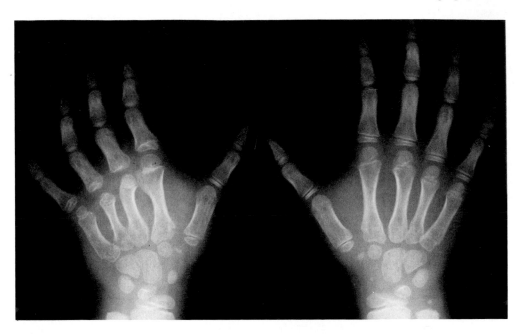

that the tips of the fingers are not growing. Radiographs disclose premature closure of the epiphyseal plates (Fig. 14-19).

Wringer Injuries

Crushing may damage growth cartilage and produce growth arrest (Fig. 14-20). Wringer injuries are discussed in greater detail on page 54.

Nerve and Tendon Injuries

There is much to be said for primary repair of injured nerves and tendons. Children with these injuries should be referred immediately to a surgeon who specializes in hand surgery. Because there are several excellent works on tendon and nerve injuries, the subject will not be discussed further.

BIBLIOGRAPHY

Dixon, G. L. Jr., and Moon, N. F.: Rotational supracondylar fractures of the proximal phalanx in children. Clin. Orthop., *83:* 151, 1972

Griffiths, J. C.: Bennett's fracture in childhood. Brit. J. Clin. Pract., *20:* 582, 1966

Hakstian, R. W.: Cold induced digital epiphyseal necrosis in childhood. Can. J. Surg., *15:* 168, 1972

Leonard, M. H., and Dubravcik, P.: Management of fractured fingers in the child. Clin. Orthop., *73:* 160, 1970

McCue, F. X., Honner, R., Johnson, M. C., and Gieck, J. H.: Athletic injuries of the proximal interphalangeal joint requiring surgical treatment. J. Bone Joint Surg., *52A:* 937, 1970

Murphy, A. F., and Stark, H. H.: Closed dislocation of the MPJ of the index finger. J. Bone Joint Surg., *49A:* 1579, 1967

15

Pelvis

The pelvis is like a suit of armor: when it is damaged there is much more concern about its contents than about the structure itself. The problems for the orthopaedic surgeon are different at each age. Osteoporotic old people sustain minor fractures in falls that pose neither visceral nor orthopaedic problems; young adults involved in road accidents suffer fractures that may be difficult to reduce in addition to life-threatening visceral injuries; children's fractures are seldom displaced much and can usually be treated by bed rest, but their other injuries may require much treatment.

A review of 100 cases of fracture of the pelvis in children between the ages of 1 and 18 years who were treated at our hospital during the past 10 years was carried out by Dr. Bernard Nolan. The greatest incidence was in children between 1 and 8 years old, who have little road sense. Ninety percent were the result of automobiles striking child pedestrians. Associated injuries were seen in 87 percent and the mortality rate was 8 percent. Blood transfusion was necessary in 30 percent, but this was mostly because there were multiple injuries: only 2 percent required transfusion for the pelvic fracture alone.

ASSOCIATED INJURIES IN 100 CHILDREN WITH PELVIC FRACTURE

Remote

Head injury—61% (caused most deaths)
Chest injury—9%
Fractures of the upper extremity—17%
Fractures of the lower extremity—17% (15 fractures, 2 hip dislocations)

Local

Hematuria—30%
Urologic injury requiring surgery—10% (3 renal, 3 urethral ruptures, 4 bladder ruptures)
Abdominal injury—11% (6 required surgery for spleen, G.I. tract, and mesentery)
Perineal/gluteal lacerations—7%

These statistics are similar to those for adults. The incidence of hematuria is the same as reported by Levine and Crampton. A similar proportion of patients required surgery, as reported by Hawkins et al. The visceral problems are not different in children.

CLASSIFICATION

A useful classification of pelvic fractures in children is based on the most serious aspect of the injury (Quinby, 1966).

Group I Uncomplicated. A minor fracture is undisplaced. Shock is absent and transfusion is not required. Signs of abdominal and urological injury are absent or settle quickly with nonoperative treatment.

Group II Fracture with visceral injuries requiring exploration are more severe, and the child is in shock and requires immediate transfusion.

Group III Fracture with immediate massive hemorrhage. The sacroiliac joint is separated, and the pulses in one leg are absent. A major branch of the internal iliac artery is torn. The child is admitted in profound shock and requires rapid transfusion of blood in massive quantities—up to 8 liters. Visceral injuries are also present. Despite energetic treatment, most of these children die.

The importance of concealed hemorrhage from fractures of the pelvis cannot be overstated. An autopsy study of 200 fatally injured pedestrians revealed that about half had sustained a fracture of the pelvis. In 21 the injuries were restricted to the pelvis; 10 had visceral injuries and 11, or 5 percent, had no visceral injuries and died of hemorrhage alone. (Many died while their doctors were obtaining sheaves of x-rays without starting fluid replacement.)

INITIAL MANAGEMENT

The possibility of a fracture of the pelvis is great in any child who has been hit by a car. The initial care is that of any patient with multiple injuries. Life-threatening injuries are treated, an I.V. infusion is started, blood is ordered for immediate use, and a nasogastric tube is passed if there is abdominal distension. The number of physicians quickly increases, and the areas of injury are mapped out and investigated as thoroughly as time permits.

Pelvic fractures may be accompanied by visceral, vascular, or neurologic injuries; so look for blood at the urethral meatus, vagina, and anus. Perform abdominal and rectal examinations. Feel the pulses, and test active movements in both legs. Test sacral sensation. The site and size of any swelling should be noted. Stability of the pelvis should be judged by compression.

The session in the radiography department may be long if urologic injury is suggested by either clinical signs or by the location of the fracture. Disruption of the symphysis or displaced fractures of the pubic ramus are most likely to cause injury to the bladder and urethra. Urethrogram, cystogram, and intravenous pyelogram may be required. The radiography department is usually the venue for a consultation among all specialists involved. While this goes on, the general condition of the child should be the first priority: in the twilight of an x-ray department the temptation is to take more and more films. But don't let the patient bleed to death.

A plan of definitive treatment is worked out for each aspect of the injury.

Visceral Injury

The investigation and treatment of urological injury is described on page 74 and of intraperitoneal injury on page 69.

Fig. 15-1. Three views of the pelvis are the minimum required to identify the degree of displacement. The fracture through the right sacral foramen is seen only in the 30-degree, down-shot view.

Hemorrhage

Hemorrhage may be intraperitoneal or extraperitoneal. Intraperitoneal hemorrhage is comparatively easily controlled at laparotomy: extraperitoneal may be massive around the sacroiliac joint, and (at operation) has terrified and defeated many surgeons (including me). Slow hemorrhage will tamponade and stop, but rapid hemorrhage requires control. Exposure of the bleeding vessels is often difficult; if packing does not control hemorrhage it may be helpful to enlist the assistance of a radiologist. King et al. have used arteriography to reveal the site of hemorrhage. An arterial

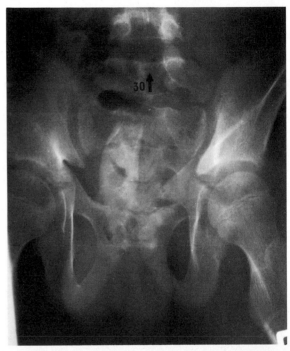

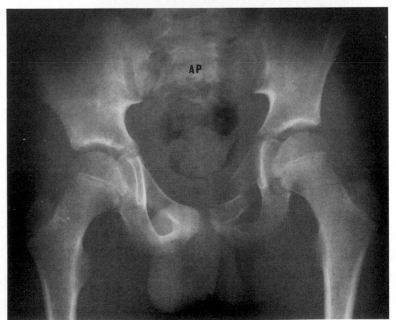

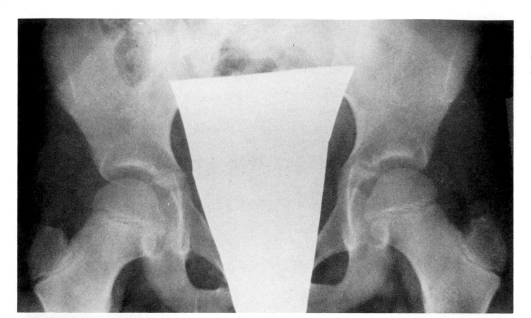

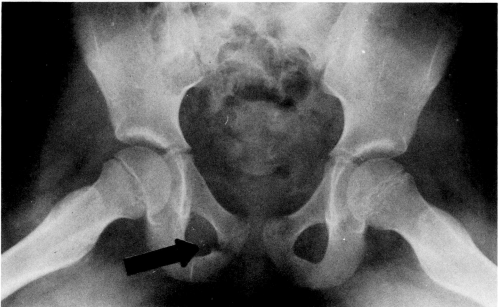

Fig. 15-2. This boy complained of pain in the (R) hip after a fall. The guard hid the fracture of the pubic ramus on the first film.

catheter is inserted through the femoral artery of the least injured side. The catheter is then manipulated into the vessel leading to the leak, usually the hypogastric artery. Autologous clot is injected which is carried to the leak by preferential flow. Successful arrest of hemorrhage is recognized by a fall in the blood requirements and by a repeat arteriogram.

Nerve Injury

Many of these injuries are missed because detailed neurological examination is neglected, and weeks later a slight limp is easily attributed to other factors. The lumbosacral plexus is closely related to the sacroiliac joint. When the sacroiliac joint is dislocated and widely separated the lumbosacral trunk, the superior gluteal nerve, and the obturator nerve may be stretched or ruptured as they cross the joint. Intradural rupture of the roots of the cauda equina may be produced by traction, particularly by transverse fractures of the sacrum. Fractures of the sacral ala can narrow the foramina and compress sacral nerves.

Huittinen who studied this subject in patients and in the autopsy room found nerve injuries in 20 of 42 dissections of fractures of the pelvis. He noted that these injuries could only be recognized by careful neurological examination. Exploration is not required. The chances of recovery are remote.

Fracture Patterns

The site and displacement of the fracture is best defined by upshot and downshot views in addition to the standard anteroposterior (Fig. 15-1). On occasion, lateral and oblique films are required. Obviously a gonadal shield should not be used; we have missed a few minor fractures of the pubic rami in children being x-rayed for a painful hip with a shield in place (Fig. 15-2).

The classification of children's pelvic fractures is essentially the same as that in adults: double fractures of the ring (Fig. 15-3); single fractures of the ring; fractures involving the acetabulum; and fractures not involving the ring (Fig. 15-4).

However children's fractures, unlike fractures due to extreme violence in adults, are seldom displaced enough to require reduction.

In our series 80 percent of fractures involved the pubic rami; 18 percent, the ilium; and 2 percent, the acetabulum, the majority were stable; only 13 percent showed radiological evidence of disruption of the sacroiliac joint.

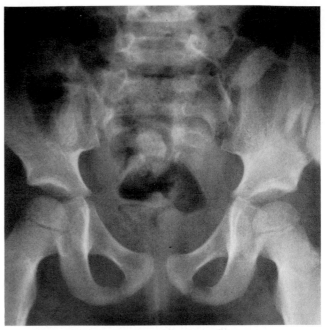

Fig. 15-4. Hit by a car, this 4-year-old sustained an isolated fracture of the (L) ilium that posed no problems.

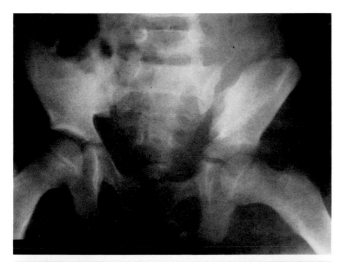

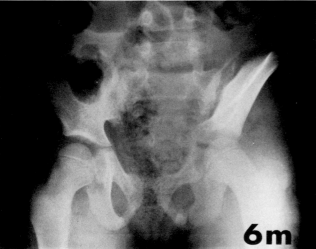

Fig. 15-3. Crushed by a car, this 8-year-old girl was admitted with hypotension, a large laceration, a left obturator, sciatic nerve palsy, and vaginal bleeding. Radiographs disclosed fracture of the left pubic ramus and disruption of the sacroiliac joint. She received 4 litres of blood, and extraperitoneal hemorrhage was controlled with packs.

Sacral fractures are difficult to see on radiographs and are usually missed. Compression fractures through the foramina of the ala are overlain by gas shadows; transverse fractures are in the wrong plane to be seen on anteroposterior films; laterals or upshots are needed. Both types of fracture may be associated with neurological lesions.

Injury through growth cartilage may occur in major and minor trauma. Everett has described avulsion of an unossified iliac apophysis resulting in intestinal obstruction due to a lumbar hernia. Rodrigues noted growth arrest following injury to the triradiate cartilage; this caused a mini-acetabulum.

Muscles spanning the hip and knee joints may pull off an apophysis during moments of extreme athletic effort. The hamstrings avulse the ischial tuberosity; rectus femoris, the anterior inferior iliac spine (Fig. 15-5); and sartorius, the superior spine.

The classic picture is represented by an athlete collapsing on the field. Radiographs confirm the diagnosis and usually show marked displacement. An apophysis is held in position by periosteum more firmly than by growth cartilage. Any displacement signifies a periosteal tear. Unlike most other Type I injuries, these are usually widely displaced.

Muscle function does not suffer as a result of fibrous union in the displaced position. However, the ischial apophysis is a weight-bearing area for sitting: an ununited apophysis leads to discomfort. Spontaneous reduction has been reported by Martin and Pipkin, but most reported cases have required reposition with a

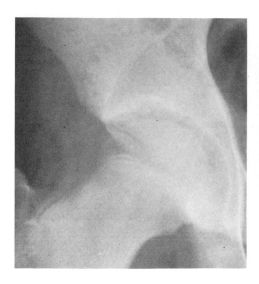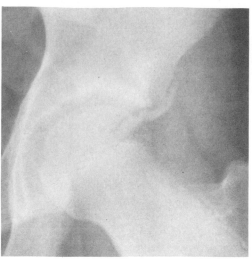

Fig. 15-5. Avulsion of the anterior inferior iliac spine, the result of a 12-year-old kicking a ball. This appearance can be confused with an accessory center of ossification.

screw using Milch's approach. Excision may be required for neglected cases.

Apophyseolysis—slight displacement due to repeated sprains—has been described as a source of local pain. Rest is suggested to prevent massive displacement.

TREATMENT

Although the same general principles apply in children as in adults, the majority of children require only symptomatic treatment. In our series 97 percent were treated by bedrest until the pain subsided and then by mobilization on crutches. Reduction was attempted in

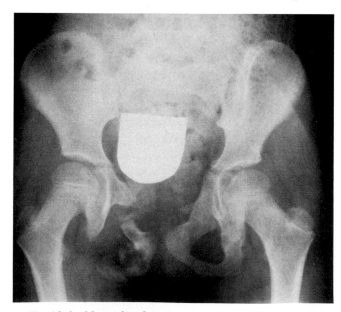

Fig. 15-6. Nonunion 2 years after bilateral fracture of the pubic rami in a 7-year-old girl. Disruption of the vagina and bladder had required repair.

3 percent. (An open fracture of the ilium with overlapping fragments was treated by open reduction. Manipulation improved another, and traction made no difference to a third.) The associated injuries require much more treatment than the fracture itself.

The long-term results have not been systematically studied, but a few minor problems have come to light. A few girls complain of assymetry of the pelvis due to malunion or to fat fracture (see p. 47). One girl has asymptomatic nonunion of an open fracture of the pubic rami (Fig. 15-6). Remodelling usually makes recognition of the fracture difficult after a year or two. In girls it is wise to obtain obstetrical views of the pelvis a year after injury (though I am not aware of any girl being left with a narrowed birth canal).

BIBLIOGRAPHY

Braunstein, P. W., et al.: Concealed hemorrhage due to pelvic fracture. J. Trauma, *4:* 832, 1964

Everett, W. G.: Traumatic lumbar hernia. Injury, *4:* 354, 1973

Hawkins, L., Pomerantz, M., and Eiseman, B.: Laparotomy at the time of pelvic fracture. J. Trauma, *10:* 619, 1970

Huittinen, V-M.: Lumbosacral nerve injury in fracture of the pelvis. Acta Chir. Scand., [Suppl.]: 429, 1972

Levine, J. I., and Crampton, R. S.: Major abdominal injuries associated with pelvic fractures. Surg., Gyne., Obstet., *116:* 223, 1963

Martin, T. A., and Pipkin, G.: Treatment of avulsion of the ischial tuberosity. Clin. Orthol., *10:* 108, 1957

Quinby, W. C.: Fractures of the pelvis and associated injuries in children. J. Pediat. Surg., *1:* 353, 1966

Ring, E. J., et al.: Arteriographic management of hemorrhage following pelvic fracture. Radiology, *109:* 65, 1973

Rodrigues, K. F.: Injury of the acetabular epiphysis. Injury, *4:* 258, 1973

16

Hip

The osteoporotic bone of an old lady is very different from the tough growing bone of a child. Great violence is required to produce a fracture in a child. For example, most trochanteric fractures are bumper injuries in children of 6 or 7 years, the age when the greater trochanter is at the level of a car bumper (Fig. 16-1).

Fractures of the hip are rare in children; we have treated only two or three patients a year during the past 20 years. Ratliff estimated that the incidence of fractures of the femoral neck in children is 0.8 percent of that in adults. Most orthopaedic surgeons will not treat more than four or five in a professional lifetime. If this were a more common injury, perhaps we would all know a lot more about the best methods of treatment and thus be able to achieve better results.

There are several important differences between hip fractures in adults and in children:

1. The periosteal tube in a child is much stronger than that in an adult, so that perhaps half of these fractures are undisplaced.

2. The blood supply of the head is different. Avascular necrosis in a child may affect the epiphysis, the epiphysis *and* the metaphysis, or the metaphysis alone. The violence of the initial injury is commonly blamed for the high incidence of avascular necrosis in children—about 40 percent in most series.

It is not clear whether avascular necrosis results from complete division of all vessels, kinking of those vessels that remain intact, or tamponade by a high-pressure hemarthrosis within the hip capsule.

3. Avascular necrosis is commonly accompanied by premature closure of the growth plate, which leaves the child with a short femoral neck.

4. The hyperemia of fracture repair may produce coxa magna and a slightly long leg.

5. Children will tolerate cast immobilization. The

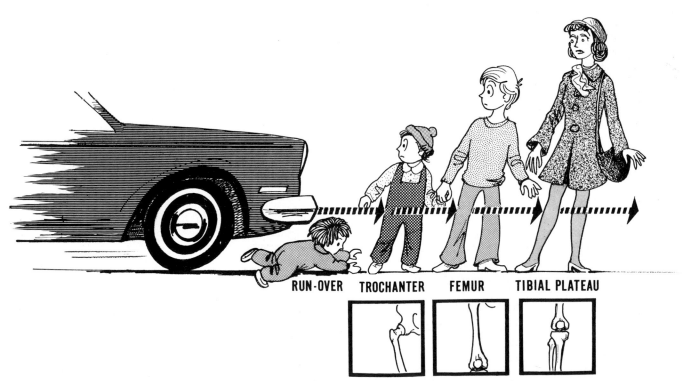

Fig. 16-1. Age determines the site of a bumper fracture.

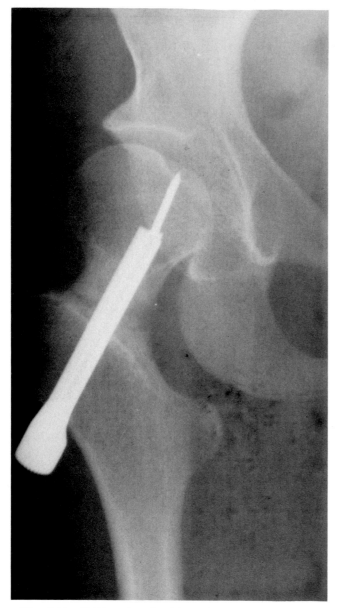

Fig. 16-2.   Triffin pins should not be used.   The fracture has been slightly distracted and the guide pin bent, preventing removal.   Stress fracture in child with cerebral palsy, aged 14.

chance of union is excellent in a young child with an *undisplaced* fracture.   In a cast he will not develop bed sores or deep vein thrombosis or lose the will to live, but malunion is a real hazard.   When a *displaced* fracture of the neck is reduced and held in a cast coxa vara is almost a certainty.

6. The hardness of a child's bone and the small size of the femoral neck are not suited to fixation with a standard Smith-Petersen nail (Fig. 16-2).   Threaded pins or screws should be used.

7. When problems arise in a child, prosthetic replacement is not available as a solution.

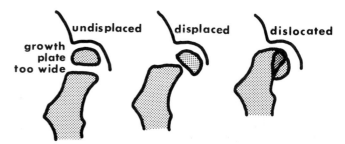

Fig. 16-3.   Classification of Type I injuries.

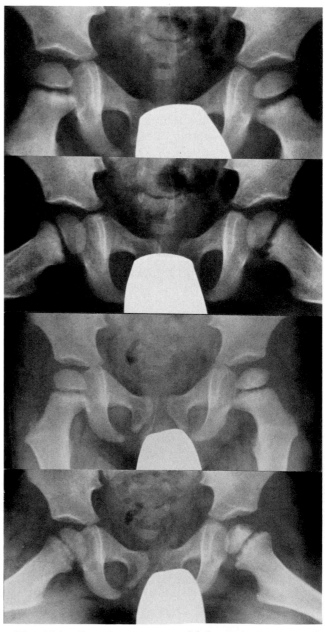

Fig. 16-4.   Type I separation of left upper femoral epiphysis of a boy of 3 years.   The growth plate is too wide. Later avascular necrosis can be recognized.

Fig. 16-5. (*A, B*) Acute slipped upper femoral epiphysis; girl aged 12. (*C, D*) Three months later, after pinning, the other epiphysis is displaced. (*E*) After further pinning. The girl was found to be hypothyroid and was placed on medication.

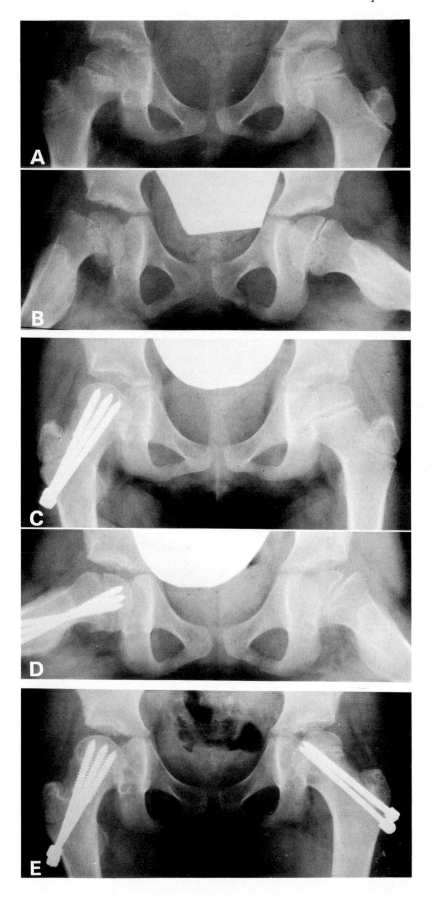

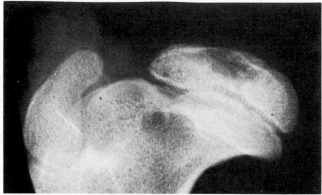

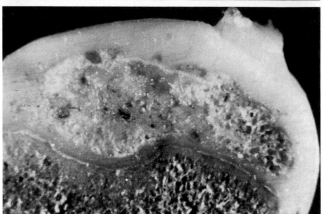

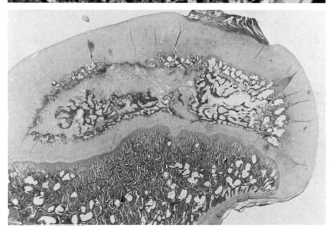

Fig. 16-6. Experimental avascular necrosis. A tight noose was placed around the femoral neck of a piglet 50 days earlier. At sacrifice the superior surface was soft and could be pushed in like a ping pong ball. (*A*) Radiograph of whole head. (*B*) Cut section. The vessels, injected with dark vinyl, can be seen, demonstrating that the head is revascularized. (*C*) Histological section. The head contains fibrous tissue and sclerotic bone, resembling a pseudarthrosis. New subchondral bone is forming.

TYPE I INJURIES

The femoral head separates from the neck through the growth plate. The various degrees of severity are shown in Figure 16-3.

In *infants,* this injury is most likely to occur when the child has been run over. It may also be seen in an abused infant. In *children,* great violence is required, and there are usually other injuries as well (Fig. 16-4). In *adolescents,* an acute Type I injury is seen which represents one end of the spectrum of slipped upper femoral epiphysis. *Pathological* slip occurs in many diseases, including renal osteodystrophy, hypothyroidism (Fig. 16-5), and neglected septic arthritis.

Traumatic Separation

Ratliff has analyzed 13 traumatic separations in children aged 9 years or under and found complications in 11: premature fusion, avascular necrosis, and nonunion. He recommends traction for those with no displacement. In displaced fractures, closed reduction is commonly easy, and the reduction should be held in a one-and-a-half hip spica. Displacement does occur occasionally in the cast, and frequent radiographs should be taken to detect this. Pin fixation is unnecessary and may aggravate the tendency to premature fusion. If the head is dislocated, open reduction will be required.

Traumatic separation of the proximal femoral epiphysis is a severe injury, and the parents should be warned that problems are more likely than not.

Slipped Epiphysis

Bobechko, at The Hospital for Sick Children, has reviewed acute slipped upper femoral epiphysis in adolescents and concludes that immediate but slow reduction using skin traction with internal rotation is safer than immediate manipulative reduction under general anesthesia. Avascular necrosis occurred in 5 of 35 children, and all these had had manipulative reduction under anesthesia. Therefore, immediate institution of gradual correction is recommended over 3 to 4 days before internal fixation is carried out.

In conclusion, use a cast for the younger child with a traumatic separation and use internal fixation for older children and when the slip is pathological.

TRANSCERVICAL AND BASAL FRACTURES

Transcervical and basal fractures are the most common hip fractures; the midcervical level is commonest. The perils of this injury may be very great. Avascular necrosis has been reported in 17 to 45 percent. Obviously much commoner in displaced fractures, avascular necrosis (Fig. 16-6) also occurs in undisplaced, even basal, fractures. A sequel to avascular necrosis is premature closure of the growth plate, which leads to a short neck and a weak lever arm for the abductor muscles, a short leg, and limitation of abduction owing to

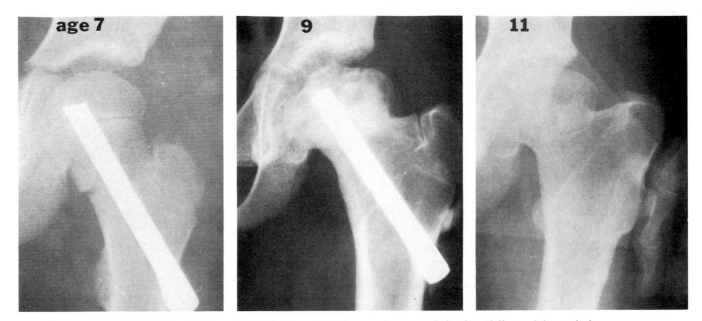

Fig. 16-7. Displaced basal fracture. Total avascular necrosis leads to failure of the capital growth plate. The neck is short. Unexpectedly, the growth of the greater trochanter stops early (probably due to a Type IV injury). Overgrowth is more common.

overgrowth of the greater trochanter (Fig. 16-7). Delayed union, nonunion, and slipping into coxa vara while in a cast carry similar penalties.

It is difficult to write much about this fracture from personal experience. It is misleading to apply the mass of information about adult fractures to children, and the small number of papers that relate specifically to children present widely varying statistics which are almost impossible to compare. But the following general observations emerge.

Fixation of the Fracture

Muscular forces across the hip joint tend to produce coxa vara in *displaced* fractures (i.e., fractures in which the periosteum has been torn). Cast fixation after reduction does not neutralize these muscular forces, and slip is almost certain. For displaced fractures the conservative approach is internal fixation. *Undisplaced* fractures in young children have some inherent stability, and the safe way to supplement it is by hip spica (safe because pinning may increase the risk of avascular

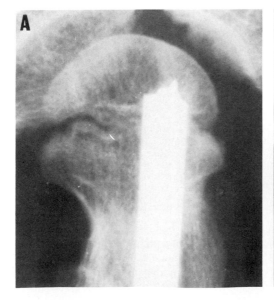
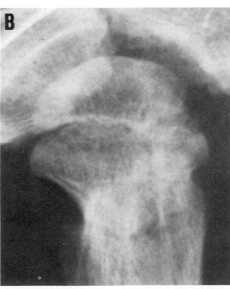

Fig. 16-8. Avascular necrosis following internal fixation in a 7-year-old boy. (*A*) On the day of hip pinning, a wedge of increased bone density extends from the top of the pin. (*B*) One year later the boy was asymptomatic.

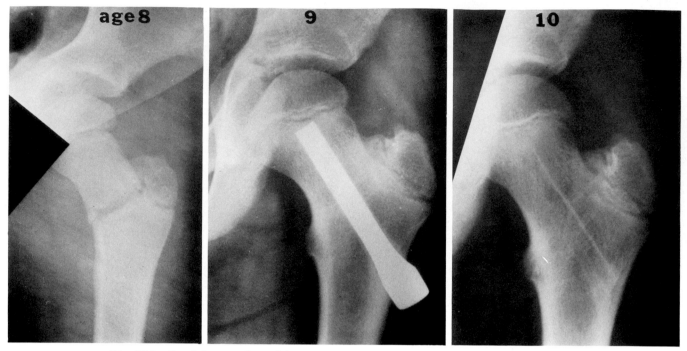

Fig. 16-9. Basal fracture in a girl aged 8 years. A short pin does not damage the head.

necrosis and carries the chance of infection and refracture at the site of pin entry). In older children pinning is technically easier and reduces the chances of displacement.

Type of Internal Fixation

One of the difficulties is that no series has been reported that used sound methods of internal fixation. Most authors condemn nails, particularly large nails, because the bone is so hard that driving nails in is difficult, and distraction is common. All the bone displaced by the nail must go somewhere; my belief is that it fills vital vascular spaces (Fig. 16-8). From the literature, it is not possible to determine the best method of internal fixation; most authors express a preference for threaded pin fixation. If multiple threaded pins are used, they should lie parallel to avoid distraction. The metaphysis is composed of hard bone, unlike the adult metaphysis, and provides a good hold. It is usually unnecessary to cross the plate, but in high fractures do not hesitate to put a pin temporarily across the plate. But when the plate is transfixed, pins should be removed as soon as possible to avoid interfering with growth.

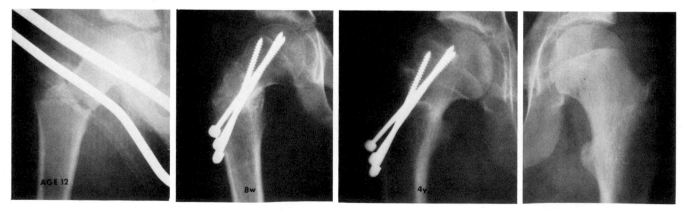

Fig. 16-10. Displaced basal fracture. In addition, this 12-year-old boy sustained a complete traumatic paraplegia. The pins were not well suited to withstand his flexor spasms and he slipped into varus. A nail plate should have been used. Growth arrest was due to threaded pins left across the plate. His paraplegia improved, and he is able to walk with crutches without trouble from the hip fracture.

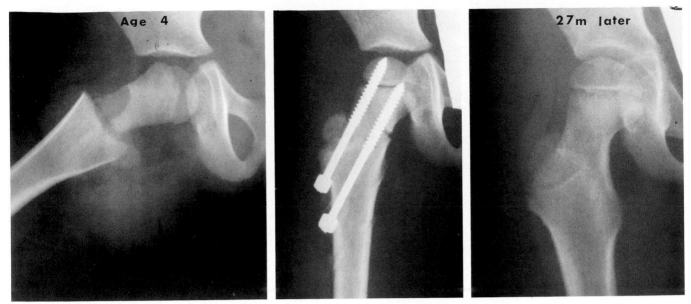

Fig. 16-11. Displaced cervical fracture. The threaded bolts could have been shorter but were removed as soon as the fracture united.

A lag screw inserted through a predrilled and tapped hole, and avoiding the growth plate wherever possible, would appear to be the strongest and least traumatic form of fixation.

TREATMENT

Undisplaced Fractures

Experience indicates that excellent results are generally, though not universally, achieved however these are treated. A one-and-one-half hip spica with the leg held in internal rotation and abduction, for 8 to 12 weeks is sufficient. The fracture should be checked for slip. In the past we have often used short pins with good results, but that is probably overtreatment (Fig. 16-9).

Displaced Fractures

The risk of coxa vara and avascular necrosis are very high (Fig. 16-10). Kay and Hall have argued that the hip should be aspirated to prevent tamponade of the vessels; this has not been evaluated. Manipulation under anesthesia will generally correct displacement (Fig. 16-11). But if a perfect reduction cannot be achieved in the older child, either an open reduction using an anterolateral approach will be needed, or an intertrochanteric osteotomy, which has been known to yield good results. A hip spica alone will not hold reduction; on this all agree. Internal fixation is needed (Fig. 16-12).

A child does not need rapid rehabilitation. Apply a hip spica for 8 to 12 weeks to protect the hip. Re-

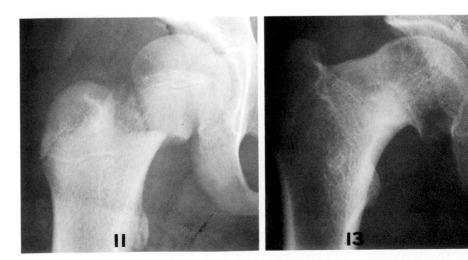

Fig. 16-12. A typical result of cast immobilization for a displaced fracture.

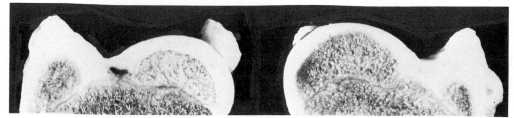

Fig. 16-13. (*Left*) Early avascular necrosis in the left hip of a pig. A month earlier a ligature was tied around the left femoral neck to occlude circulation of the head. (*Right*) The right hip was untouched. The left ossific nucleus has not grown, and the surface cartilage is thicker because it has not ossified.

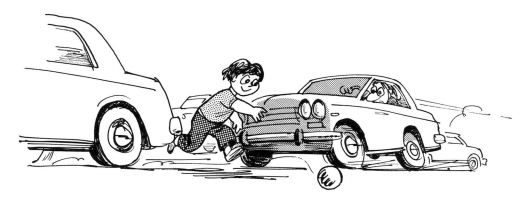

Fig. 16-14. When a child runs across the road, he is more likely to be hit by cars in the nearside lane. The cars in the opposite lane have more warning. In countries that drive on the right there is a preponderance of left-sided injuries.

member the load on the hip imposed by straight leg raising is just the same as that imposed by walking. A belt-and-suspenders approach is needed to prevent coxa vara.

Avascular necrosis is best detected with a scan early but is usually apparent radiographically within the first few months, and probably always within a year. Radi-

ographs should be obtained every two months during the first year. The first signs of avascular necrosis are as follows: the head does not become osteoporotic; it does not grow; and the cartilage space becomes wider (Fig. 16-13). These signs are present long before signs of gross density, fragmentation, and deformity of the head. Slight disturbance of circulation produces coxa

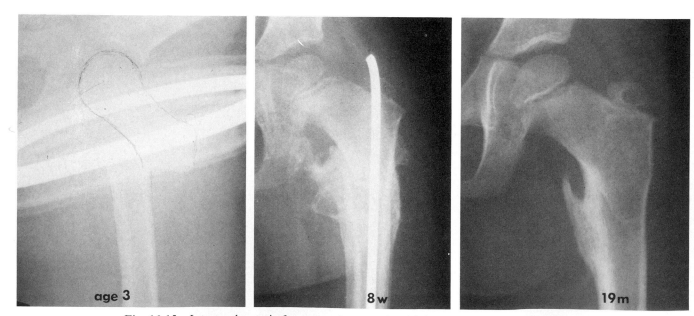

Fig. 16-15. Intertrochanteric fracture. A severe head injury made her very restless, and the fracture could not be controlled. A vertical pin provided simple and effective fixation.

Fig. 16-16. Intertrochanteric fracture in a girl of 2½ years. She had concomitant severe injuries, and this fracture was maintained in traction without much expectation that she would survive. Four years later she has a left spastic hemiplegia; the leg is 1 inch short. There is excellent re-modelling, but bone has not crossed the site of capsular interposition.

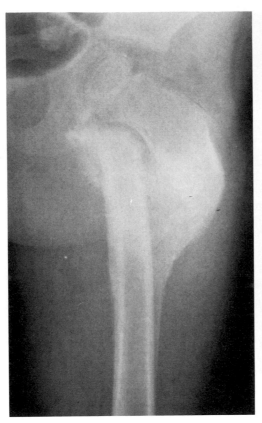
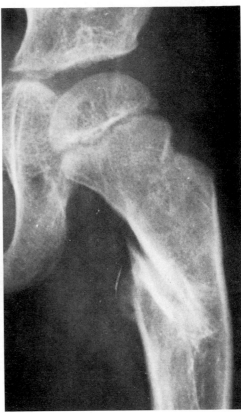

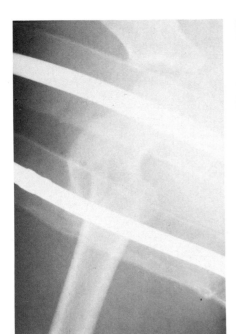
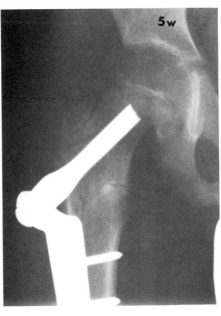
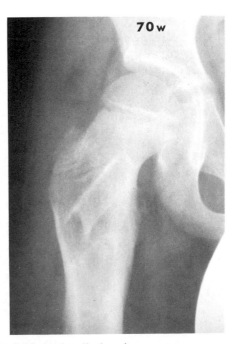

Fig. 16-17. Intertrochanteric fracture in a boy aged 7. Even a child-sized nail-plate is very bulky. Though this is a good result; a similar result could probably have been obtained with traction.

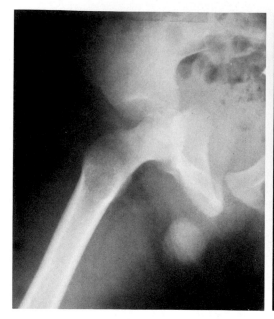
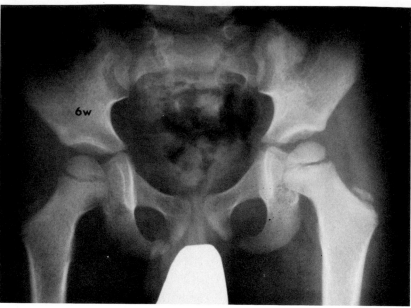

Fig. 16-18. Anterior dislocation of the hip. Six weeks after reduction the right hip is osteoporotic by comparison with the left. The circulation must be intact to permit this; avascular necrosis is most unlikely. Even in this boy, aged 6 years, the anterior and posterior lips of the acetabulum are cartilaginous.

magna luxans. The large head is poorly covered by the acetabulum. Both these conditions may be treated by innominate osteotomy.

TROCHANTERIC FRACTURES *

Between 1962 and 1972, 20 nonpathological fractures of the trochanteric region of the femur were treated at The Hospital for Sick Children. All fractures between the base of the neck and a line 1 cm. below the lesser trochanter of the femur were included.

The average age at time of injury was 7 years; 80 percent were produced by motor vehicle accidents; the remainder by falls and toboggan accidents. The majority of fractures were left-sided (Fig. 16-14). Associated soft tissue injuries were noted in all patients, 65 percent sustained other fractures, [e.g., skull, pelvis, clavicle], and 55 percent had significant craniocerebral injuries, leaving 4 of these patients with residual posttraumatic hemiplegia or other neurological deficit.

Treatment of Intertrochanteric Fractures
(Figs. 16-15 to 16-17)

Most intertrochanteric fractures can be reduced and held in skin traction. When callus is present at 3 to 4 weeks a one-and-one-half hip spica should be applied. The chief indication for internal fixation is ir-

*Based on a review by Dr. Barry Malcolm.

reducibility or inability to hold the fracture in traction because of other injuries. Operative treatment can be extremely difficult, because considerable comminution or separation of the greater trochanter may be present without being obvious on radiographs. Always obtain first quality films before starting surgery.

Avascular necrosis is not a hazard, and the tendency to varus deformity is more easily overcome than in more

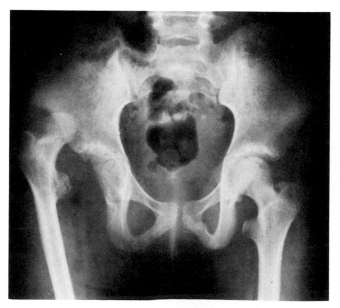

Fig. 16-19. Dislocation in Down's syndrome.

Fig. 16-20. Traumatic dislocation of the left hip in a baby of 9 months. The dislocation was not recognized for several months. An open reduction was performed, and avascular necrosis followed. The result at the age of 6 years was good.

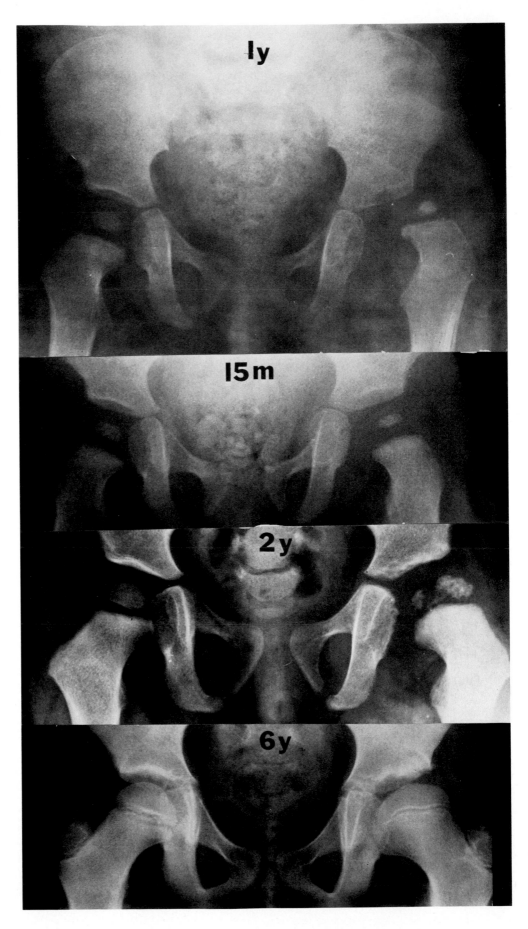

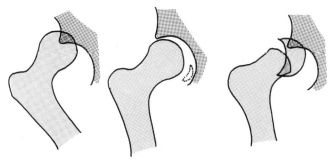

Fig. 16-21. Complications recognized after reduction. An acetabular fragment may block complete reduction. A type I injury may become evident.

proximal fractures. The only consistent late finding in 5 cases we reviewed was overgrowth—an average of 1.2 cm.

Subtrochanteric fractures will be considered in the next chapter.

DISLOCATION OF THE HIP

Dislocation is commoner than fracture of the femoral neck, and it carries fewer problems. (The hip, metacarpophalangeal joint, and patellofemoral joint are the only sites at which dislocation occurs with any frequency in children).

The hip of a child under the age of 5 is usually dislocated by a fall. Trauma is minimal. At this age the acetabulum is largely cartilaginous and therefore soft; joint laxity is common. If all the muscles around the hip are relaxed, little force is required to dislocate the hip. As age increases, so the degree of violence escalates to athletic injuries between the age of 6 and 10, and to automobile accidents thereafter. Greater violence is more likely to be associated with fracture of the acetabulum or femur and sciatic nerve damage.

Posterior dislocation, the commonest sort, produces a flexed, adducted, internally rotated leg. Anterior dislocation produces the reverse deformity (Fig. 16-18).

A recent traumatic dislocation can hardly be confused with a long-standing paralytic dislocation for which the treatment is entirely different. But recurrent dislocation of the hip in Down's syndrome may be confusing (Fig. 16-19). The bone looks normal, and only the appearance of the facies makes the diagnosis. In a survey, I found that 2 percent of patients with Down's syndrome (in all age groups) have dislocatable hips.

Treatment

It is not merely kind to reduce a dislocated hip as soon as possible. Early closed reduction will almost always succeed, but each passing day makes the need for open reduction more likely. Prompt reduction will reduce the incidence of avascular necrosis. At our hospital avascular necrosis has only been seen when reduction was delayed beyond 12 hours (Fig. 16-20).

Reduction is easy if you ask the anesthetist to use relaxants. A posterior dislocation is reduced by flexing the hip and the knee to 90 degrees and applying traction while the leg is internally rotated. Anterior dislocation is best reduced by pulling the leg in extension, abduction, and internal rotation. After reduction, the hip should move freely without crepitus. A radiograph should be obtained to check that the hip is concentrically reduced.

After reduction, we nurse the child in Buck's traction with a pillow under the knee for a few days and then apply a hip spica, in which the child should remain for 4 to 6 weeks to allow capsular healing. Movement usually returns quickly, and myositis ossificans is rare. A scan should be obtained to assess the vascularity of the head. Radiographic review should continue for a year to detect avascular necrosis.

Complications

Problems are unusual (Fig. 16-21). During reduction an unrecognized epiphyseal separation may become manifest. The neck, not the head, reduces into the acetabulum. Open reduction and pinning will be required.

Trapped Interarticular Fragment

It is commonly at a later stage that a trapped interarticular fragment becomes recognized (Fig. 16-22). When the cast is removed, the hip is painful and never regains very much movement. Retrospective examination of the radiographs reveals that the head was never completely reduced. An arthrogram will show the reason—commonly a radiolucent cartilaginous fragment from the acetabulum, which can only be removed by arthrotomy. If this complication is borne in mind at the time when the hip is reduced, it should be possible to make the diagnosis and remove the loose fragment immediately.

Recurrent Dislocation

Recurrent dislocation of the hip is a rare sequel except in Down's syndrome. Information on the management of Down's dislocation is little better than anecdotal. I treated one child after an acute episode with abduction casts, and 4 years later the hip was satisfactory: I know of another child who required bilateral capsulorrhaphy.

Fig. 16-22. A year after reduction of a traumatic dislocation, the right hip was stiff and painful. The distance between the teardrop and the femoral head is increased. The femoral head is displaced laterally. At arthrotomy a fibrocartilaginous body was removed from the floor of the acetabulum. A year later the hip was excellent clinically. Hyperemia has increased the size of the right head compared with the left.

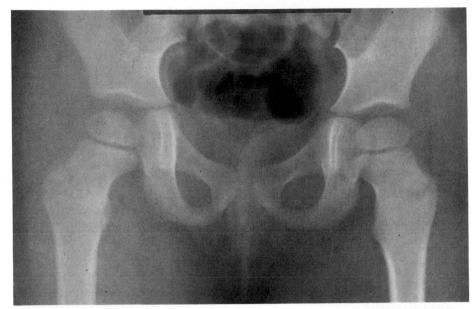

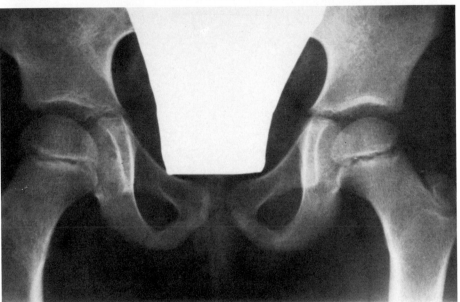

Avascular Necrosis

The overall incidence of avascular necrosis in the literature is 10 percent or less (Fig. 16-21). Delayed reduction and severe injury are the most important causes. Prolonged avoidance of weight-bearing after dislocation does not influence the incidence.

RESULTS

In each of two series that reported the results in children followed to maturity, about one-third were found to have some abnormality of the hip. Simple dislocations of the hip in children under the age of 6 years almost always had a good result. A poor result was commonest when treatment was delayed beyond 24 hours, when severe trauma produced associated injuries, and when the situation necessitated open reduction. The results are better than those in adults.

REFERENCES

Fractures

Casey, B. H., Hamilton, H. W., and Bobechko, W. P.: Reduction of acutely slipped upper femoral epiphysis. J. Bone Joint Surg., *54B:* 607, 1972

Ingram, A. J., and Bachynski, B.: Fractures of the hip in children. J. Bone Joint Surg., *15A:* 867, 1953

Kay, S. P., and Hall, J. E.: Fracture of the femoral neck in children and its complications. Clin. Orthop., *80:* 53, 1971

Lam, S. F.: Fractures of the neck of the femur in children. J. Bone Joint Surg., *53A:* 1165, 1971

Miller, W. E.: Fractures of the hip in children from birth to adolescence. Clin. Orthop., *92:* 155, 1973

Ratliff, A. H. C.: Fractures of the neck of the femur in children. J. Bone Joint Surg., *44B:* 528, 1962

Ratliff, A. H. C.: Traumatic separation of the upper femoral epiphysis in young children. J. Bone Joint Surg., *50B:* 757, 1968

Ratliff, A. H. C.: Complications after fractures of the femoral neck in children and their treatment. J. Bone Joint Surg., *52B:* 175, 1970

Schatzker, J., and Barrington, T. W.: Fractures of the femoral neck associated with fractures of the same femoral shaft. Can. J. Surg., *11:* 297, 1968

Weiner, D. S., and O'Dell, H. W.: Fractures of the hip in children. J. Trauma, *9:* 62, 1969

Zolczer, L., Kazar, G., Manninger, J., and Nagy, E.: Fractures of the femoral neck in adolescents. Injury, *4:* 41, 1973

Dislocation

Gaul, R. W.: Recurrent traumatic dislocation of the hip in children. Clin. Orthop., *90:* 107, 1973

Pearson, D. E., and Mann, R. J.: Traumatic hip dislocation in children. Clin. Orthop., *92:* 189, 1973

Pennsylvania Orthopaedic Society: Traumatic dislocation of the hip in children. J. Bone Joint Surg., *50A:* 79, 1968

17

Femoral Shaft

As it is easily aligned on a splint, without much need to demonstrate skill in manipulation or surgical technique, femoral fracture has generally good results. Slight shortening is made up by overgrowth. Bayonet apposition is very common; in other bones, it produces an ugly lump, but in the femur, the covering muscle hides the lump from parent's probing fingers. A fracture of the femur is generally a low-key injury, but

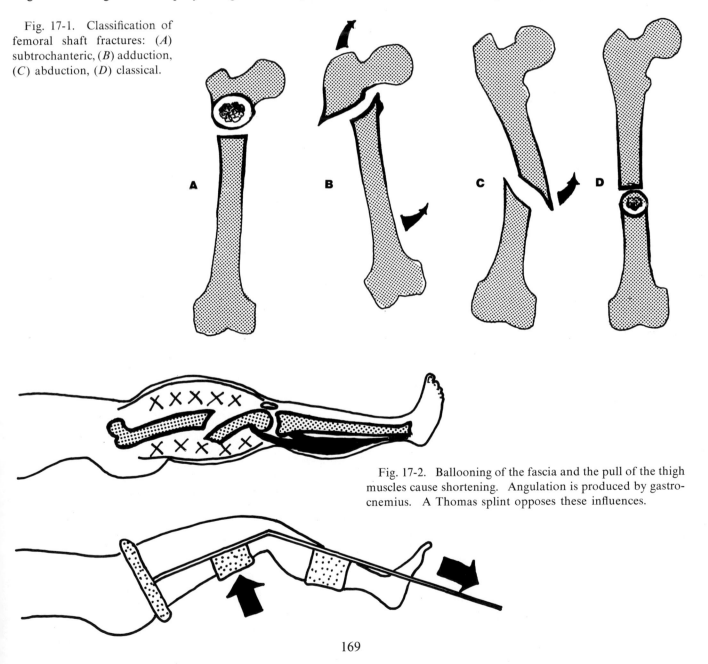

Fig. 17-1. Classification of femoral shaft fractures: (A) subtrochanteric, (B) adduction, (C) abduction, (D) classical.

Fig. 17-2. Ballooning of the fascia and the pull of the thigh muscles cause shortening. Angulation is produced by gastrocnemius. A Thomas splint opposes these influences.

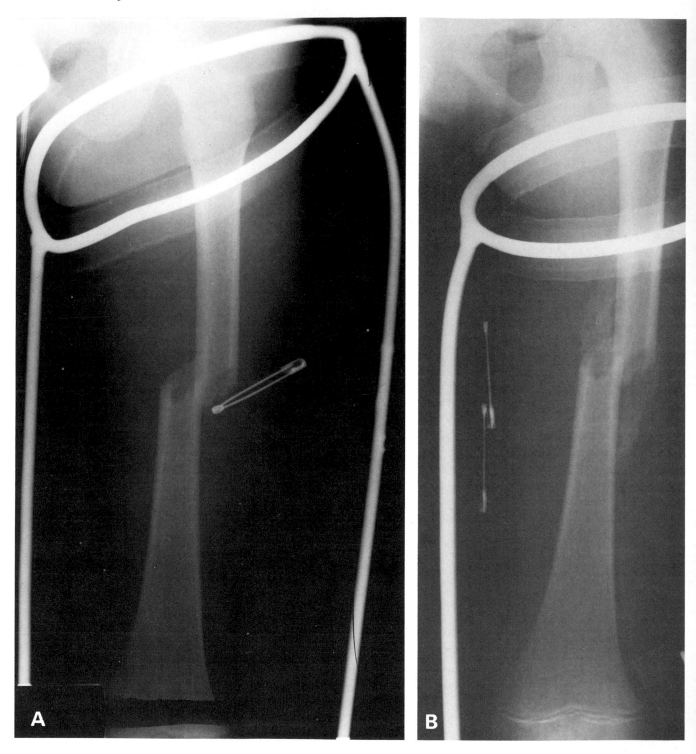

Fig. 17-3. A typical fracture of the midshaft of the femur in a boy aged 10 years. (*A*) Initial appearance. Note that the diagnosis was made on clinical signs and the splint was applied before radiographs were taken. (*B*) At 17 days the fracture is clinically united and ready to go into a spica. (*C*) At 10 weeks. (*D*) The lateral view shows that the normal anterior bow of the femur has been maintained.

problems can arise. The most common difficulties are aligning high fractures; managing fractures when there are other major injuries; and ischemia.

INITIAL EXAMINATION

It does not require a physician to diagnose a fractured

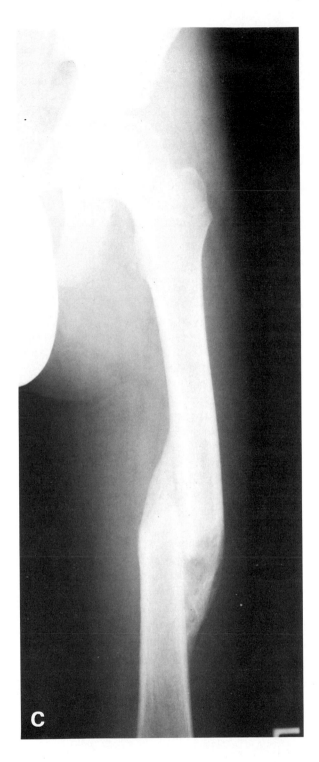

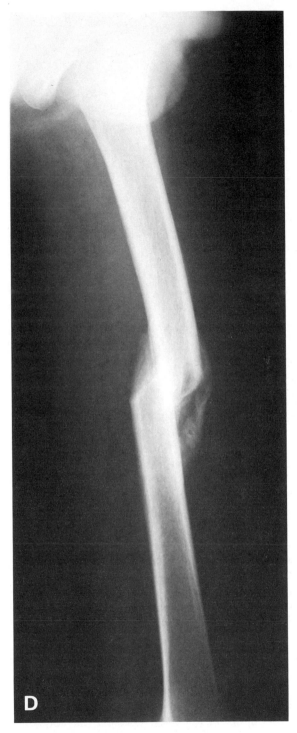

femur. The patient can do this. It does require a physician to appreciate that, after the pedal pulses have been palpated, the leg should be splinted before radiographs are taken. Look for other injuries. Determine the blood pressure. Shock is never the result of a fractured femoral shaft in children; it is always due to internal hemorrhage, e.g., a ruptured spleen. The radiograph should include the hip and knee joints otherwise the patient may be lying with a uniting fracture and an unrecognized dislocation of the hip that will cause a lot of red faces next week and white faces later.

CLASSIFICATION

Classical Midshaft Fractures

Whether oblique or transverse, a midshaft fracture

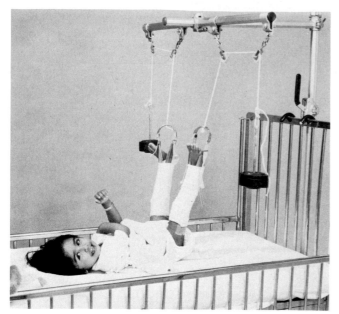

Fig. 17-4. Gallows traction for children under 2 years of age.

shortens owing to the pull of the thigh muscles and ballooning of the investing fascia of the thigh by swelling. The distal fragment displaces posteriorly owing to gravity and the pull of gastrocnemius (Fig. 17-2). The aim of treatment is union with about a centimeter of shortening and with correct rotation and no angulation (Fig. 17-3).

Children Under 2 Years of Age (Fig. 17-4). Gallows traction for about 2 weeks is sufficient to produce clinical union. For infants this may be all that is needed, but for toddlers a short time in a hip spica afterwards may give more peace of mind. The risk of ischemia has discouraged us from using gallows traction for older children. John Hall found a high incidence of ischemia when older children were managed in this way; even the uninjured leg was affected.

Children 2 Years and Over (Fig. 17-5). Fixed skin traction using a Thomas splint on an inclined Bradford frame provides comfortable fixation. It is wise to lift the end of the frame only a few inches for the first few days. Later it can be elevated about 18 inches. This reduces the chance of ischemia. Be sure that the band behind the calf is causing no excessive pressure.

Radiographs should be taken the day after injury to see that the position is adequate. Then radiograph each week to check alignment. Malunion is only malposition that has been neglected; at this site malposition is easily corrected by adjusting the traction. Length is best assessed with a tape measure, because radiographs can be misleading (Fig. 17-6). If more than 1 cm. of over-riding is present raise the foot end of the Bradford frame; lower the foot end to correct distraction.

During the course of the third week a mass of callus can be felt, then towards the end of that week the fracture sets overnight and movement is no longer possible. A hip spica can be applied without an anesthetic. I apply a hip spica with a foam rubber sole for walking and have found no problems from this. The hip and knee are flexed about 40 degrees—without abduction—so that the apparent length of both legs is the same. A 1-inch raise is applied to the shoe of the opposite foot. Not all children learn to walk, but at least they can stand and sit.

As soon as the cast is hard the child goes home; the cast is removed in clinic in 6 to 8 weeks. It has been helpful to provide parents with a printed handout when their child is admitted to explain this pattern of care. From the outset they appreciate that the child will be on crutches for about 2 weeks after the cast comes off, and will go on limping for about 3 months.

There is little to be gained by advising definite periods of nonweightbearing after cast removal. Mothers cannot enforce your advice and only worry. Tell mother that children have an unfailing sixth sense to protect them from putting too much weight on the leg or discarding crutches too soon. Leave it to them. Children should be seen about a month after the cast is removed; a few who are making very slow progress require physiotherapy at this stage. Leg length should be assessed a year after injury.

Recently cast bracing has been used for children instead of a spica to reduce stiffness and muscle wasting. The early results are so promising that the spica may soon be superceded.

Alternative Methods. Methods used in other institutions include: (1) *Hamilton Russell traction,* which I have always found requires constant adjustments; (2) *Perkin's traction,* which is excellent for adults, but does not offer sufficient immobilization for children to be comfortable; and (3) *immediate hip spica.* In two large series reported recently (Irani and Burton and Fordyce) the results of

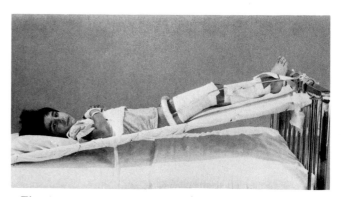

Fig. 17-5. Fixed Thomas traction on a Bradford frame. Skin tapes are tied to the end of the splint, which is tied to the bed end.

cast fixation are just as good as those obtained with traction, in children between the age of 2 and 10 years. Spica fixation may be the method of choice because it saves hospital beds. Irani applies a single hip spica (with the sole of the foot cut out to prevent the child pushing up) without admission and without an anesthetic. The leg should be cast with an almost extended knee and hip. Though setting the leg with the hip and knee flexed may seem to give better control I have seen this produce a slough in the popliteal fossa with disastrous results. Judet noted unsatisfactory results in half the patients treated in casts with the hip and knee flexed to right angles. Cast treatment can supplant traction for all these fractures, but it must be done well.

Adducted Fractures

When the fracture is subtrochanteric and oblique, the pull of the abductors proximally and the pull of adductors distally tend to produce an outward bow. Often this will correct in routine traction. If it does not correct, either apply a little pad at the site of the bow, or put blocks under the side of the bed as well as the end to increase abduction of the distal fragment.

Extended Fractures

The degree of displacement of a subtrochanteric fracture depends on the direction of the fracture line (Fig. 17-7). Psoas tends to flex the proximal fragment if the direction of the fracture line permits. Some transverse fractures may be so flexed that they produce a bone-on-end appearance on anteroposterior radiographs.

If angulation is slight, raise the end of the Thomas splint. If angulation is gross, the distal fragment should be flexed using 90–90 traction maintained with a supracondylar pin (Fig. 17-8).

While an assistant holds the leg in this position, a Steinmann pin is inserted from the medial side. Do not put the pin in with the knee extended if you wish to avoid impaling and trapping tensor fascia lata. Try to get the pin square to the leg. Because it is easier to be sure where the pin goes in than where it will come out, the medial approach is recommended to avoid risk to the femoral artery.

After 3 to 4 weeks in traction the pin is removed and a hip spica is applied.

Abducted Fractures

This is unusual except in low fractures with a suitably oblique fracture line. The medial bow may be corrected with a medial pad or by putting a little traction on the normal leg to level the pelvis and reduce the pull of the adductors.

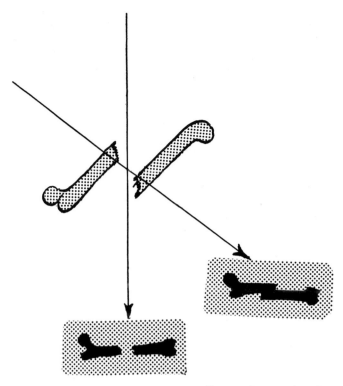

Fig. 17-6. A fracture may appear distracted or overlapping depending on the angle at which the radiograph is taken. Judge length with a tape measure.

EARLY PROBLEMS

Multiple Injuries

Many children with fractures of the femoral shaft have head injuries. Most children with severe, life-threatening multiple injuries sustained in traffic accidents have a fracture of the femur. This is because the femur of a child is at car bumper level (Fig. 17-9).

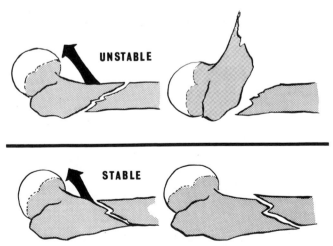

Fig. 17-7. The direction of the fracture line determines whether a subtrochanteric fracture will be unstable or stable. Unstable fractures require 90–90 traction; stable fractures are managed in a Thomas splint.

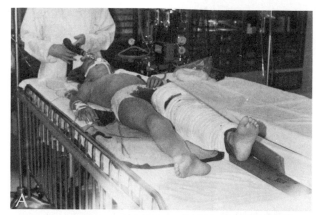

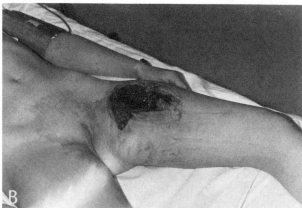

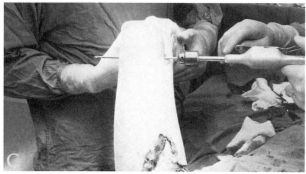

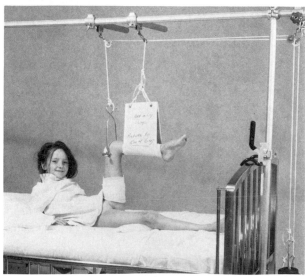

It has already been remarked that shock in a child with apparently nothing more than a fracture of the femur *always* indicates internal hemorrhage; most commonly, a ruptured spleen.

Management.   Look after serious injuries first and immobilize the femur temporarily in a Thomas splint with the patient flat.   Head injuries render the head-down position undesirable.   The skin against the ring should be checked and treated several times a day by the nurses to prevent pressure areas.   This is usually safe for a day or two.   If the child cannot go into head-down traction at this time, choose another form of definitive treatment.

Traction.   Hamilton Russell traction or 90–90 degree traction works well if the child lies fairly still and does not require turning.

Intramedullary Fixation.   Though rarely indicated, intramedullary fixation greatly facilitates nursing care for children with prolonged decerebrate restlessness or those with chest or spinal injuries (Fig. 17-10).   Nailing should be done early because vascular spasm may be precipitated if overlap is corrected at a week.   After nailing, the fracture can be forgotten.   The main objection to nailing is the risk of sepsis.   The special objections in childhood are the risk of slight disturbance of growth in the greater trochanter at the site of entry of the nail, and an over-long leg due to bringing the fracture out to length.   I wish I had used this method in a child with bilateral diaphyseal fractures who convulsed for a week after a head injury.   When he came out of 90–90 traction—at about 6 weeks—he refractured both femora during spasms.   His radiographs, taken during convulsions, were permanently left up on the view box in the ICU by the nurses, in an attempt to make me change my ways.   Every doctor on the staff who had ever treated a fracture of the femur offered me advice.   Massive callus left him with a quadriceps contracture, which, happily, resolved after 6 months before his legs became perfect.

Fractures of the Femur and Tibia on the Same Side

This subject is discussed on page 197.

Fig. 17-8.   Open subtrochanteric fracture. (*A*) This girl arrived well splinted. Only when she was anesthetized was the wound inspected. After debridement (*B*) a pin was placed through the distal femur for 90–90 traction. (*C*) The anesthetist's view of the insertion. Ask the anesthetist to tell you to raise or lower the handle of the drill to obtain a horizontal pin. (*D*) Five days later she was surprisingly comfortable.

Fig. 17-9. *Waddell's Triad.* When a child is struck by a car always look for three injuries.

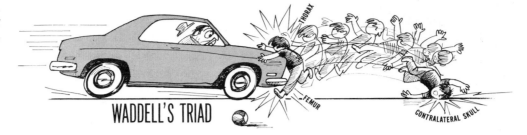

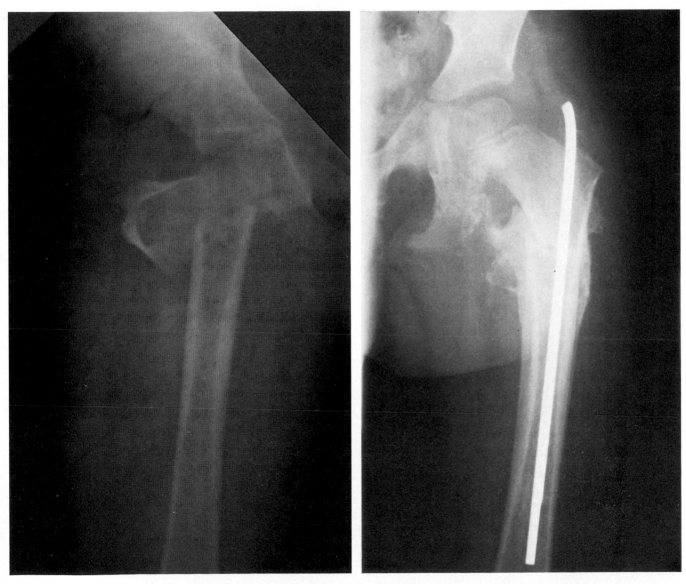

Fig. 17-10. Subtrochanteric fracture in a girl of 3 years. She shows the bone-on-end appearance, because the proximal fragment is flexed 90 degrees. The fracture could not be held in any sort of traction because of severe protracted decerebrate rigidity. She was on a respirator for a week. The fracture was pinned on the third day after injury when it was obvious that the fracture could not be treated by traction and that the decerebrate rigidity was going to last. She started to walk independently after 6 months and has a residual hemiplegia and some intellectual impairment.

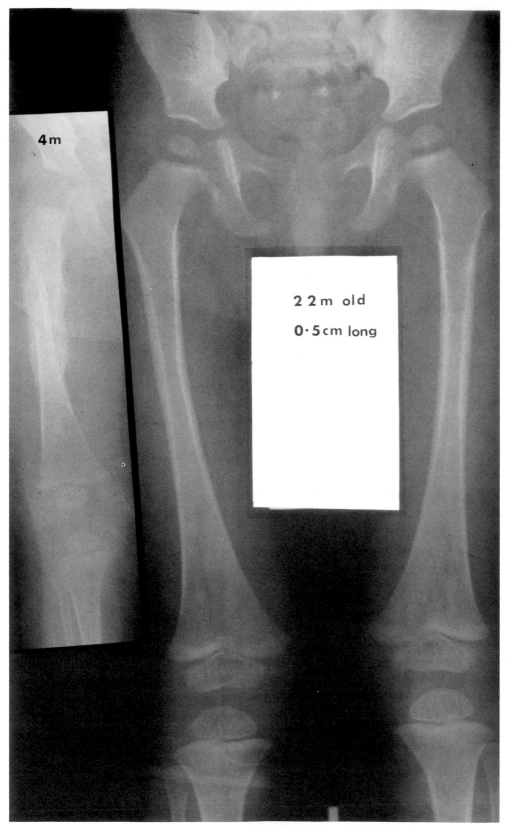

4 m

22 m old
0·5 cm long

Fig. 17-11. Remodelling is excellent after fractures of the femur. At 3 weeks this fracture is united with 0.5 cm. overlap. The right lower extremity is 0.5 cm. long 18 months later.

Ischemia

Individual experience with ischemia will be limited. Early recognition is a prerequisite to successful care in every patient. Feel the pedal pulses; test toe movement and sensation; and look for an ischemic cause of unexpected pain.

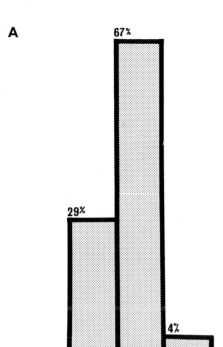

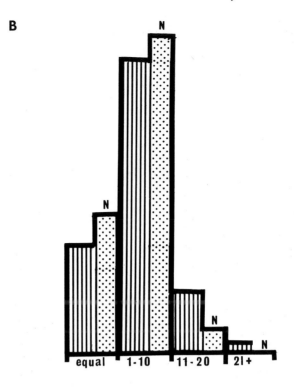

LEG LENGTH DISCREPANCY
in 100 fit soldiers (Rush & Steiner, 1946)

Fig. 17-12. (*A*) Leg length discrepancy in a population of young fit soldiers. (*B*) Relationship between backache and leg length discrepancy. Leg length was measured radiographically in soldiers with nonspecific backache (striped column) and compared with fit soldiers (stippled column). In those with discrepancies greater than 1 cm., more had backache than were fit. (*C*) Leg length discrepancy in one series of children's fractures. Perhaps a quarter of these children have a greater risk of backache in later life.

Early ischemia may be due to a lesion of the artery or to displacement of the fracture. I well remember a child with a fracture at the level of Hunter's canal. Pedal pulses could not be felt on admission very soon after the accident. Within an hour the foot became cold and the girl lost toe movement and sensation. When the fracture was reduced under general anesthesia, the foot suddenly became warm and the veins filled. As soon as the girl awoke after the anesthetic her toes moved and were sensitive, but it was about 2 weeks before her pulses returned. Her artery was not explored because the peripheral circulation was adequate.

If the circulation does not return as well as this, the artery should be explored and the fracture fixed internally.

Late Ischemia. Tight bandages over skin traction or inelastic bandages supporting the calf are the main causes. The risk of ischemia is greater in the presence of hypotension due to other injuries. If the patient is unconscious, ischemia passes unnoticed. Arterial exploration with a Fogarty catheter and fasciotomy will be needed (see Chap. 4).

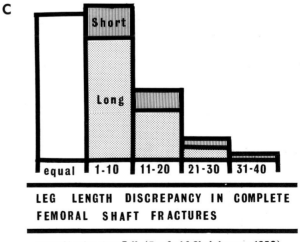

LEG LENGTH DISCREPANCY IN COMPLETE FEMORAL SHAFT FRACTURES

83 patients: 2 yr F.U. (Barfod & Christensen, 1958)

Fat Embolism

Approximately half the children with a fractured femur in a series we studied showed biochemical evidence of fat embolism. Clinical fat embolism, though unusual, resembles that of the adult form (Weicz, Rang & Salter).

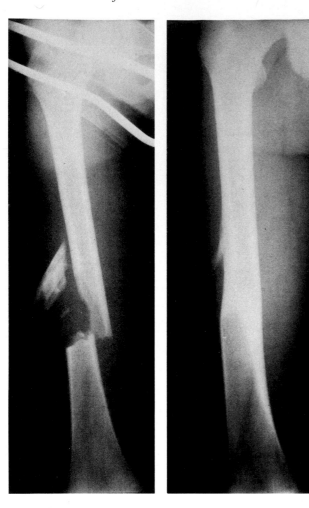

Fig. 17-13. This 11-year-old has a large butterfly fragment. After 4 weeks in traction the shaft united leaving the isolated butterfly fragment as a lump under the skin. It was excised before she was placed in a spica. Two years later a spur was easily palpable and occasionally painful.

LATE PROBLEMS

The incidence of late complications is low. Most potential problems are related to leg length inequality.

Leg Length

After any diaphyseal fracture longitudinal growth is accelerated. In the femur this amounts to about 1 cm. and occurs during the 18 months after injury. No further growth acceleration or equalization takes place after this time (Banerjee and Bobechko). Overgrowth is useful because most fractures of the femur resist pulling out to length exactly. One centimeter of overriding is ideal (Fig. 17-11).

A short leg is the result of excessive overriding or gross bowing.

A long leg occurs if there is end-to-end apposition

(particularly if this is obtained with intramedullary fixation). Refracture stimulates growth again, and the greatest overgrowth I have seen was due to refracture of an undisplaced fracture.

In a small child, a leg length discrepancy of 1 cm. may produce a limp because the legs are short and the pelvis is narrow. As the child becomes taller the discrepancy becomes insignificant.

Lawyers are very interested in possible sequelae of leg length discrepancy. In reports I usually deal with the problem under these headings.

Limp. 1 cm. and under produces no limp in an adult, but it may in a small child.

Backache. Rush and Steiner measured leg length very accurately in 100 fit soldiers and a hundred soldiers with backache due to no apparent cause (Fig. 17-12). They concluded that a leg length discrepancy exceeding 1 cm. may be a cause of backache.

Osteoarthritis of the Hip. On the side of the long leg the femoral head is less well covered by the acetabulum, a circumstance that may cause osteoarthritis of the hip. The importance of this is unknown.

Spurs

On two occasions I have seen children with butterfly fragments in the vastus lateralis, or under the skin. One of these was so prominent that it was removed. Bony spurs may form that are painful when stuck and may require excision (Fig. 17-13).

Quadriceps Contracture

Quadriceps contracture in children is much less common than in adults. The same management is required.

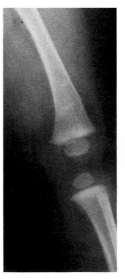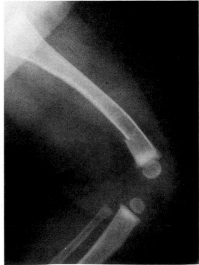

Fig. 17-14. Greenstick fractures in infants may present as sudden refusal to walk.

Fig. 17-15. A stress fracture of the femur.

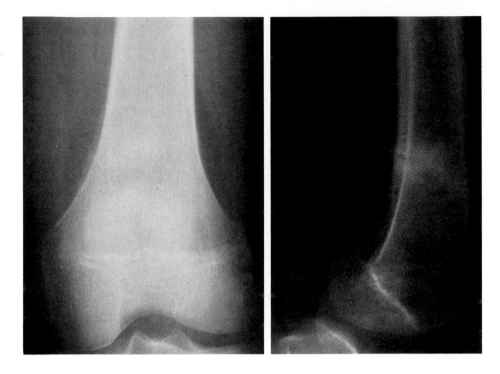

Malrotation

Perhaps because the hip is a ball-and-socket joint, malrotation is an uncommon problem. However, if femoral anteversion is measured after a fracture of the femur, alterations are commonly found. Burton and Fordyce found malrotation in 37 percent—usually loss of external rotation.

The Three-Week-Old Case From Elsewhere General Hospital

Fame may bring you a child whose fracture is healing with gross angulation or overlap. When the fracture is no more than 4 weeks old angulation is easily corrected by manipulation under anesthetic. A rotatory force will loosen things up. After this time manipulation becomes more strenuous but still possible. A drill osteotomy leaves little scar and facilitates correction. Overlap may be corrected by manipulation followed by skeletal traction, with the child at a steep angle. One case was treated effectively using a leg-lengthening apparatus.

SUPRACONDYLAR FRACTURES

Buckle Fractures

Buckle fractures occur in preschool children and in older children with osteoporosis. The young will pro-

tect these fractures themselves. A padded stovepipe cast will allow the older child to move about (Fig. 17-14).

Stress Fractures

Stress fractures should be protected to relieve pain (Fig. 17-15).

Displaced Fractures

If there is sufficient violence to fracture the femur, the periosteum usually tears, allowing the fracture to displace, with the risk of arterial damage. I find a displaced uncomplicated fracture very hard to treat because it is a very unstable fracture and angulates in every direction. Malunion carries the penalty of obvious deformity and prolonged knee stiffness. It is possible to hold position with a Thomas splint, but an inordinate amount of adjustment is required. My solution to this problem is to leave the resident to treat the fracture with the misleading suggestion that the fracture is easy to treat requiring only a little intelligence and aptitude. Only when failure is inconceivable will union in an adequate position be achieved by placing a little pad here or there, adjusting the degree of knee flexion, and fiddling a little bit every day. Some transverse fractures are most easily managed by manipulation and immobilization in a hip spica.

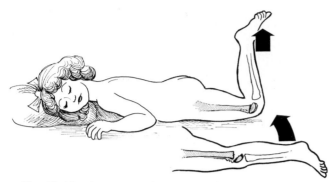

Fig. 17-16. A separated lower femoral epiphysis is usually anteriorly displaced. Gravity will help rather than hinder reduction if the child is prone.

Internal fixation is technically difficult. Steinmann pin traction—with the pin through the distal fragment—does not prevent the fragment from spinning. An efficient and elegant method of treating this rare injury in children has yet to be developed. After the growth plate has closed, there should be no hesitation about inserting an ASIF blade plate.

Separation of the Distal Femoral Epiphysis

In the days when children stole rides on buggies these injuries were common and often accompanied by vascular injury. Children caught the leg in the spokes of the wheel as they fell off. Today, hyperextension injuries of the leg are unusual.

The epiphysis together with a small metaphyseal fragment is usually displaced anteriorly. Reduction is most easily obtained under anesthesia with the child *prone.* Lift up the foot, maintaining traction as the knee is flexed to about 110 degrees, just as you would reduce a supracondylar fracture at the elbow. This is much easier than trying to reduce the fracture with the patient supine. A well-padded above knee cast is applied in this position. After three weeks, flexion is reduced to about 60 degrees, and, three weeks later, the cast can be removed. Movement is usually slow to return (Fig. 17-16).

Rarely, the reduction is unstable. Do not hesitate to insert two Kirschner wires through each condyle into the shaft of the bone. The secure hold will allow the leg to be immobilized in about 30 degrees of flexion.

Fractures due to valgus or varus forces are sustained during football and may masquerade as injuries of the collateral ligaments (see Fig. 2-13); stress films make the distinction. Rest the leg in a splint until the swelling recedes before applying a stovepipe cast.

Intraarticular fractures of the distal femur are discussed in the knee section.

The following story was published over a hundred years ago:

SENTENCE ON A FRENCH BONE-SETTER. On August 26th, 1859, an infant aged 15 months, in the department of Mayence in France, fell from the arms of a little girl who was carrying it. A bone-setter, named Lefaux, a farmer, was called in. He declared the thigh to be fractured, employed extension and violent pressure, and, after wrapping the thigh in a handkerchief soaked in soap and water, he left, promising to return in a fortnight, but first receiving a fee of sixteen *francs.* At the end of the fortnight, he did not come, and messages were sent to him in vain. In the meantime, a large abscess had formed, and the ends of the bone had become exposed. A medical man was then called in, and succeeded in procuring union of the bone only at the end of five months, and at the expense of considerable shortening of the limb. An action was brought by the father of the child against Lefaux; who, on February 25th, was condemned to a fortnight's imprisonment, to a fine of two hundred *francs,* and to the payment of a thousand *francs* damages to the child, and the expenses to which the father had been put in the course of the illness.

BIBLIOGRAPHY

Femoral Shaft

Banerjee, S., and Bobechko, W. P.: Growth acceleration after femoral shaft fracture in children. Canadian J. Surg., [In Press]

Barfod, B., and Christensen, J.: Fractures of the femoral shaft in children with special reference to subsequent overgrowth. Acta Chir. Scand., *116:* 235, 1959

Burton, V. W., and Fordyce, A. J. W.: Immobilization of femoral shaft fractures in children aged 2–10 years. Injury, *4:* 47, 1973

Burwell, H. N.: Fractures of the femoral shaft in children. Postgrad. Med. J., *45:* 617, 1969

Griffin, P. P., Anderson, M., and Green, W. T.: Fractures of the shaft of the femur. Orthop. Clin. N. Amer., *3:* 213, 1972

Irani, R. N., Nicholson, J. T., and Chung, S. M. K.: Treatment of femoral fractures in children by immediate spica immobilization. J. Bone Joint Surg., *52A:* 1567, 1972

Judet, J., and Judet, R.: Traitement des fractures de cuisse chez l'enfant. Rev. Chir. Orthop., *39:* 658, 1953

Rush, W. A., and Steiner, H. A.: A study of lower extremity length inequality. Amer. J. Roent., *56:* 616, 1946

18

Knee Joint

When an old lady injures her knee, she is most likely to sustain a bumper fracture. A football-playing undergraduate tears a cartilage or ligament. Children are spared most of these injuries because:

1. Articular cartilage and growth cartilage are thick and absorb energy which otherwise may injure bone or ligament.
2. Ligaments are stronger than growth plates. Epiphyseal separations replace ligamentous disruption.
3. Osteoporosis comes later in life.

The pattern of children's injuries is different. For example, if mother says the child's leg was bent through a right angle or that she heard it crack, you must find something amiss. It is most unlikely to be a ligamentous tear; much more likely it is a spontaneously reduced separation of the femoral epiphysis which may show only on stress films (Fig. 2-13).

Always take obliques and skyline radiographs (even an arthrogram) if there are clinical signs of a major injury without radiographic confirmation on the initial pair of films. Unfortunately arthroscopy does not help when the knee is full of blood. It is impossible to see anything but blood.

The following intraarticular injuries are seen in children.

TRAUMATIC HEMARTHROSIS

Traumatic hemarthrosis is an unsatisfactory diagnosis; translated, it means "something is injured in this bloody joint and I don't know what it is." After you have tested ligaments, patellar stability, and menisci, and studied oblique films and stress films, you will still find many patients who fall into this category. Aspirate the hemarthrosis if it is tense and painful; fat in the aspirate suggests a fracture. Apply a Robert Jones bandage, send the patient, on crutches, to physiotherapy for isometric quadriceps exercises. If you were right in concluding that the injury is no more than a synovial tear they will be well again within a month.

TIBIAL SPINE

Injuries that rupture the anterior cruciate ligament of an adult will avulse the tibial spine of a child. The spine repairs by bone when reduced and yields much better results than a complete tear of the ligament (Fig. 18-1). The majority of fractures are produced in road accidents, particularly falls from bicycles. If a child presents with a swollen knee after falling from a bicycle he should be presumed to have a fracture of the tibial spine until proved otherwise.

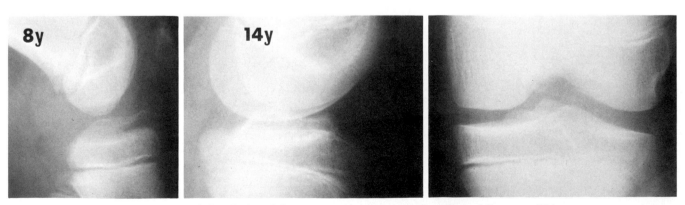

Fig. 18-1. Partially displaced fracture of the tibial spine in a boy of 8 years. This was reduced by extending the knee. Six years later the knee is clinically normal, but the tibial spine is large, and the medial tibial plateau has a turret.

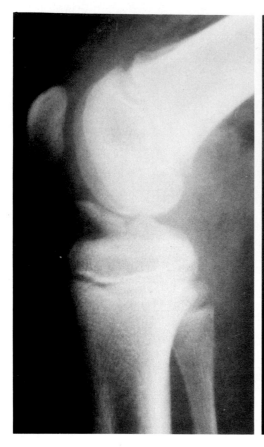
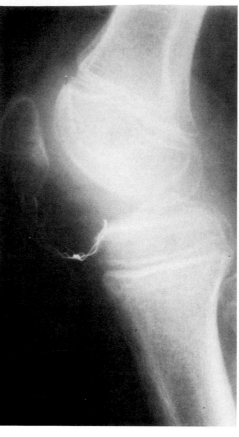

Fig. 18-2. Complete fracture of the tibial spine. Closed reduction failed. At open reduction holes were drilled through the epiphysis (avoiding the plate) to hold the fragment in place. The wires later required removal. Boy aged 9 years.

Some patients are unaware that anything is seriously wrong until the following day, when the hemarthrosis has become tense and painful. The radiological diagnosis is easy. But the radiograph only shows a little of the damage. Above the small ossific spine are wide radiolucent wings of articular cartilage from the weight-bearing surface of the tibia. Much more than the spine is lifted up. The fragment is usually partially detached. The anterior part lifts; the posterior part hinges. The femoral condyles will usually ram the

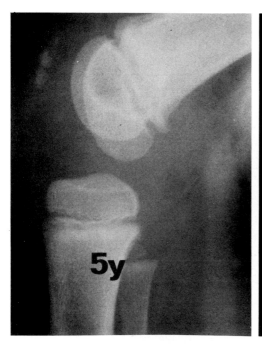
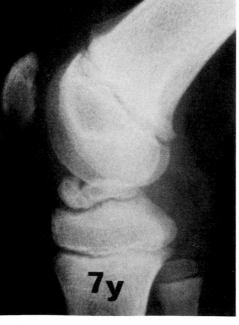

Fig. 18-3. At the age of 5, this boy sustained a traumatic hemarthrosis. The roentgenogram was interpreted as normal. He was never able to extend the knee fully, and a roentgenogram made 2 years later shows the reason: a displaced ununited fracture of the tibial spine. This was excised with good result. At the time of the initial injury the cartilage model of the tibial spine was avulsed. Could this have been diagnosed by testing the range of movement of the knee?

Fig. 18-4. Acute dislocation of the patella. Usually the dislocation reduces before the radiograph is taken. Girl aged 13 years.

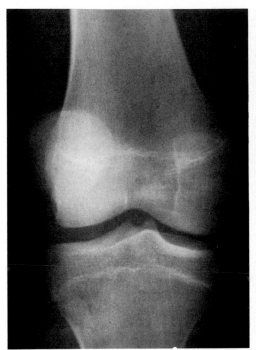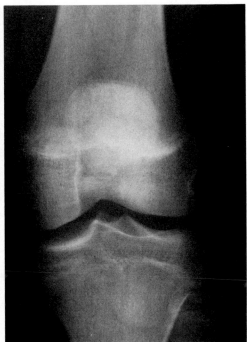

wings of articular cartilage back into position when the knee is extended. When the fragment is completely detached, interposed meniscus or rotation of the fragment may prevent closed reduction.

In our series of 15 patients with this injury, eight fractures were reduced by extension of the knee (often accompanied by aspiration), usually under anesthesia, and immobilization in a stovepipe cast for about 4 to 6 weeks.

Five out of 15 were treated by open reduction, because the fractures could not be reduced by closed means. The knee is opened through a medial parapatellar incision. Two holes are drilled through the epiphysis, and the fragment is tied down (Fig. 18-2). Closed reduction had failed in one patient because the medial meniscus was trapped in the fracture and in another because the fragment had rotated. Good results were obtained.

Two patients who were left unreduced lost full extension. The diagnosis was missed in one other patient (Fig. 18-3).

DISLOCATION OF THE PATELLA

In some children dislocation of the patella is an episode in the history of recurrent dislocation. In others, it is the result of injury (Fig. 18-4). Most dislocations are reduced before the child comes to hospital, either spontaneously or by the child or a buddy. Certain

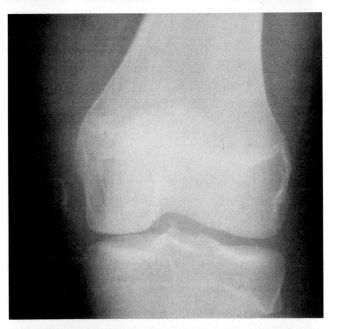

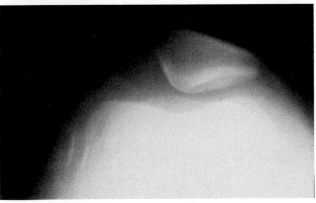

Fig. 18-5. Osteochondral fragment associated with acute dislocation of the patella. This was removed at arthrotomy.

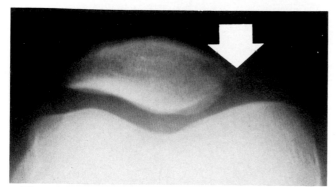

Fig. 18-6. New bone along the medial border of the patella.

diagnosis is not always easy. The signs are hemarthrosis, tenderness along the medial border of the patella, and increased lateral movement of the patella.

Always look for a loose fragment knocked off the lateral femoral condyle or medial aspect of the patella during the process of recoil (Fig. 18-5). Boys produce fragments more often than girls. If a loose fragment is present it should usually be removed. Occasionally, a large fragment merits replacement with Smillie pins or ASIF small fragment screws.

First Dislocations

There is much argument about the treatment of first dislocations. Should they be managed by immobilization in extension for 4 weeks, or should they be repaired surgically? We have always been conservative, aspirating the effusion and applying a Robert Jones bandage reinforced with medial and lateral slabs, and the results have been satisfactory. If radiographs are taken some weeks after injury, new bone can be seen along the medial border of the patella on the skyline view (Fig. 18-6). Others have argued in favor of repairing first dislocations when there is arthrographic evidence of a capsular tear. I have been unable to trace any review comparing operative with nonoperative methods. It is our impression that a dramatic acute dislocation occurs in a normal knee, and the dislocation does not recur. Recurrent dislocation, on the other hand, begins "not with a bang but a whimper," because the cause is anatomical and not traumatic.

Recurrent Dislocations

Recurrent dislocations in growing children should be managed by semitendinosus tenodesis (Baker et al.). This is preferable to transfer of the tibial tubercle, which frequently produces genu recurvatum due to growth arrest of the anterior part of the tibia. Transfer of the tendon of semitendinosus into the patella has excellent results.

FRACTURES OF PATELLA

These are unusual and are often comminuted. In older children some transverse fractures have been treated by the ASIF technique (parallel Kirschner wires and a tension band), but the majority are not sufficiently displaced to require anything more than aspiration of a tense effusion and a Jones bandage reinforced with medial and lateral slabs. After a week or two, this is

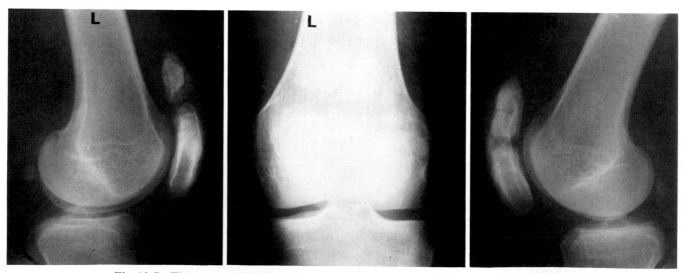

Fig. 18-7. The result of fractures of the patellae in a boy aged 2 years when he was dragged on his knees behind a milk van losing much of the skin off his knees. At the age of 16 both patellae were enormous, and painful. A bilateral patellectomy has produced a good result.

Fig. 18-8. Separation of the posterior part of the femoral condyle. This is an unstable injury. It was held with threaded Steinmann pins inserted through the nonarticular surface of the femur. Girl aged 14 years.

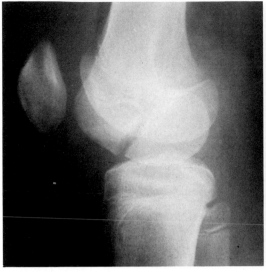
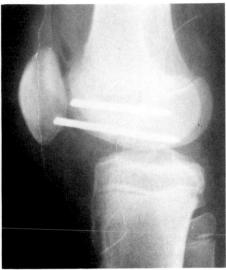

changed to a cast. Total immobilization time need not exceed 4 weeks. Occasionally marked overgrowth follows injury in infancy (Fig. 18-7). Excision is occasionally indicated.

A bipartite patella is occasionally confused with a fracture. The ossicle is always in the upper outer quadrant, has rounded edges, and is not tender.

INTRAARTICULAR FRACTURES OF THE FEMUR

The posterior part of a femoral condyle may be displaced. This may be replaced with a compression screw; through a long posterolateral approach one of the heads of gastrocnemius is lifted from the femur. The fragment must be replaced without devascularizing it (Fig. 18-8). Type III injuries are unusual and should be anatomically reduced with a transepiphyseal screw. Type IV injuries will produce partial growth arrest and a disturbed joint if not reduced and held with internal fixation (Figs. 18-9 and 18-10).

FRACTURES OF THE TIBIAL PLATEAU

Tibial plateau fractures are rare, except in children with osteoporosis. Oblique radiographs may be re-

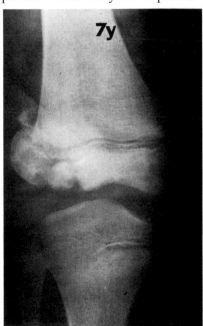
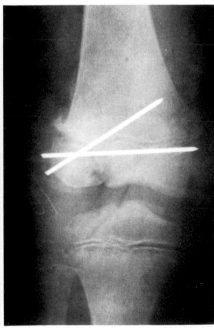
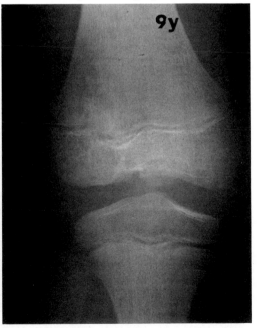

Fig. 18-9. Comminuted Type IV injury. Without open reduction this would certainly have undergone growth arrest. Two years later the knee is slightly enlarged but functions well. Some crushing of the growth plate must have occurred but slight enough for growth to continue. (Courtesy Dr. T. Barrington)

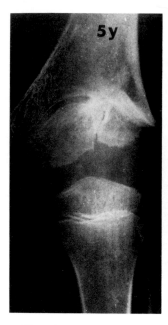 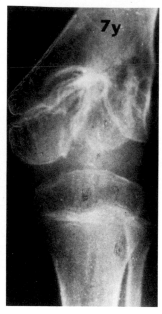

Fig. 18-10.   Neglected Type IV injury sustained at age 2½ years.   A bony bridge between epiphysis and metaphysis partially arrests growth.   (Courtesy Dr. Lipmann Kessel, who collected it from a source he was sworn not to divulge)

quired to see these fractures; gentle stress examination films under anesthesia and arthrography may assist in assessment.   Aspiration eases pain.   Protection in a three-point molded stovepipe cylinder for 6 to 8 weeks has been sufficient, in my slight experience.   Warn the parents to expect a slight valgus deformity (Fig. 18-11).

AVULSION OF THE TIBIAL TUBERCLE

This injury occurs in soccer playing boys aged between 14 and 16 years.   Soccer is not popular in

Fig. 18-11.   An unusual Type V injury of the tibial plateau.   Initially this was thought to be an avulsed tibial spine. When the medial tibial plateau failed to grow the original films were reviewed.   The medial plateau had been depressed and crushed.   This child will require corrective osteotomy and leg equalization procedures.

Toronto, and this may be the reason I have never seen this injury.   Watson-Jones described 3 types:

Type I.   The tubercle is hinged up without displacement of the proximal base.   Closed reduction and a stovepipe cast is sufficient treatment.

Type II.   A small portion of the tubercle is avulsed and retracts proximally.

Type III.   The tubercle, together with a portion of the articular surface of the tibia, is displaced.

Hand et al. report good results from open reduction and internal fixation of Types II and III.   Pins, wires, or screws can be used with equally good effect.

LIGAMENTOUS AND CAPSULAR INJURIES

Complete ligamentous disruption occurs only after growth plate closure.   However, many skiing children with torsional fractures of the tibia complain of pain and tenderness along the medial joint line, probably an indication of partial injury of the medial collateral ligament.   When the cast is removed the knee is asymptomatic.   This follows the general rule that torsional fractures anywhere are accompanied by irritability of the neighboring joint.

THE MENISCUS IN CHILDHOOD*

Meniscal pathology is the second most frequent indication for arthrotomy in the growing child.   (Patellar stabilization is the most common.)   In the past 10 years at H.S.C., 96 meniscectomies were performed for torn and discoid menisci.

The typical patient was a 12 or 13-year-old athletic boy with a history of sport trauma.   Girls were not immune to meniscal problems, but more often had patellofemoral pathology.   Tears presented with a history of 8 to 9 months; discoid menisci had been troublesome for years.   Specific complaints, such as buckling and locking, occurred in a minority.   Physical examina-

*The following two sections were contributed by Dr. Robert McMurtry.

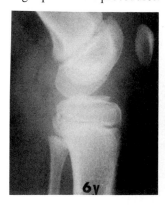 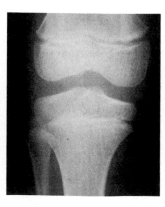 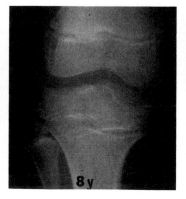 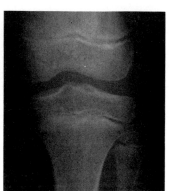

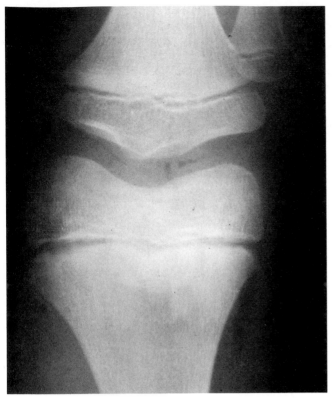

Fig. 18-12. No one suspected that a small laceration over the front of the knee was deep. But the air arthrogram effect on a routine film indicates a penetrating injury.

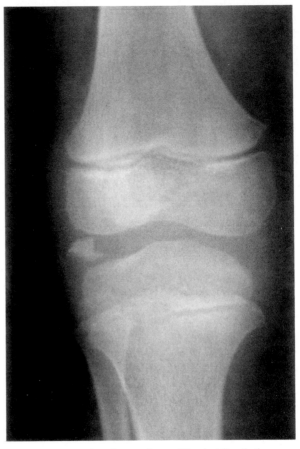

Fig. 18-13. Another laceration. The habit of always requesting a radiograph resulted in the disclosure of a piece of lead glass.

tion proved more useful. Quadriceps wasting and joint line tenderness were seen in most, but the traditional signs, McMurray's locking and effusion, were seen in less than half.

Diagnosis by implication was difficult. Errors, we feel, are best avoided by deferring judgment in acutely injured knees and by the use of arthrography. The latter achieves 80 to 90 percent accuracy. Additional information may be gained from arthroscopy. This tool in the hands of the experienced is nearly as good as arthrotomy and carries considerably less morbidity.

Fig. 18-14. This girl had no idea there was a needle in her knee. Presumably it had entered while she was crawling around the floor. Removal can be difficult when the needle lies hidden under a meniscus.

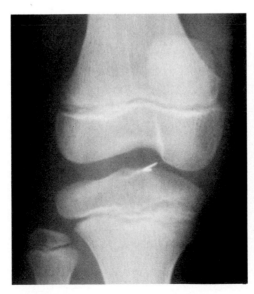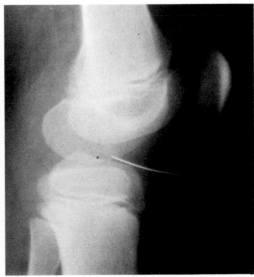

Treatment

With an established diagnosis of a torn meniscus, removal is warranted. A word of caution: hypermobile menisci or discoid menisci should be left in until a tear and significant disturbance of function is proven. At surgery much the same type of tear seen in adults can be anticipated, but a bucket-handle tear is more frequent in children. Discoid menisci account for one-third of our meniscectomies. Usually they are not a problem until they tear, which they are more prone to do than a normal semilunar meniscus.

We have conducted studies of late embryonic and fetal knees and concluded, as have others, that a discoid meniscus is *not* a persistence of a normal stage in fetal development.

The outcome of meniscectomy for established tears in children is good. Our long-term follow-up review of 61 knees indicated that most had excellent results. Infection did not occur, nor did neuromata or numbness. Quadriceps rehabilitation was shown to appreciably reduce postoperative morbidity.

In summary, meniscal problems do occur in children, but diagnosis can be elusive. Appropriate treatment yields very good results.

LOCKING

The hallmark of a locked knee is incomplete extension due to mechanical obstruction. True locking, however, must be distinguished from apparent locking.

Intraarticular mechanical obstruction is due to bone, cartilage, or both, being displaced and jamming between the articulating surfaces of the femur and tibia. This may occur with a dislocated patella which has caused an osteochondral fracture; after reduction, full extension is not restored. Torn meniscus and other internal derangements also occur, but less commonly.

Apparent locking is characterized by painful resistance to extension due to hamstring spasm. The distinction between true and apparent locking can only be established by relieving pain so that the patient can relax. Generally this requires traction, time, and sedation, or even anesthesia.

"Benign locking of childhood" is a condition we have confronted quite often. It is the commonest cause of "locking" in children under the age of 10 years. There is a vague history of trauma after which the child limps about on a flexed knee. The only physical sign is block to full extension. After a few days in traction, full extension returns, and the child becomes normal again. The cause is unknown.

SUBLUXATION OF THE PROXIMAL TIBIOFIBULAR JOINT

The proximal tibiofibular joint may be disrupted as an isolated injury or in association with a fracture of the tibia. Ogden reviews this subject well. As in disruption of the sternoclavicular joint, the diagnosis is easily overlooked if too much reliance is placed on radiographs. Closed reduction is usually successful.

PUNCTURE WOUNDS AND FOREIGN BODIES

Hopefully most physicians will debride, irrigate, and close obvious open knee injuries. But some are easily missed. The knee is a subcutaneous joint. Small cuts may enter the knee; the wise emergency surgeon radiographs these for intraarticular air to make the diagnosis. Children also drive needles into their knees as they creep about on the broadloom (Figs. 18-12 to 18-14).

BIBLIOGRAPHY

Abrams, R. C.: Meniscal lesions of the knee in young children. J. Bone Joint Surg., *39A:* 194, 1957

Baker, R. H., Carroll, N., Dewar, F. P., and Hall, J. E.: The semitendinosus tenodesis for recurrent dislocation of the patella. J. Bone Joint Surg., *54B:* 103, 1972

Hand, W. L., Hand, C. R., and Dunn, A. N.: Avulsion fractures of the tibial tubercle. J. Bone Joint Surg., *53A:* 1579, 1971

Myers, M. H., and McKeever, F. M.: Fracture of the intercondylar eminence of the tibia. J. Bone Joint Surg., *41A:* 209, 1959

Ogden, J. A.: Subluxation and dislocation of the proximal tibiofibular joint. J. Bone Joint Surg., *56A:* 145, 1974

Roth, P.: Fracture of the spine of the tibia. J. Bone Joint Surg., *29:* 509, 1928

19

Tibia

These fractures heal so much more readily in children than in adults that they should be a joy to treat. The majority of children have a cast applied without an anesthetic and only require a pair of crutches, a lift on the shoe, and a note to arrange transportation to school. However, there is more variation to these fractures than is generally realized. If foresight is to be used to prevent problems, the fracture should be classified first. The classification scheme for proximal tibial injuries is depicted in Figure 19-1.

PROXIMAL GROWTH PLATE INJURIES

Growth plate injuries are more common in the distal femur than in the proximal tibia, because of the arrangement of the ligaments. The medial collateral ligament of the knee is attached to the tibial *metaphysis* and the femoral *epiphysis,* protecting the tibial growth plate from valgus injuries. Bohler, in 1951, could trace only 12 authentic cases of separation of the proximal tibial epiphysis in world literature. The rarity of the injury is fortunate because 2 of the 3 separated epiphyses at our hospital produced vascular problems due to the proximity of the popliteal trifurcation.

Stress views are sometimes needed to demonstrate these injuries (Fig. 19-2). The separations unite quickly.

PROXIMAL METAPHYSEAL FRACTURES

Masquerading as innocent little cracks with no particular reputation for evil, proximal metaphyseal fractures are among the worst. In the course of treating about 1000 tibial fractures in children we have found that fractures in this region have been responsible for amputation (a late result of a Volkmann's ischemia) and the only corrective osteotomies. Two distinct types of fracture occur in this region.

Arterial Hazard Fracture

The anterior tibial artery passes over the proximal

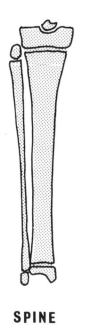 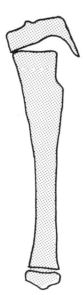 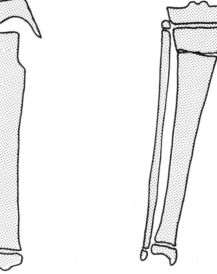 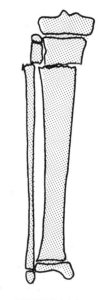

SPINE   **TYPE 1**   **VALGUS GREENSTICK**   **ARTERIAL**

Fig. 19-1. Classification of high tibial fractures.

189

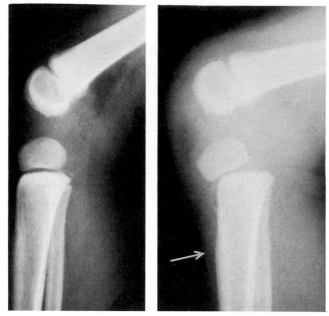

Fig. 19-2. Stress films were required to demonstrate this injury.

edge of the interosseous membrane into the anterior compartment and is closely applied to the tibia (Fig. 19-3). Because of this fixed position, the artery may be compressed, stretched, or torn. If it is stretched, the posterior tibial artery may also be occluded. The initial sign of vascular damage may be a cold, pale, pulseless leg that in about an hour, becomes anesthetic and

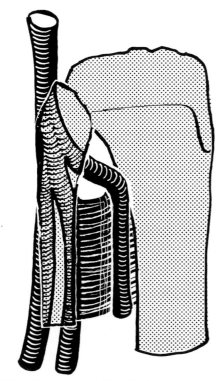

Fig. 19-3. Fractures of the tibial metaphysis can easily injure the trifurcation.

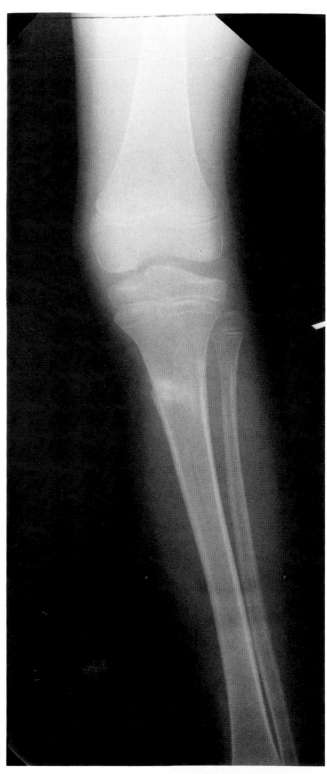

Fig. 19-4. The fracture of the proximal tibial metaphysis was not reduced, and union was slow. Initial deformity and overgrowth have produced marked valgus deformity. This 9-year-old boy may well require osteotomy.

paralyzed. Muscle ischemia alone is less dramatic; a warm skin has misled many.

When there is a high fracture of the fibula, the temp-

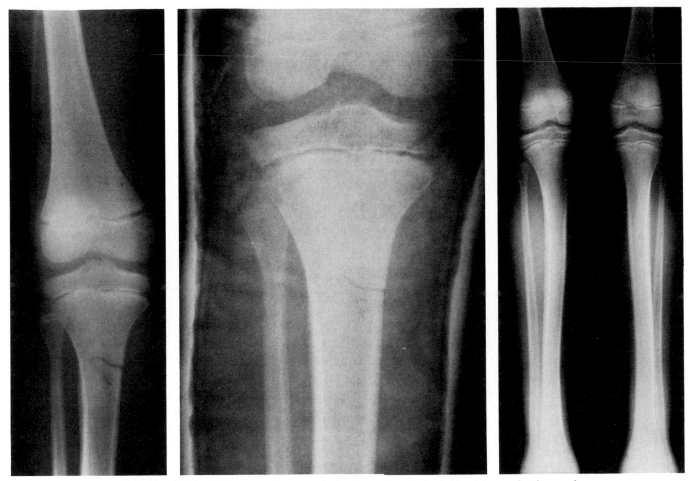

Fig. 19-5. This degree of valgus angulation is easily overlooked. After reduction under anesthesia the position is improved. Four years later the right tibia has slight valgus deformity and is slightly longer.

tation to blame the neurological signs of ischemia on local lateral popliteal nerve damage should be resisted. Treatment is urgent. Realignment of displacement and angulation may restore the circulation. If not, the vessels must be explored. Ideally, a vascular surgeon and an orthopaedic surgeon should collaborate.

Valgus Greenstick Fracture

In children between the ages of 3 and 10 years, greenstick fractures are occasionally seen. The cortex is slightly open on the medial side of the tibia. On radiographs, the amount of angulation is very unimpressive, and most of these fractures are accepted as undisplaced and casted in situ. When the cast is removed an unacceptable degree of knock-knee comes as an unpleasant surprise (Fig. 19-4). It does not improve with time. But if anyone had taken the trouble to look at the leg itself initially in the fully extended position, the deformity would have been apparent. Unfortunately, children hold the injured leg flexed, and in the flexed position the deformity is not apparent. The deformity

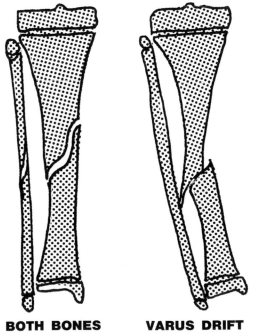

BOTH BONES   **VARUS DRIFT**

Fig. 19-6. In children the fibula is commonly intact.

Fig. 19-8. (*Opposite*) Most beginners, believing that the leg should look straight, produce valgus deformity. The cast should have a concave medial border. The medial part of gastrocnemius is mobile, so the cast should be molded to the medial border of the tibia. The muscles of the lateral compartment are less mobile. Feel this for yourself.

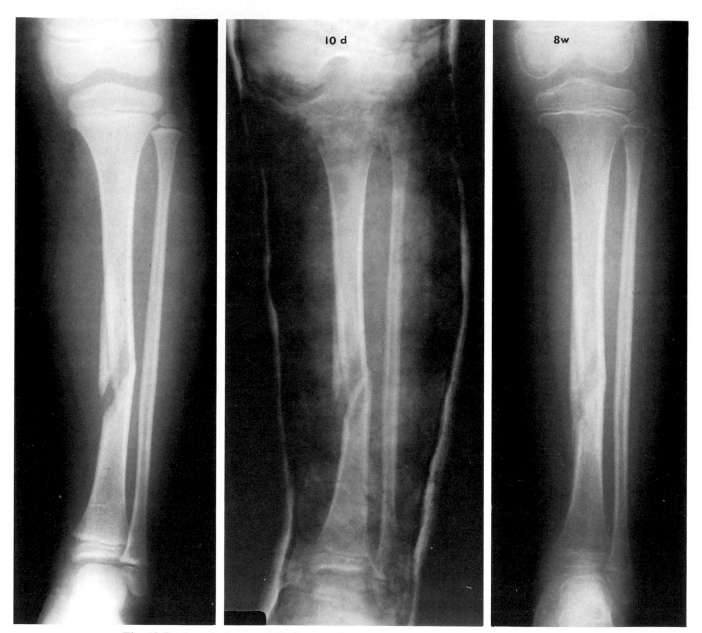

Fig. 19-7. A typical varus drift fracture due to an intact fibula. An artless cast has done nothing to help. A new cast with valgus molding was applied under anesthesia to produce a good result.

should be corrected under anesthesia, and the leg should be immobilized in extension with varus molding (Fig. 19-5). Pollen (1973) advises wedging the cast.

Taylor (1963) drew attention to this injury and suggested that valgus was due to the overgrowth of the tibia (because of fracture hyperemia) while the intact fibula acted as a tether. Overgrowth plays a part, but it has been our experience that if the fracture is reduced, the leg remains straight.

Osteotomy to correct the established deformity has

Fig. 19-9. (*Opposite*) This high oblique fracture in a child with transient decerebrate rigidity was difficult to control. Pins held the position firmly with the leg in slight varus. Despite this precaution, overgrowth has produced slight valgus.

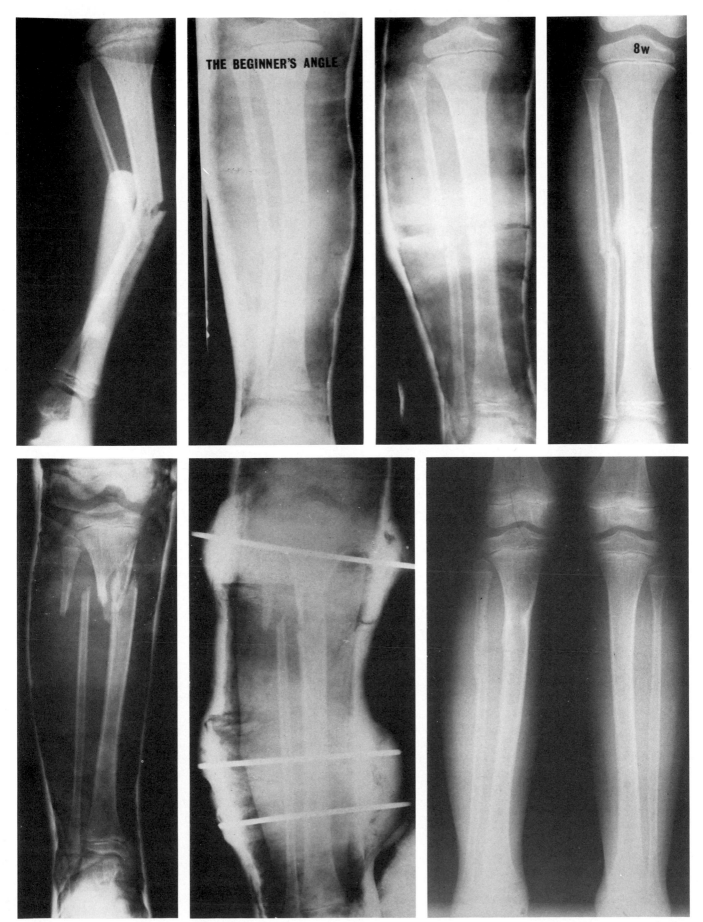

THE BEGINNER'S ANGLE

8w

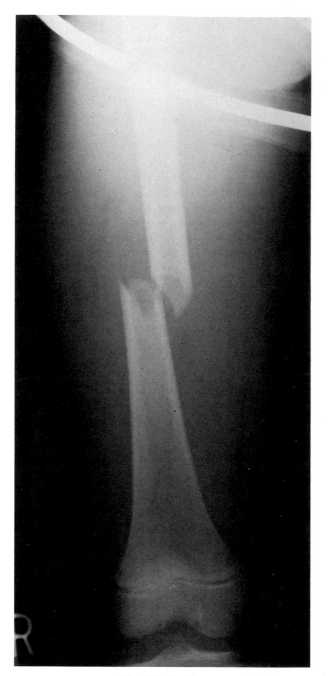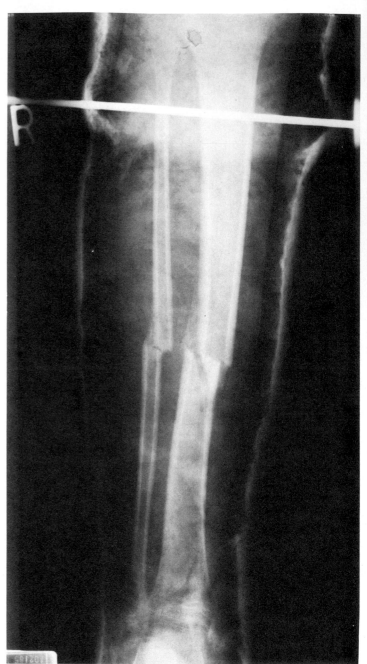

Fig. 19-10. Fracture of the femur and tibia in the same leg. Skeletal traction is applied through a tibial pin placed distally enough to avoid the growing tibial tubercle. A Thomas splint controls the femoral fracture, and a below-knee cast incorporated around the pin controls the tibial fracture. A hip spica was applied at 4 weeks and the child went home. Orthoroentgenogram (*opposite*) at 1 year shows that the right leg is 3 mm. short.

been only moderately successful. The correction has been inadequate in some, and these children have required a second osteotomy. The fibula should be divided.

DIAPHYSEAL FRACTURES

Diaphyseal fractures are common and easy to treat in children. Last year, for example, we treated 101 fractures of the tibia. In the majority of children (70 percent) the fibula was intact (Fig. 19-6).

Most of the fractures (80 percent) were stable and undisplaced, because periosteum is more resilient than bone in a child; in the adult, bone is stronger than periosteum, so that the periosteum is almost always torn when the bone is broken. In a child, the recoil of the

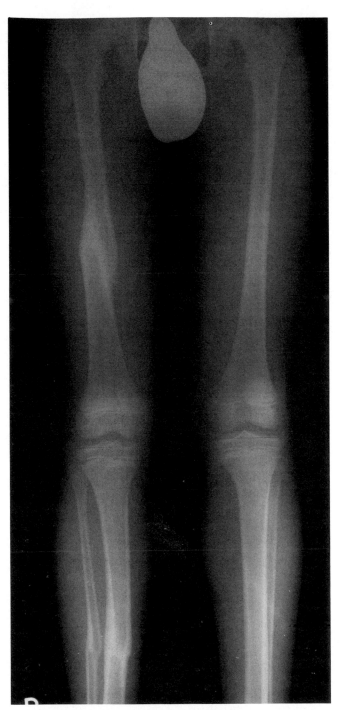

Fig. 19-10. *Continued.*

by molding the cast, but a few children with gross displacement required an anesthetic. Only 5 percent of children redisplaced in the cast and required further correction. Only 10 percent of children were admitted.

Children of all ages were seen: babies who had been dropped, infants who had fallen down stairs, teenagers injured in sports or road accidents.

Treatment

Because a fracture of the child's tibia unites certainly and quickly and does not lead to knee stiffness, we use an above-knee cast and do not feel bound to encourage early weight bearing. Only when reduction is necessary do we admit these children to hospital.

Ensure that the rotation is correct; in very young children we have done this by applying a cast with the knee flexed to 90 degrees and ensuring that the alignment of the feet is symmetrical. This will certainly prevent weight bearing. For stable fractures we apply a cast with the knee slightly flexed and expect to apply a walking heel after a week or two. A cast change is seldom needed. The cast is removed after about 6 to 8 weeks; but in infants the bone unites in 2 to 3 weeks while in some teenagers it will take about 10 to 12 weeks.

When the cast is removed some children will start to walk unaided immediately, but others need crutches for a week or two. Leave the children to decide for themselves.

A limp, due to calf wasting, persists for several months after the cast is removed. Warn the parents about this to save many anxious phone calls.

There is almost no place for open reduction. "The trouble with the tibia," said someone, "is that it is so subcutaneous that it's easily opened to abuse." During the past 8 years I can trace only three patients who have been treated with internal fixation; one had a gross degloving injury of the leg with an unstable fracture. Fixed with two screws, he had a superb result, but the bone fractured through a screw hole 6 years later. Another, with much shortening, was referred late; open reduction and internal fixation was selected to improve the position. The third patient was an Olympic skier with bilateral oblique fractures which, in some way, were thought to justify a single screw in each tibia. Despite much shaking of heads, he made an excellent recovery and was skiing in 9 weeks!

COMMON VARIATIONS

The Intact Fibula

The fibula is a bone that will bend without obvious fracture. If you doubt this, radiograph the normal leg when next you see a child with an angulated fracture

intact periosteum holds the fracture in good position so that the majority of fractures can be casted without an anesthetic and without hospital admission. Only one child, who had been sent home, required admission the next day because of edema.

The remaining 20 percent of children had displacement that required correction. Displacement was much more common when both bones were fractured than when the fibula was intact (50 percent compared with 5 percent). The displacement could often be corrected

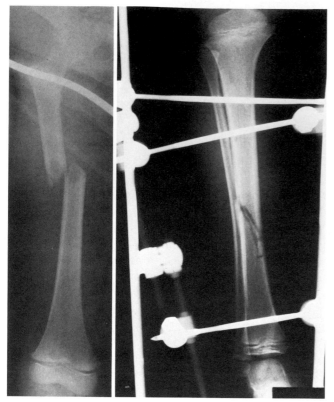

Fig. 19-11. This seven-year-old cycled into the side of a bus. The back wheels went over this leg. The accident was so sudden that the driver did not have time to apply the brakes sparing the boy an avulsed, degloved flap. The fracture of the tibia was open and unstable. He was treated by closing the wound with a skin graft over a rotated muscle flap and with Roger Anderson apparatus (to which traction was applied to control the femur). The arrangement was so rigid and permitted such ready inspection of the skin that his care was free of anxieties.

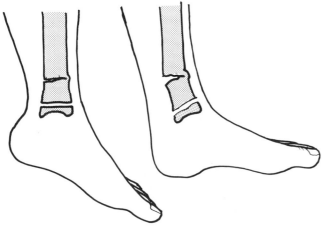

Fig. 19-12. Robert Gillespie's fracture. Placing a fracture of this type in a cast with the ankle at a right angle produces deformity.

of the tibia alone, and compare the shape of the fibula on each side. Fracture of the tibia in children is more commonly associated with an intact, if bent, fibula than with a fractured fibula.

The intact fibula struts the bone ends apart. Varus deformity with posterior bowing is a common sequel unless the cast is molded into valgus (Fig. 19-7). The bowing may not be apparent in initial films but commonly develops in the course of 2 or 3 weeks if the cast is not suitably molded. It is a deformity more easily prevented than corrected.

Fractures of the Tibia and Fibula

Longitudinal stability can be achieved in almost all fractures involving both bones of the leg, because segmental fractures, butterfly fragments, and comminution are infrequent in children. Usually the bone ends can be locked, leaving only the problem of angulation and rotation to manage (Fig. 19-8). A good position can usually be obtained. But, if a good position cannot be obtained initially, or if the fracture slips, it is easy to correct rotation and angulation at 2 to 3 weeks when the fracture is sticky. If longitudinal instability is a problem, it is most easily controlled with Steinmann pins above and below the fracture, incorporated in the cast (Fig. 19-9). Leg lengthening apparatus has been used for children who presented late with more than a centimeter of shortening.

The Limping Infant

Children under the age of 2 years may present with a painful limp due to a healing fracture a week old. Three per cent of our fractures last year were in this category. Apply a cast for a week or two if this appears helpful.

UNCOMMON VARIATIONS

During the past 8 years we have admitted 143 children with fractures of the tibia. Although there are no exact figures for the total number of fractures treated, by extrapolation, these represent the problems from about 1,000 injuries.

Open Fractures

Open fractures (2.3 percent of all fractures) are usually the result of being hit by a car. The wounds are usually small and represent punctures from within. They are easily debrided and we have had no infection whether antibiotics were used or not. Three patients had runover injuries of the foot; two required skin grafting; and the third required Syme's amputation.

Associated Injuries

Head injuries (2.8 percent)—fractures of other bones, and visceral injuries occur but do not influence treatment except for—

Fractures of the Femur and the Tibia in One Leg (0.6 percent)

A child usually sustains fractures of the tibia and femur in an auto wreck. Half of the children had parents killed in the accident, and this circumstance provided a major challenge in management. Five of the 6 patients had major wounds elsewhere (Figs. 19-10, 19-11).

The middle fragment must be held with a pin through which traction can be applied to the femoral fracture while the tibial fracture is held in a cast. Where should the pin go? There is no doubt in my mind that the pin should go in the tibia. The pin can easily be incorporated with a below-knee cast. Two out of three femoral pins allowed the tibial fracture to slip, and one of these children needed osteotomy for knock-knee deformity. Three out of three tibial pins were satisfactory.

Pathological Fractures (0.4 percent)

Local lesions in this series included chronic osteomyelitis, nonossifying fibroma, and an undiagnosed area of sclerosis. Not included, though quite common, were fractures in osteogenesis imperfecta, meningomyelocele, polio, and muscular dystrophy.

Miscellaneous Associations

Battered babies (0.2 percent). The signs closely mimic those of osteomyelitis.

Coagulopathy (0.2 percent). If replacement therapy is provided for the first few days, the fractures heal normally. One boy had trouble with recurrent knee effusions afterward.

COMPLICATIONS AND PROBLEMS

Vascular Problems

We have not encountered vascular problems with diaphyseal fractures. Ischemia has only occurred with injuries through the proximal growth plate or metaphysis. But that does not stop us looking for it.

Nerve Palsies

If the cast is tight over the fibular head, a lateral popliteal nerve palsy may occur. Avoid this with padding.

Remanipulation

Some fractures will slip in the cast and require correction (3 percent). Angulation is easily corrected, but serious loss of length is more difficult. The choice lies between the use of a leg lengthening apparatus and open reduction with internal fixation.

ROBERT GILLESPIE'S FRACTURE OF THE DISTAL TIBIAL DIAPHYSIS

This little-known fracture is worth recognizing, as it is a potential source of grief. The injury appears to result from landing on a dorsiflexed foot. The anterior border of the tibia is crumpled while the posterior surface opens, producing slight posterior angulation. Seemingly innocent at first, by the time the cast is removed the angulation has increased to an unacceptable degree. Cast the leg with the foot in equinus to prevent this problem (Fig. 19-12).

METAPHYSEAL FRACTURES

Buckle fractures occur in the young child or the osteoporotic older child. It is customary to cast these for about 4 to 6 weeks.

Ski boot fractures occur at the level of the top of the boot. These are compression failures of bone. There may be some comminution, but the periosteum is intact so that displacement is slight and easily held in a cast.

BIBLIOGRAPHY

Bohler, L.: The treatment of fractures. New York, Grune & Stratton, 1956

Haas, L. M., and Staple, T. W.: Arterial injuries associated with fractures of the proximal tibia following blunt trauma. Southern Med. J., *62:* 1439, 1969

Jackson, D. W., and Cozen, L.: Genu Valgum as a Complication of Proximal Tibial Metaphyseal Fractures in Children. J. Bone Joint Surg., 53A: 1571, 1971

Salter, R. B., and Best, T.: The pathogenesis and prevention of valgus deformity following fractures of the proximal metaphyseal region of the tibia in children. J. Bone Joint Surg., 55A: 1324, 1973

Steel, H. H., Sandrow, R. E., and Sullivan, P. D.: Complications of tibial osteotomy in children for genu varum or valgum. J. Bone Joint Surg., 53A: 1629, 1971

Taylor, S. L.: Tibial overgrowth: a cause of genu valgum. J. Bone Joint Surg., 45A: 659, 1963

20

Ankle

In 1898 John Poland made an extensive study of epiphyseal separations about the ankle. He noted that injuries in children differed from those in adults in three important ways.

1. The growth plate forms a plane of weakness directing fracture lines in patterns different from those of adults.

2. Ligaments are stronger than bone so that ligamentous injuries are almost unknown.

3. Certain injuries will affect growth.

To Poland's observations the following should be added:

4. Fractures rarely disturb the talotibial relationship, so that persistent disability due to incongruity is unusual (Fig. 20-1).

5. From the age of 14 to 15 years onward, when the growth plate has closed, the adult pattern of fractures emerges.

APPLIED ANATOMY

The three major groups of ligaments are each attached to an epiphysis (Fig. 20-2). When the foot is

Child **Adult**

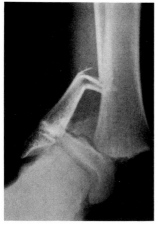 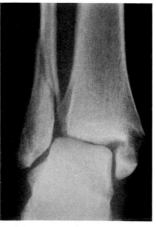

Fig. 20-1. The ankle joint is less often disrupted in children (*left*) than in adults (*right*).

Dr. Alex Finsterbush did much of the work for this chapter and assisted with the follow-up review on which it is based.

forced into an abnormal position, tension and compression forces are generated. The structure of the ankle appears to permit tension injuries most frequently with the result that avulsion injuries of the epiphysis are commoner. Compression injuries producing Type IV or Type V fractures are unusual.

PROBLEMS OF DIAGNOSIS

Many people assume that there is no fracture if the radiograph appears normal. However, undisplaced epiphyseal separations show no fracture. The clinical signs and localized soft tissue swelling on the radiograph should be sufficient to sustain the diagnosis. Disregard

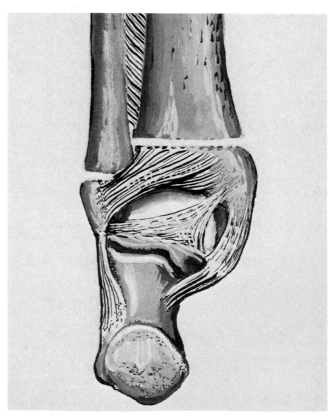

Fig. 20-2. Strong ankle ligaments attached to the epiphyses account for epiphyseal separation being more frequent than epiphyseal fractures.

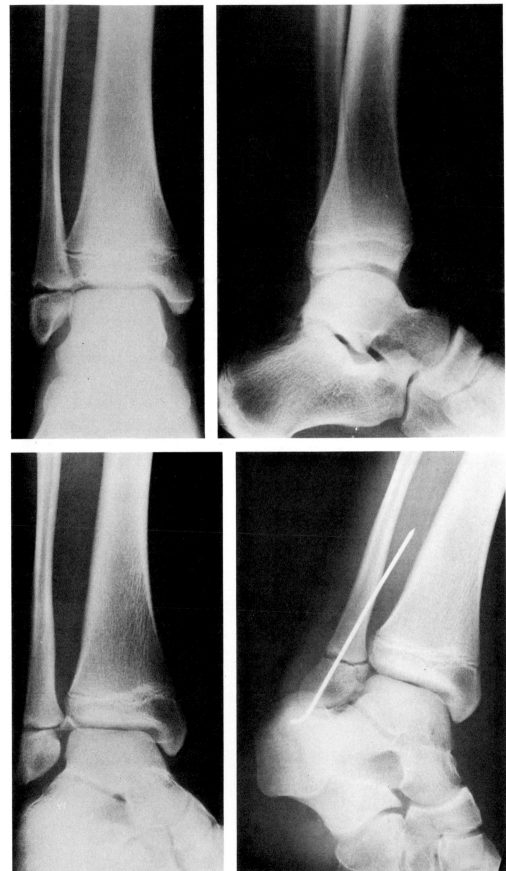

Fig. 20-3. The ankle was swollen laterally; these two views show the fibular growth plate was wide, indicating a Type I injury. An oblique view was required to avoid missing the rest of the diagnosis (see Fig. 20-4).

Fig. 20-4. The oblique view shows a displaced fragment of the fibular epiphysis. This was replaced at open operation and a pin was used to hold the mobile fibular epiphysis in place.

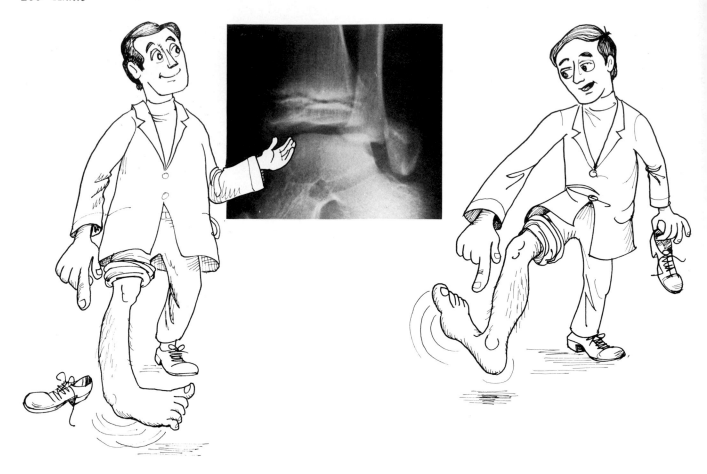

Fig. 20-5. One surgeon demonstrating to another the mechanism of an ankle injury.

the radiologist's report if he fails to recognize the injury. We have missed some fractures about the ankle when we relied on only two views of the ankle (Fig. 20-3, 20-4). Always take an oblique view.

FRACTURE PATTERNS

Customarily ankle fractures are classified on the basis of divination of the direction of force at the time of injury. This method is so conjectural that it is unusual for two people to agree about the classification of any particular injury (Fig. 20-5). Furthermore, this specification does not guide treatment, and we prefer the Salter-Harris method.

Type I Injury of the Fibula

Type I is by far the commonest injury to the fibula. It is recognized by swelling and tenderness over the growth plate; the radiographs are usually normal. Stress films under anesthesia will demonstrate injury (see Fig. 1-1) but are unnecessary as a routine, and we neither use nor advocate this technique.

A walking cast for 3 weeks reduces disability. If no cast is applied, the injury will heal, but the parents, watching their child hop around on crutches, will be an endless source of trouble to you because of their unrelieved concern. When the cast is removed, there is nothing to be gained by further radiographs, because nothing abnormal will be seen. Movement quickly returns, and sequelae are almost unknown.

Type II Injury of the Tibia

Plantar flexion and eversion injuries may produce gross displacement of the distal tibial epiphysis accompanied by a greenstick fracture of the fibula (Fig. 20-6). Gross displacement sometimes produces ischemia of the foot, which can be relieved, as a first aid measure, by partially reducing the fracture gently without anesthesia. The fractures are easily reduced by closed manipulation with the knee flexed. Because growth cartilage lies in the fracture line, no bony crepitus is experienced during reduction. The radiological degree of reduction is usually much better than clinical impressions would suggest. We have not had to operate on these fractures. Up to 20 degrees of valgus can be accepted in the expectation that remodelling will reduce the valgus

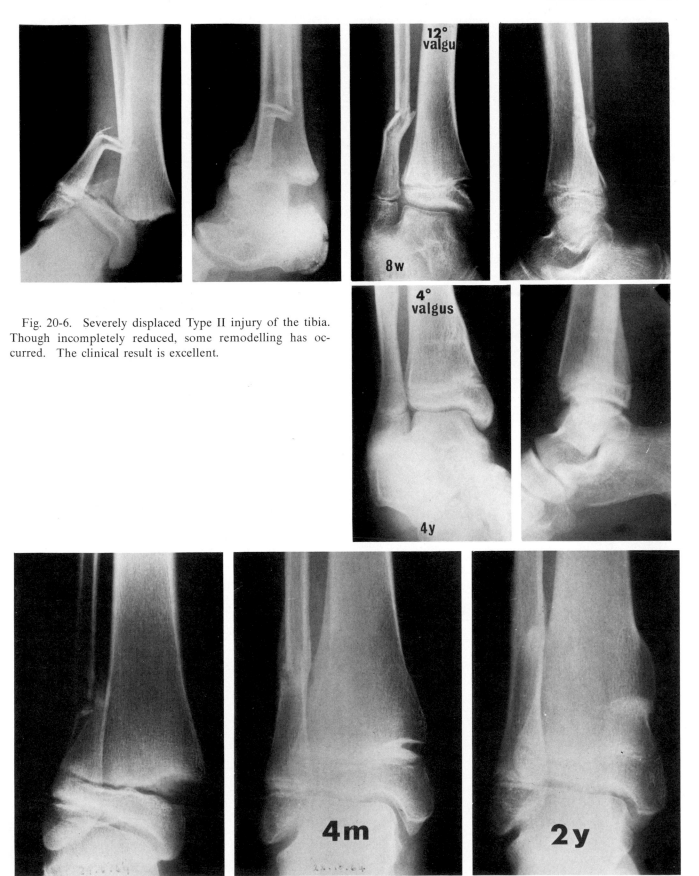

Fig. 20-6. Severely displaced Type II injury of the tibia. Though incompletely reduced, some remodelling has occurred. The clinical result is excellent.

Fig. 20-7. Soft-tissue interposition in a Type II injury (from Mr. Lipmann Kessel).

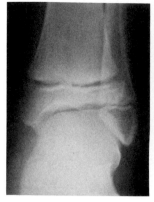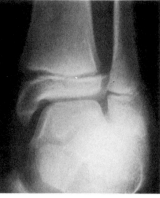

Fig. 20-8. Type I injury of the tibia. This only showed in the oblique view.

Fig. 20-9. (*Top, right*) Paul Jules Tillaux 1834–1904 (Courtesy the Wellcome Trustees). (*Below, left*) Anatomy of the Tillaux fracture. Characteristically the fracture is difficult to see (*center, right*). Frequently the fracture line is overlaid by the fibula. (*Bottom, right*) The Tillaux fragment has locked in the displaced position producing diastasis. The fibula shows a rotatory fracture. When the fragment is fixed back, the mortise closes. The young fibula is pliable and rarely fractures. In the usual Tillaux fracture, the fibula probably bends and then springs back, returning the fragment into place.

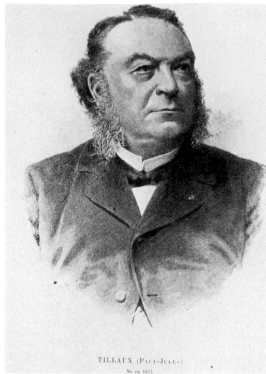

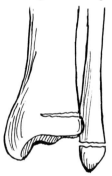
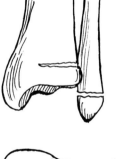

ant. t.f. lig.

post. t.f. lig.

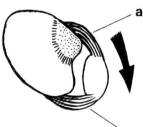

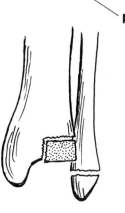

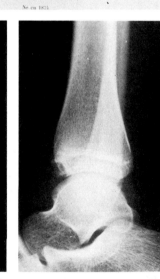

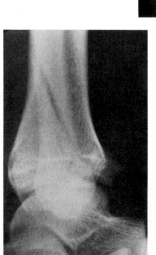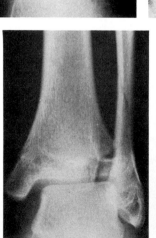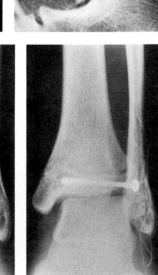

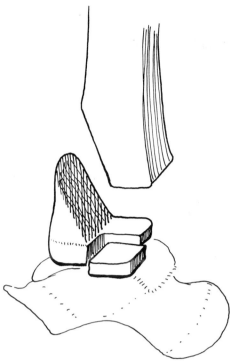

Fig. 20-10. The triplane fracture.

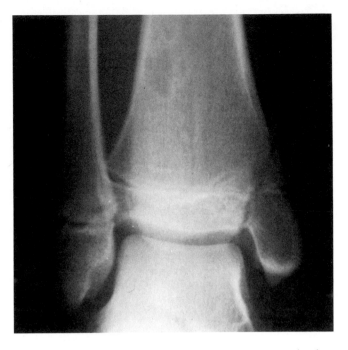

Fig. 20-12. A Type IV injury. Accurate open reduction and internal fixation are required to prevent growth arrest.

Fig. 20-11. A variant of the triplane fracture. The antero-medial portion of the plate has closed, preventing separation. Surprisingly, anatomical position was achieved with closed reduction. At follow-up 2 years later the ankle was perfect.

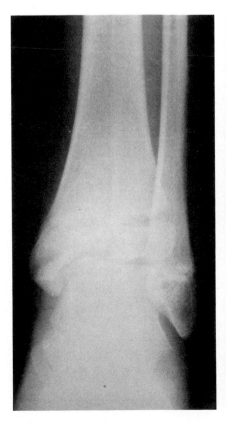

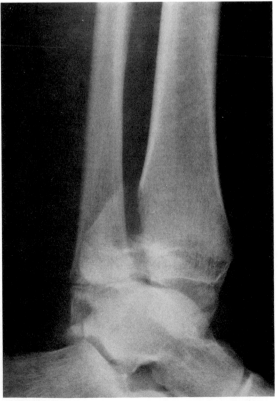

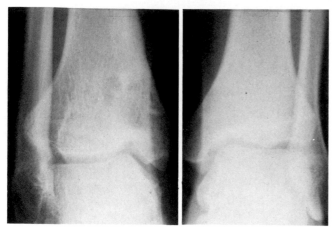

Fig. 20-13. This Type IV injury sustained at the age of 9 years was treated as a sprain by a chiropractor. Here, 5 years later, the result after tibial osteotomy and fibular epiphyseodesis can be seen. There is tenting of the articular surface and ankle varus.

to insignificance. A long-leg cast with a walking heel for a period of 6 weeks provides sufficient immobilization. Because the talotibial joint has not been disturbed in any way, recovery is speedy.

Growth disturbance is unusual. In our series of 14 children with this fracture who were followed up to maturity, only two demonstrated shortening, and that was so slight as to be clinically insignificant. Siffert has described avascular necrosis after this injury. Soft-tissue interposition may produce a bizarre appearance later (Fig. 20-7).

Type I injuries of this epiphysis do occur but are exceptional (Fig. 20-8).

Intraarticular Fractures of the Tibia

This group, including the Tillaux fracture, Frost's triplane fracture, and fractures of the medial malleolus, cause most of the problems in ankle fractures.

The Tillaux Fracture

A Type III injury of the lateral part of the tibial epiphysis, this fracture was originally drawn on a scrap of paper by Tillaux. The drawing was found after he died by Chaput, who made the best of the ambiguous sketch. Kleiger and Mankin (1964) have written comprehensively on the fracture.

At the age of 13 or 14 years, when the medial half of the distal tibial growth plate is closed, the lateral portion remains open. The anterior tibiofibular ligament links the tibial epiphysis with the fibular metaphysis. An external rotation force may avulse the anterior quadrant of the tibial epiphysis. This injury appears to be the adolescent equivalent of diastasis (Fig. 20-9).

In our experience of about 30 such fractures, we have considered the majority to be so minimally displaced that no reduction is required, and that immobilization in a below-knee cast is sufficient. A small number have required open or closed reduction. A follow-up review of eight patients indicated that pain and stiffness was common for up to 2 years after injury, despite well-healed fractures. Kleiger and Mankin noted that rotatory instability, detectable by an examination under general anesthetic, is a feature of this fracture, and for this reason they applied a long-leg cast with the foot in full medial rotation. Their published results, from a very few children, appear better than those that we have obtained, and in the future I intend to follow their teaching.

The Triplane Fracture

This uncommon fracture (Fig. 20-10) marries a Type II injury to a Tillaux fracture. The radiographs are

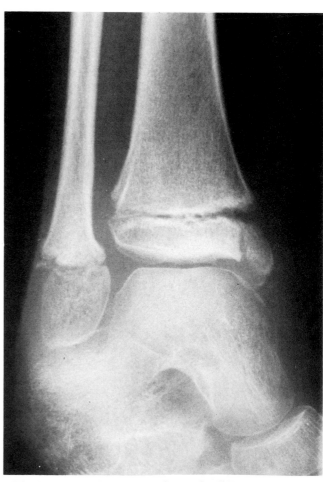

Fig. 20-14. In a young child it may be difficult to be certain whether the fracture extends into the metaphysis or not. This was a Type III fracture of the medial malleolus with a Type I fracture of the fibula. A cast was applied; healing was sound.

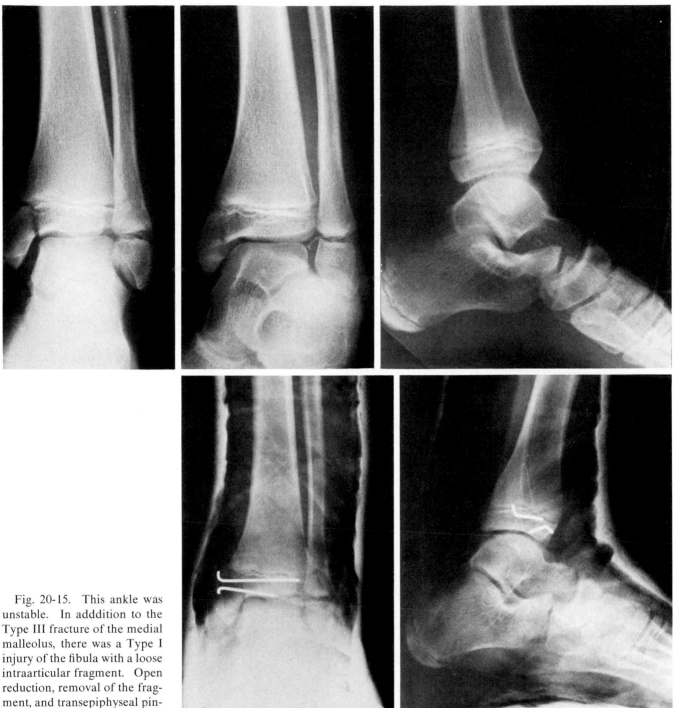

Fig. 20-15. This ankle was unstable. In adddition to the Type III fracture of the medial malleolus, there was a Type I injury of the fibula with a loose intraarticular fragment. Open reduction, removal of the fragment, and transepiphyseal pinning is needed.

hard to interpret. We have treated two children with this injury by closed reduction, and maintained position with an above-knee cast for about 8 weeks (Fig. 20-11). If closed reduction fails, operate.

Fractures Around the Medial Malleolus

Growth plate damage is common around the medial malleolus (Figs. 20-12 to 20-15), and will produce a varus deformity of the ankle and a short tibia, accompanied by relative overgrowth of the fibula.

In theory, the radiograph should allow the fracture to be classified into Type III, IV or V, so that appropriate treatment and prognosis may be determined. In practice, the interpretation is seldom clear because a little comminution is common, and because the medial margin of the growth plate is poorly defined. Exact reduction of the large fragment is essential and transepiphys-

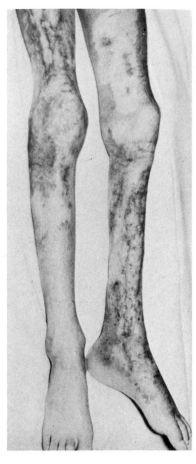
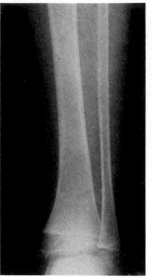
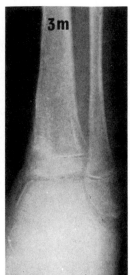
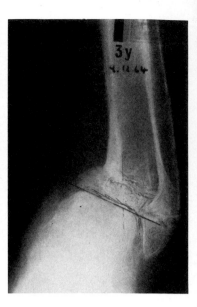

Fig. 20-16. Type VI injury. At the time of a runover injury with massive degloving, the medial side of the growth plate was exposed. Within 3 months the plate closed partially, and varus deformity followed. (Courtesy Mr. Lipmann Kessel)

eal pins should be used to achieve this. Reduction may be hindered by trapped, loose fragments that will require removal.

Grossly comminuted fractures usually do not appear displaced and are treated in an above-knee cast. Growth disturbances of varying degrees have ensued in some. In the teenager, tenting of the epiphysis will be unimportant, whereas in the younger child it will cause a major problem.

Type VI Injuries—Ablation of the Perichondrial Ring

Lawn mower- and degloving injuries may remove the perichondrial ring. Lipmann Kessel has shown that this permits a callus bridge to form between the epiphysis and metaphysis with resulting varus deformity and failure of growth. (Fig. 20-16; for further discussion, see p. 17.)

MISCELLANEOUS INJURIES

Battered Baby Syndrome

The ankle is commonly affected. The heat, swelling, and redness may simulate osteomyelitis.

Epiphyseal Fractures

The very tip of either malleolus is occasionally avulsed. As healing occurs, an ossicle forms, and the entire epiphysis may become a little larger (Fig. 20-17).

Fracture of the Fibula with Intraarticular Fragment

The fragment may require operative reduction (Fig. 20-3).

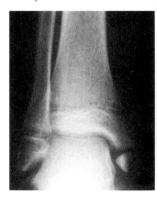
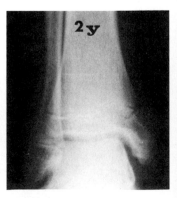

Fig. 20-17. Horizontal fractures of the medial malleolus are rare and require open reduction and internal fixation. This fracture in a 12-year-old was held temporarily with a screw. Two years later function was excellent.

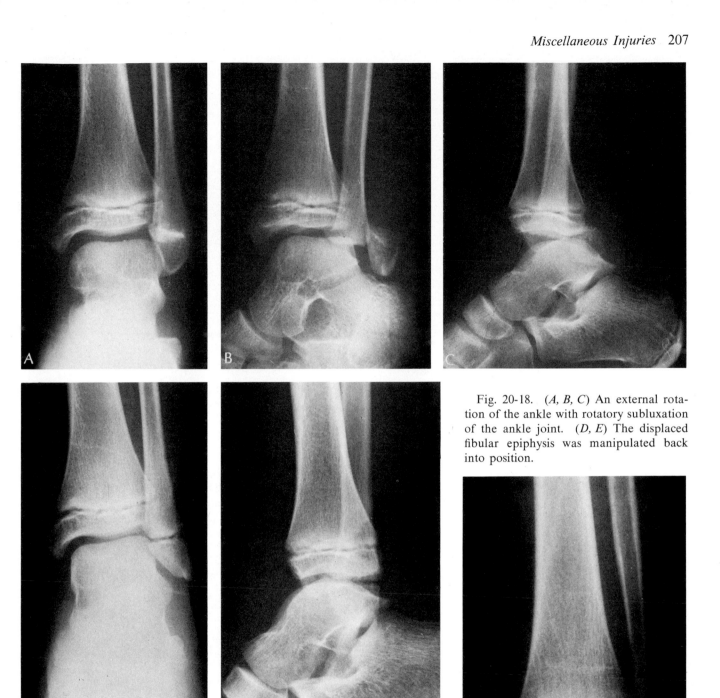

Fig. 20-18. (*A, B, C*) An external rotation of the ankle with rotatory subluxation of the ankle joint. (*D, E*) The displaced fibular epiphysis was manipulated back into position.

Fig. 20-19. Two years before, at the age of 4, this child lost the end of the fibula in a street accident. Though the foot is in varus, owing to loss of peroneal power, the ankle is in valgus and the talus is subluxed laterally. Repeated osteotomies and ankle fusion are likely to be required.

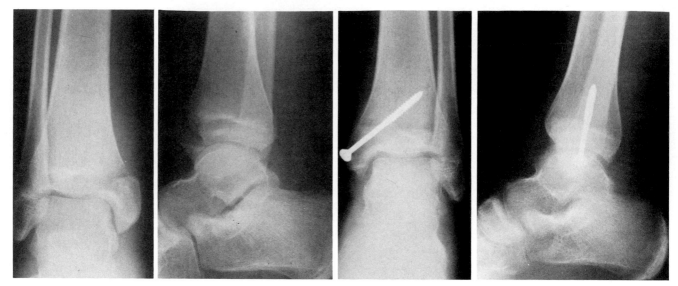

Fig. 20-20.   Adolescents with closing plates sustain fractures of the adult type.   Use internal fixation if stable, accurate closed reduction cannot be achieved.   Boy aged 15.

Rotated Fractures

The tibial epiphysis may be rotated through 90 degrees.   I have seen two examples in which the separated fibular epiphysis was displaced completely posteriorly (Fig. 20-18).

Loss of Fibula

A valgus deformity develops when the fibula is short due to growth retardation or loss of part of the bone (Fig. 20-19).

Adult Fractures

Young people with closed plates who sustain fractures may come to a children's hospital.   Their fractures are of the adult-type, and they may require open reduction and internal fixation (Fig. 20-20).

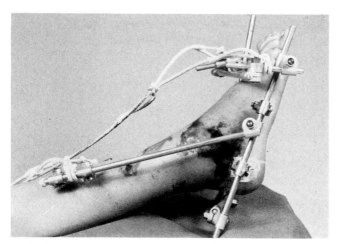

Fig. 20-21.   Like many people involved in industrial accidents, it was Patrick's first day at the car wash; the foot was almost torn off through the distal tibial growth plate by the continuously moving chain on the floor.   The posterior tibial nerve, artery, and tendon were divided.   The circulation to the foot was precarious for a time.   The leg was debrided and the fracture was held with Roger Anderson apparatus. A wound extending halfway around the circumference of the leg was closed.   Some skin subsequently became necrotic and was replaced with grafts.   Rigid external fixation greatly facilitated the care of the soft tissues.

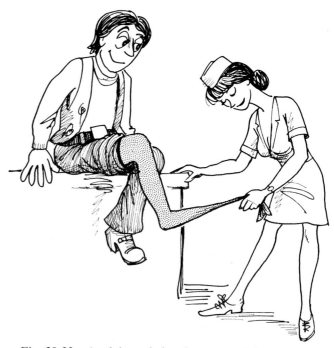

Fig. 20-22.   Applying a below-knee cast.   The easiest way to hold the ankle at a right angle is to have an assistant control the foot with the stockinet.

Open Fractures

The skin over the ankle is thin, and there is little fat or fascia to cover tendons and nerves. Holding a fracture reduced is difficult when the overlying skin is damaged by degloving or by the bone bursting through. Figure 20-21 shows one method of management.

BIBLIOGRAPHY

Aitken, A. P.: The end results of fractured distal tibial epiphysis. J. Bone Joint Surg., *18:* 685, 1936

Bishop, P. A.: Fractures and epiphyseal separation fractures of the ankle. A classification of 332 cases according to the mechanism of their production. Am. J. Roentgenol., *28:* 49, 1932

Carothers, C. O., and Crenshaw, A. H.: Clinical significance of epiphyseal injuries at the ankle. Amer. J. Surg., *89:* 879, 1955

Gill, G., and Abbott, L.: Varus deformity of ankle following injury to distal epiphyseal cartilage of tibia in growing children. Surg., Gynecol., Obstet., *72:* 659, 1941

Johnson, E. W., and Fahl, J. C.: Fractures involving the distal epiphysis of the tibia and fibula in children. Amer. J. Surg., *93:* 778, 1957

Kaplan, L.: Epiphyseal injuries in children. Surg. Clin. Amer., *17:* 1637, 1937

Kleiger, B., and Mankin, H. J.: Fracture of the lateral portion of the distal tibial epiphysis. J. Bone Joint Surg., *46A:* 25, 1964

Lynn, M.D.: The triplane distal epiphyseal fracture. Clin. Orthop., *86:* 187, 1972

Marmor, L.: An unusual fracture of the tibial epiphysis. Clin. Orthop., *73:* 132, 1970

McFarland, B.: Traumatic arrest of epiphyseal growth at the lower end of the tibia. Brit. J. Surg., *19:* 78, 1931

Robertson, D. E.: Post-traumatic osteochondrosis of the lower tibial epiphysis. J. Bone Joint Surg., *46B:* 212, 1964

Siffert, R. S., and Arkin, A. M.: Post-traumatic aseptic necrosis of the distal tibial epiphysis. J. Bone Joint Surg., *32A:* 691, 1950

21

Foot

Injuries to children's feet, despite all the little bones and joints, are remarkably uninteresting. Very few fractures will be encountered that display any subtleties or tricks; few are even displaced.

TALAR FRACTURES

Fractures of the talus are unusual in children. In 10 years we have been able to trace only 12 examples.

Neck

The majority are undisplaced fractures of the neck of the talus which heal in casts without avascular necrosis. The only sequel in one case followed to adult life was that the talus was slightly smaller than its counterpart in the opposite foot. When the head is superiorly displaced in relation to the body, the foot should be immobilized in plantar flexion to avoid malunion (Fig. 21-1). Fracture of the neck accompanied by subtalar dislocation usually can be reduced by closed manipulation (Fig. 21-2).

Body

Displaced fractures through the body require open reduction. This may be difficult because wide exposure is required in order to demonstrate the fracture adequately and yet, to minimize the risk of avascular necrosis, care must be taken to avoid removing any soft tissue attachments from the bony fragments. Multiple Kirschner wires across the fracture and across the subtalar joint will provide fixation. Subsequently, the subtalar joint remains stiff, and avascular necrosis of the body, a complication that requires protection with a patellar tendon bearing brace for a year or two, is a real hazard (Fig. 21-3).

Lateral Wall

Lateral wall fracture, probably representing an osteochondral fragment avulsed by the anterior talofibular ligament, is seldom recognized initially. Persisting pain and point tenderness just in front of the lateral malleolus should indicate the need for oblique radiographs and perhaps tomograms, to show the small loose body. Excision may be needed (Figs. 21-4 and 21-5).

OS CALCIS FRACTURES

Children seldom fracture the os calcis. Displaced fractures involving the subtalar joint that require reduction are very unusual. Fractures in the sagittal plane are easily missed if axial views of the os calcis are omitted.

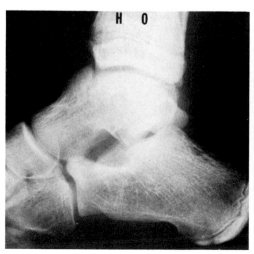 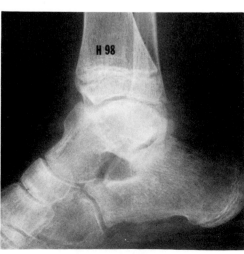

Fig. 21-1. Displaced fracture of the neck of the talus. This was not reduced. Ninety-eight days later the fracture was solidly malunited, and he was never able to put his foot flat on the ground again.

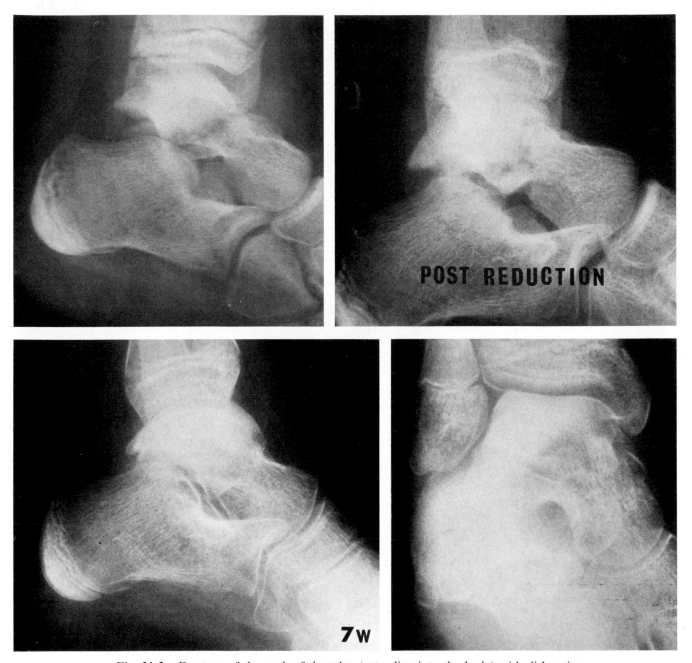

Fig. 21-2. Fracture of the neck of the talus (extending into the body) with dislocation of the subtalar joint. This was manipulated into good position. At 7 weeks the fracture was united, but the density suggests avascular necrosis. Bone scan showed normal uptake throughout the talus.

Most children require admission to elevate the leg for a few days and start early movements. The child should not bear weight on the heel until the fracture is united, so use a cast. Open reduction yields worse results than this technique in our hands. The os calcis has a predilection for simple bone cyst, which may initiate a pathological fracture and require a bone graft (Figs. 21-6 and 21-7).

MIDTARSAL INJURIES

Mechanisms that simulate a well-applied Thomas wrench can disrupt the midtarsal area. Valgus or varus deformities may be more apparent on clinical examination than on radiographs. Whether reduction is needed or not, the child should be admitted for elevation of

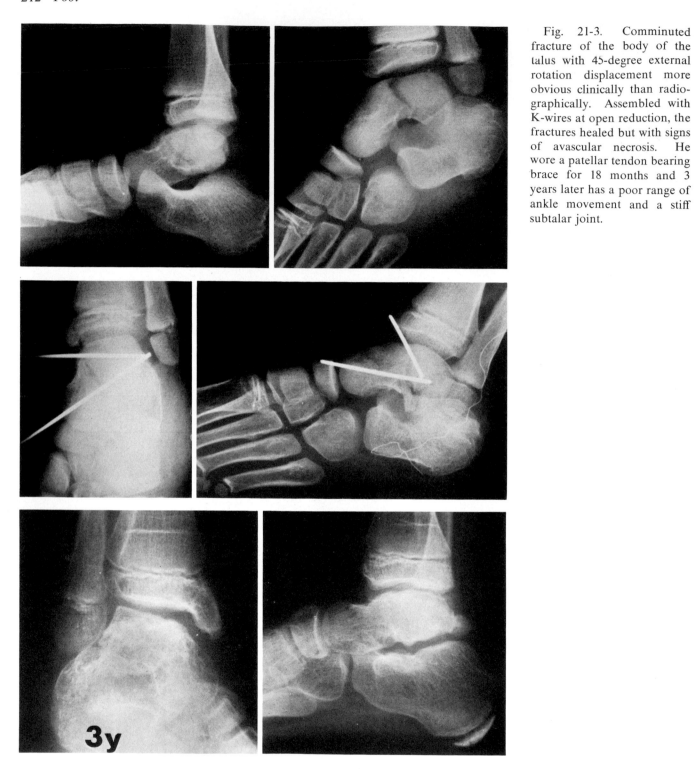

Fig. 21-3. Comminuted fracture of the body of the talus with 45-degree external rotation displacement more obvious clinically than radiographically. Assembled with K-wires at open reduction, the fractures healed but with signs of avascular necrosis. He wore a patellar tendon bearing brace for 18 months and 3 years later has a poor range of ankle movement and a stiff subtalar joint.

the foot and observation, since massive swelling is usual, and vascular impairment has been described. Decompression through the dorsum of the foot may be necessary when skin viability is threatened. Displacement should be corrected and held with percutaneous Kirschner wires. A well padded soft bandage is the only safe means of support for the first week, after which a cast should be used (Fig. 21-8).

METATARSAL FRACTURES

Robert Jones Fracture of the Base of the Fifth Metatarsal

Fracture is distinguished from a normal growth plate by the direction of each (Fig. 21-9). The injury is common and painful; a walking cast for 4 weeks lessens mor-

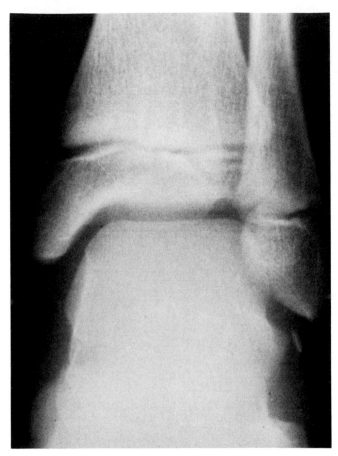

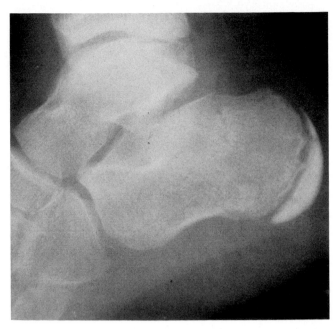

Fig. 21-6. Fracture of the os calcis. Boy aged 11. After elevation of the foot for a few days he was immobilized in a cast for a month.

Fig. 21-4. A fracture of the processus lateralis. Probably not uncommon, this fracture is only recognized on a 10-degree internal rotation oblique film. Boy aged 12 years.

bidity. Frequently, local bony tenderness persists long after the cast is removed.

Solitary Fractures

Seldom much displaced, solitary fractures are treated in a walking cast for comfort.

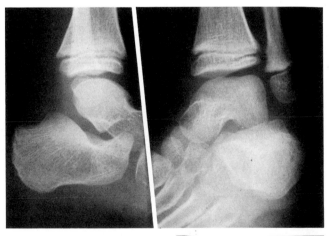

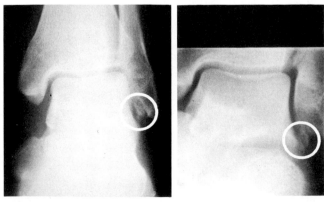

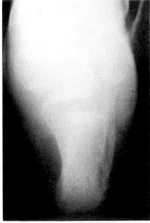

Fig. 21-5. Ossicles due to an old fracture of the processus lateralis were excised because of pain. Boy aged 15.

Fig. 21-7. This fracture of the lateral wall of the os calcis could easily have been missed if the axial view had been omitted. Boy aged 8 years.

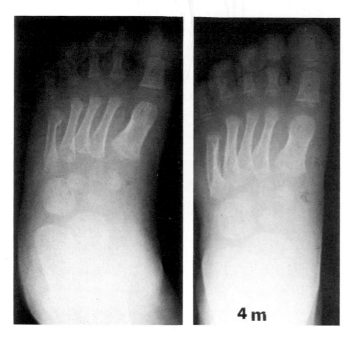

Fig. 21-8. Midtarsal joint injury in a 2-year-old child due to a car running over his foot. There was massive swelling. Hemorrhage in the fat of his foot produced a mottled appearance on the radiograph. Undisplaced fractures of the fourth and fifth metatarsal bases were barely perceptible. The foot was elevated for 10 days before he could safely be allowed home in a well padded light cast. Callus 4 months later defines the fractures more clearly.

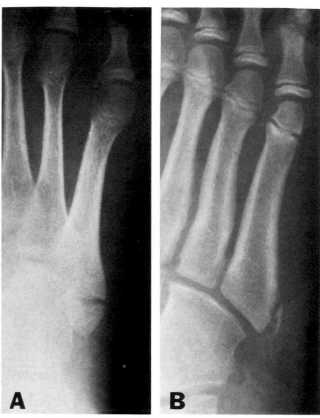

Fig. 21-9. (*A*) Fracture of the base of the fifth metatarsal bone contrasted with (*B*) normal growth plate. Note the different direction of the line.

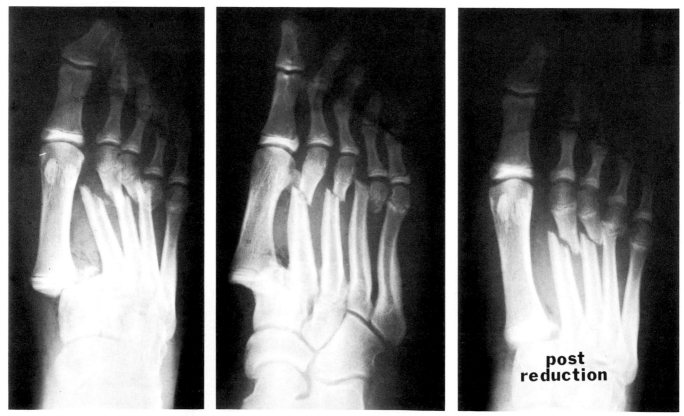

Fig. 21-10. Fracture-dislocation of the forefoot. After elevation for a few days closed reduction was effected and maintained. Boy aged 14.

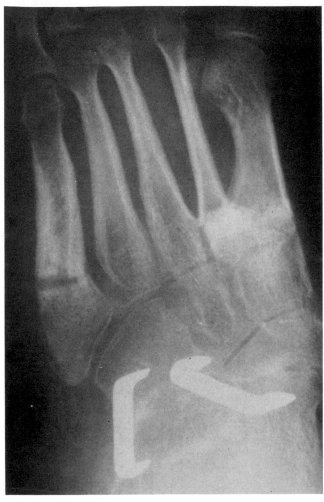

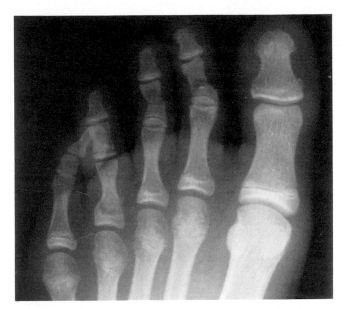

Fig. 21-12. Fractures of the middle phalanges of the second and third toes and of the proximal phalanx of the fourth toe. The displacement does not look great on the radiograph, but the boy's toes were pointing in all directions like the roots of a tree. He required reduction and immobilization. Perhaps this point has been made often enough: If the appearance of the patient suggests that a fresh fracture should be put straight, put it straight irrespective of the radiograph.

Fig. 21-11. This 15-year-old with an incompletely corrected club foot complained of pain due to a stress fracture of the fifth metatarsal. The deformity was corrected by a triple arthrodesis, and the stress fracture is beginning to heal.

Multiple Fractures

Considerable swelling is universal in multiple fractures. The foot should be aligned, not only to prevent valgus, varus, or splayfoot deformities, but to prevent depression of a metatarsal head. As the swelling recedes, alignment may improve. If it does not, intramedullary fixation with Kirschner wires is required, because nonunion may occur. Nonunion results in a short toe and irregularity of the metatarsal heads with painful metatarsalgia (Fig. 21-10).

Stress Fractures

March fracture in children is unusual, but stress fractures of the fifth metatarsal are seen in partially corrected club feet (Fig. 21-11).

PHALANGEAL FRACTURES

Phalangeal fractures seldom require more than protection and sympathy (Fig. 21-12). Intraarticular fractures of the big toe require accurate reduction, if necessary by open pinning, in order to avoid prolonged painful stiffness. Growth arrest is occasionally encountered after stubbing the big toe (Fig. 2-19).

BIBLIOGRAPHY

Davidson, A. M., Steele, H. D., Mackenzie, D. A. and Penny, J. A.: A review of twenty-one cases of transchondral fracture of the talus. J. Trauma, *7:* 378, 1967

Harrison, M.: Fractures of the metatarsal head. Can. J. Surg., *11:* 511, 1968

Hawkins, L. G.: Fracture of the lateral process of the talus. J. Bone Joint Surg., *47A:* 1170, 1965

Spak, I.: Fractures of the talus in children. Acta. Chir. Scand., *107:* 553, 1966

Thomas, H. M.: Calcaneal fracture in childhood. Brit. J. Surg., *56:* 664, 1969

22

Spine and Spinal Cord

GENERAL FEATURES

Vertebral fractures and spinal cord injuries are less common in children than in adults. Only 5 percent of cases of traumatic paraplegia occur in children (Gehrig

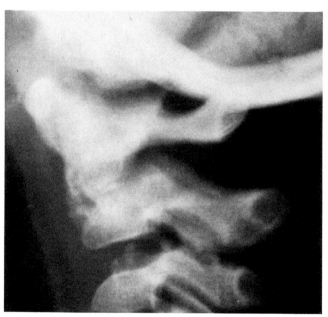

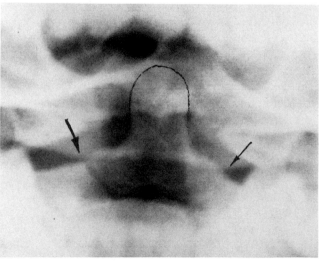

Fig. 22-1. Separation of the dens from the right neural arch (*indicated by arrows.*) Boy aged 4 years.

and Michaelis). The child's spine is more mobile than that of an adult, so that the force is dissipated more easily and over a greater number of segments. Dislocations of the spine are rare, because the ligaments are stronger than bone. The line of the growth plate may mimic a fracture or may cause *special types* of fractures. Separation of the epiphyseal end-plate of a vertebral body—a Type I injury—is the commonest birth injury of the bony spine. Here is another type: Adam fell over the bannisters and landed on the top of his head. His neck was rigid, but radiographs were normal. There was little improvement after halter traction for 3 weeks. He went home in ruffs only to return with a mildly spastic gait after another fall. Eventually, tomograms disclosed an epiphyseal separation at the base of the odontoid (Fig. 22-1). He went home in a Minerva cast and was soon normal again.

The rarity of spinal cord injuries in children does not mean that back injuries should be taken less seriously. I can well remember the piping voice of a 12-year-old describing how she had hurt her back in a field. Her brother-in-law picked her up in his arms. "I felt a terrible pain in my back, and after this I could not move my legs. I have never been able to move them since." Perhaps only once in your life will you be at the scene of such an accident, but when you are, stand guard over the patient to organize the onlookers. Move the patient on a board or on a door.

Only a small proportion of paraplegic children owe their lesion to trauma. During a 12-year period, approximately 450 children have been admitted to the Ontario Crippled Children's Centre with a diagnosis of paraplegia. Of these cases, 12 percent were traumatic, 2 percent were due to acquired disease, and the remainder were due to meningomyelocele. The major cause of traumatic paraplegia is car accidents; occasionally falls from trees and buildings and diving accidents are responsible. Traumatic paraplegia outnumbers traumatic quadriplegia by 3 to 1.

CLASSIFICATION

Comparatively little is written about spinal injuries in children, and I have drawn mostly on our experience at The Hospital for Sick Children. During a 15-year period, approximately 85 children have been admitted with injuries to the cord or vertebrae. Table 22-1 shows the composition of the group.*

Trauma to the spine in children falls naturally into three groups: (1) cord injury without fracture; (2) cord injury with fracture or dislocation; and (3) fracture or dislocation alone. A cord injury without fracture is perhaps the most interesting entity. Though a rare combination in adults, apart from hyperextension injury of the cervical spine, it represents about one-quarter of all injuries to children with neurological damage.

CORD INJURY WITHOUT FRACTURE OR OPEN INJURY

It is perhaps a mistake to look for one cause when there is cord injury but no fracture or open injury. Concussion, contusion, and infarction of the cord appear to produce the neurological disorder. But what damages the cord? This is a matter for conjecture. A displaced Type I injury of the cartilaginous epiphysis may spring back into position. This is seen in the leg and can be produced in the spine. These will heal without any radiographic signs. Another possible mechanism for this injury is excessive bending of the young spine, which has a more rubbery disc and more growth cartilage than bone. Traction is thought to be the commonest mechanism in birth paraplegia (Stern and Rand). We have treated 11 patients with this condition. Concussion accounted for five injuries, contusion for four, and infarction for two (see below).

David Burke (1971) described seven children with permanent complete traumatic paraplegia with no radiographic signs of gross injury. (Fractures of ribs were present in three, fractured transverse process in one, and slight forward subluxation of L2 on L3 in another). The paraplegia was spastic in five and flaccid in two young children with high thoracic lesions who had been run over.

Concussion

After a fall or blow, transient, incomplete neurological signs without bladder involvement are present for a matter of hours up to 2 days. All are due to cervical injuries. Rest and observation are all that is required, because recovery is quick and complete.

Contusion

A contusion of the cord is defined as a lesion that results in some degree of permanent local destruction.

*Dr. George Weicz took the initiative to review these patients, and this chapter is based on his work.

Table 22-1. Classification of Spinal Injuries in 86 Children

Skeletal Injury Without CNS Signs		
Compression fractures	31	
Rotatory fixation C1-2	6	44
Miscellaneous subluxations	7	
Skeletal Injury with CNS Signs		31
CNS Signs Without Obvious Skeletal Injury		
Concussion	5	
Contusion	4	11
Infarction	2	

Contusions occurred at all levels and showed the spectrum of severity seen in adult paraplegics. All patients improved, but to varying degrees. All required correction of lower limb spastic deformities, and one required surgical correction of scoliosis.

Infarction

A complete, permanent, flaccid paraplegia below the midthoracic region is the characteristic feature of infarction. In one patient, the onset was delayed for a day. Arterial damage was confirmed as the cause of the paraplegia in one patient. The blood supply of the thoracic cord depends on the arteries of Adamkiewicz, the spinal branches of the first and the eleventh intercostal arteries. Anastomosis between these vessels is said to be poor, and there is little supply from intervening intercostal arteries. If the eleventh intercostal artery is damaged, infarction of the cord up to the midthoracic level may follow. Because the whole cord is not functioning, the paraplegia will be flaccid, in contrast with the spastic paraplegia produced by a segmental lesion.

CORD INJURY WITH VERTEBRAL FRACTURE OR DISLOCATION

We have seen 31 children with cord injury concomitant with fracture or dislocation, which range from birth

Table 22-2. Fractures with Cord Damage in 31 Children

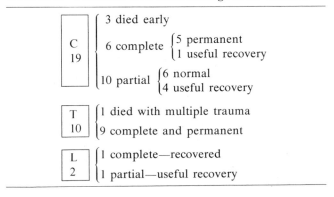

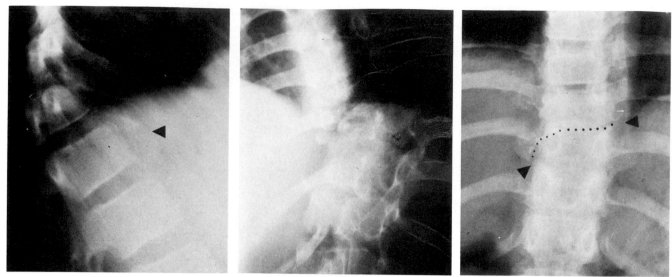

Fig. 22-2. Gary fell out of a tree at the age of 14 years, sustaining a fracture-dislocation of T9 and T10 and a total paraplegia. The dislocation was reduced and a laminectomy performed. The spinal lesion remained complete, and he required a fusion to correct kyphosis. Eight years later he is attending college in a wheelchair.

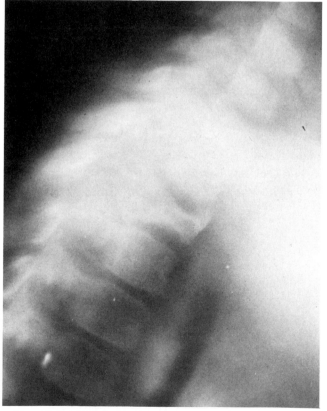

Fig. 22-3. Bursting fracture of T3. This girl sustained grossly displaced fracture of the pelvis, and inability to move the legs was attributed to plexus lesions. The high thoracic spine shows up poorly on radiographs. Only when she was transferred to another hospital and reassessed was it realized that her legs were spastic, as distinct from stiff. Tomographs revealed the spinal fracture. She has recovered sufficiently to walk with aids after hip and ankle releases.

injury to injuries sustained by 14-year-olds in car accidents or falls. I am not going to write a treatise on traumatic paraplegia; you can read many papers on this subject. But the pattern of childhood injuries shows some important differences from that in adults, and children have special long-term problems (see Table 22-2).

PATTERN OF INJURY RELATED TO PROGNOSIS

Thoracic Injuries

The prognosis for recovery in thoracic injuries is hopeless. The majority of injuries were fracture dislocations, and it may be assumed that the cord was transsected initially. Some of these children were nursed in bed, some had fusions, and some had laminectomies, but nothing made any difference. When the cases were reviewed some years after their injury, it was found that the patients were all alive, they were all at school or college, and all were in wheelchairs (Figs. 22-2, 22-3).

Cervical Injuries

By contrast with the thoracic injuries, the cervical injuries showed considerable variation in the extent of initial damage. Three children died; one was apneic after a forceps delivery, one was apneic after a C1-2 dislocation and fractured skull, and the third had multiple injuries. However, most of the lesions in patients who survived long enough to be admitted to hospital were incomplete with a hemiplegia (rather than para-

Fig. 22-4. Fracture of odontoid with retropharyngeal hematoma. Boy aged 5 years injured in car accident. He had a complete right motor hemiplegia without sensory loss, which recovered to a great extent. He was treated in a Minerva cast.

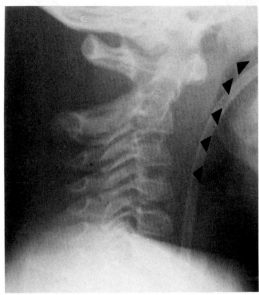
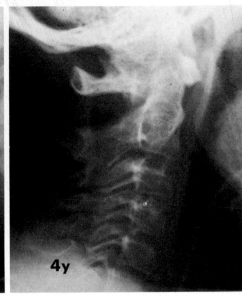

plegia or quadriplegia) occurring in 50 percent of the group (Figs. 22-4, 22-5).

Injury occurred at all levels in the cervical spine; the only striking feature was that locked facets, so common in adults, were not seen in children. Only one child in this group had an underlying congenital bone anomaly, but this is a recognized predisposing cause.

The majority of children were treated in traction until the fracture was stable, and then placed in a Minerva cast. Very few were fused.

Lumbar Injuries

Both injuries were high lumbar lesions, and both showed recovery. One child who had a complete lumbar lesion recovered after laminectomy.

Long-Term Problems

In this group of spinal injuries, only one child has died. She died of pneumonia about 1 year after a complete C5 quadriplegia. The remaining children are active and are in educational programs.

Spinal Problems

In our series about half the children with complete thoracic paraplegia required spinal fusion for deformity. Of 14 children, five were treated by Harrington instrumentation, and two more were treated by long fusions at the time of their injury (Figs. 22-6, 22-7).

There are a number of papers on this subject (Kilfoyle 1965, Audic and Maury 1969, Bedbrook 1969). All draw attention to the frequency of scoliosis in children and adolescents. Progressive angular kyphosis may damage cord function in partial lesions, and early fusion

is indicated. In complete lesions the incidence of spinal deformity (lordosis, kyphosis, or scoliosis) is higher when: (1) the lesion is high, (2) there is muscle imbalance, (3) the onset of paraplegia was early in life, and (4) when laminectomy has been carried out. Bracing is difficult, and spinal fusion is usually required. The

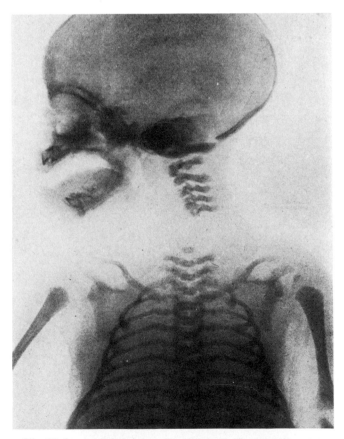

Fig. 22-5. A birth injury. Truesdell, E. D.: Birth Fractures and Epiphyseal Dislocations. (New York, Hoeber, 1917).

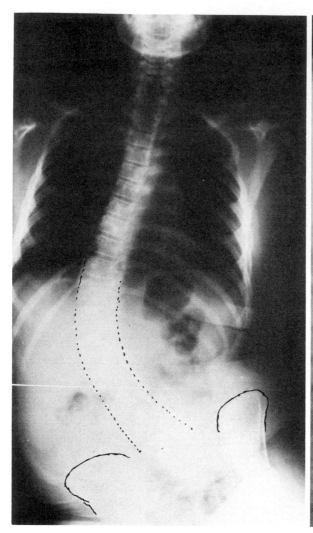

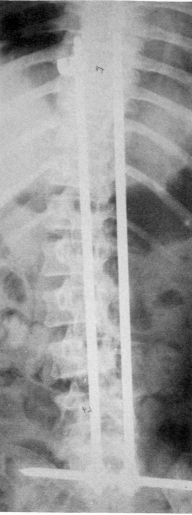

Fig. 22-6. This curve with pelvic obliquity was present 3 years after a complete thoracic paraplegia. Harrington fusion corrected this, though her pelvic obliquity has recurred since because of pseudarthrosis. Correction of paraplegic scoliosis tends to be transient.

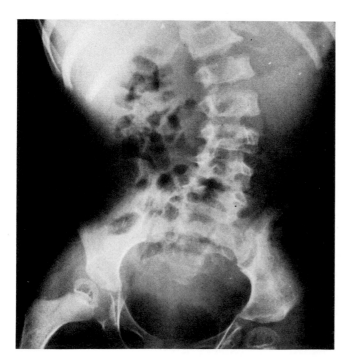

aim should be to abolish pelvic obliquity so that the risk of ischial pressure sores is reduced and to produce a stable balanced spine. This is easier said than done.

The fusion should always go down to the sacrum. It may be wise to correct pelvic obliquity with a Dwyer instrumentation and fusion and then use a Harrington instrumentation and fusion to accomplish the lumbosacral fusion and hold the thoracic spine. This is a lot of surgery, but a review of our cases shows that there is no place for half measures.

Fig. 22-7. At the age of 3 years this boy suffered a complete and permanent paraplegia due to a fracture dislocation at T12–L1. This radiograph at age 6 years shows a scoliosis and an interesting head-within-a-head appearance of the femoral heads representing disuse atrophy followed by activity. A Harrington fusion was carried out at the age of 7 years which must be repeated because of pseudoarthrosis. He has also had release surgery for leg contractures. He is mostly in a wheelchair at the age of 16 years.

Fig. 22-8. Gunshot wound of C5 in a boy of 9 years. He had a partial cord lesion which recovered to a partial left hemiplegia. He shows a scoliosis and has required tendon releases around the left ankle.

Lower Limb Problems

A smaller proportion of children required releases at the hip, knee, or ankle for spastic deformities (Fig. 22-8).

Urological Problems

The urological problems are formidable and require specialist care. None of our patients remained free of infection.

VERTEBRAL FRACTURES AND OTHER INJURIES

During this period, 45 fractures without neurological signs were seen. The injuries were evenly distributed throughout the spine.

Cervical Spine

Children with pain in the neck after a fall are a common challenge to diagnosis. If they have a torticollis, the radiographs are difficult to understand. Furthermore, radiographs of the child's cervical spine are more difficult to interpret than those of the adult. Everyone should read a paper by Cattell and Filtser on Pseudo-subluxation and Other Normal Variations in the Cervical Spine in Children. They note that normal children commonly show changes that could be mistaken for signs of injury. Apparent subluxation of C2 on C3 occurs in 19 percent of normal children. The spine has no lordotic curve in about 15 percent. Epiphyseal plates may be mistaken for fracture. Remember that if a child receives a blow sufficient to damage the neck, he usually has a bruise or cut somewhere on his head.

The following injuries are commonly encountered:
Rotatory Fixation of the Atlantoaxial Joint (Fig. 22-9). Because the name suggests a chiropractic diagnosis the very existence of this condition may be doubted by the few who have heard of it. But experience is a great teacher. Wortzman and Dewar drew attention to the essential features of rotatory fixation in 1968.

Usually beginning with a minor accident such as a blow to the head or a rear-end automobile collision the child complains of pain and stiffness in the neck and occipital neuralgia. There is torticollis, which may be so slight as to be barely discernable.

Open-mouth AP radiographs show that the odontoid is asymmetrically placed between the lateral articular

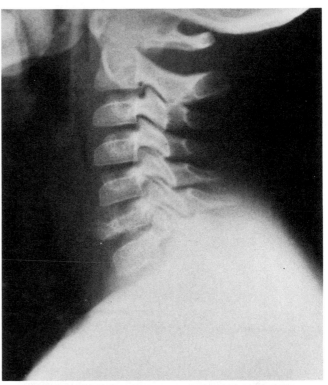

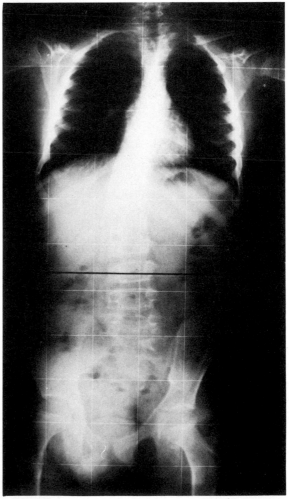

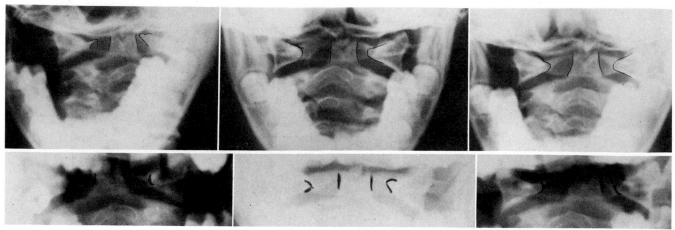

Fig. 22-9. Rotatory fixation: boy aged 7 years. The radiographs are taken looking 10 degrees to the right, looking straight ahead, and looking 10 degrees to the left. (*A*) The odontoid is displaced to the left in all views. (*B*) After 7 days in traction the odontoid is more central, and movement is taking place.

masses of the atlas. The diagnosis is confirmed by further open-mouth views taken with the head rotated 10 to 15 degrees to the right and left, which show no alteration of the asymmetry. This radiological abnormality does not occur in normals and it is not an artifact produced by torticollis.

The pathology of rotatory fixation has not been demonstrated. It may be looked on as locking of one of the lateral joints between the atlas and axis, perhaps due to a capsular tear and trapped synovial fringe.

If nothing is done, rotatory fixation tends to persist, though in the end most children will improve symptomatically, whether there is radiographically demonstrable improvement or not. A few patients with unremitting symptoms have required a Gallie fusion between C1 and C2 after it has been shown that their pain can be relieved by infiltration of the lateral atlantoaxial joints with local anesthetic under x-ray control.

Treatment. When rotatory fixation is recognized early, the child should be admitted to hospital and placed on continuous halter traction until the fixation has reduced on x-ray examination. Traction for about a week is required, and this should be followed by protective ruffs for a few weeks.

Whiplash Injuries. Affecting principally asthenic long-necked, teenage girls who have been involved in rear-end automobile collisions, the symptoms run a protracted course. Radiographs are normal. A collar and medication with diazepam seem to make little difference. The parents usually grow tired of your failure to effect a cure and move on to other doctors.

The following injuries are rare.

Subluxation or Dislocation C1 on C2. We have seen this condition only once in a child, perhaps because the ligaments are stronger than the bone. Hunter describes the nontraumatic variety in children.

Jefferson's Fracture of the Lateral Mass of C1 certainly occurs in children.

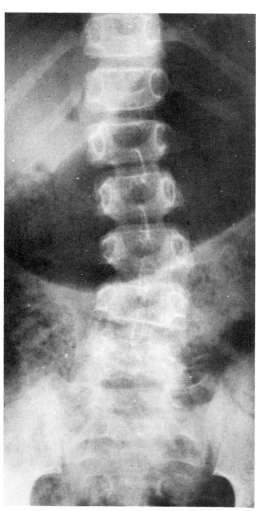

Fig. 22-10. Lateral wedge compression of L3 and L4 producing a persisting scoliosis. The extreme gastric dilatation occurring immediately after major trauma is well seen. Girl aged 6 years.

Fractures of C2. In distinction from adult injuries, the odontoid is rarely fractured. The majority of odontoid anomalies are congenital. Fractures of the odontoid are uncommon; union can be obtained in skull traction. Obviously fusion is required for those that do not unite.

Lower Cervical Spine Fractures. Compression fractures with dislocation may occur without cord injury. Fractures of the articular facets are also seen.

Treatment of Cervical Fractures. In our experience, traction, followed by Minerva cast, has given good results. Instability is unusual and fusion is seldom required.

Lumbar and Thoracic Spine

Minor wedge fractures are seen at all levels and require no more than bed rest for about 2 weeks. Relief of pain is usually rapid (Fig. 22-10).

There is some controversy over whether there is such an entity as traumatic spondylolysis. I have seen three children with what looks like a fresh fracture of the pars interarticularis. One united in a unilateral hip spica body cast, one required fusion, and the other became asymptomatic. Recent work by Krenz and Troup and Wiltse and Widell support the idea that it is not unrealistic to work toward union of recent fractures.

Fractures of the Sacrum and Coccyx

Direct violence will produce these injuries. They are difficult to recognize on radiographs. However, displacement of an intercoccygeal joint is recognizable on radiographs, and causes pain on bimanual examination. The pain usually settles when a cushion (disguised as a canvas book bag) is placed on the school chair.

A BRIEF GUIDE TO THE CARE OF SPINAL INJURIES IN CHILDREN

Assessment

Detailed neurologic examination is a must. Finding some intact function in an otherwise apparently complete lesion will provide hope for recovery. In a partial lesion increasing signs may require action, and improvements are very encouraging. Children with apparently purely vertebral lesions should be examined carefully for signs of root injury or minimal long tract signs.

Radiographs must be good enough to show the exact nature of the lesion. Order AP and lateral tomograms if they may help. Decide, using Holdsworth's criteria, whether the fracture is stable or unstable. If unstable, the position must be held by traction or (rarely) by internal fixation. Because ligamentous rupture is rare in children, most fractures occur without rupture and will stabilize by bony healing. Instability produced by congenital anomalies usually requires fusion.

Curative Measures

It is an unhappy fact that the cord is maximally damaged at the moment of impact when the spine is maximally displaced. The role of persistent bony compression, edema, thrombosis, and hematomyelia is small in clinical practice.

Correction of Deformity. For cervical injuries, persistent deformity is corrected by skull traction; for thoracic and lumbar injuries pillows are usually enough though fusion may be needed for gross displacements, particularly with partial lesions.

Myelography and Laminectomy. For centuries laminectomy has had appeal, because it is the only alternative to doing nothing for what is, after all, the worst possible injury. Indiscriminate laminectomy is disappointing or harmful, except for the occasional miracle.

Laminectomy, in our opinion, is only indicated if there is a myelographic block. Myelography is generally indicated only for the rare case in which a partial lesion worsens, but sometimes it is indicated for cases with partial lesions that do not improve. Morgan *et al.* were strongly opposed to laminectomy for incomplete lesions, because half the patients were worse afterwards. Complete lesions are usually considered a contraindication. None of four children with complete thoracic paraplegia who came to laminectomy recovered. But one lumbar complete lesion with lateral subluxation and wedging at L1, in a battered 10-month-old child recovered completely after laminectomy and fusion.

Other Measures. Steroids are very effective in cerebral edema, and this has encouraged their use in spinal injury, though without any convincing efficacy. Tator reviews the place of local hypothermia, hyperbaric oxygen, diuretics, myelotomy, and monoamine oxidase synthesis blockade.

Preventive Measures

Prevention of pressure necrosis of skin, prevention of contractures, and prevention of renal infection require the same vigilance as in adults.

Rehabilitation

Children with traumatic lesions are usually placed in rehabilitation with those who have meningomyelocele. By comparison, the former shine.

REFERENCES

Audic, B., and Maury, M.: Secondary vertebral deformities in childhood and adolescence. Paraplegia, *7:* 10, 1969

Bedbrook, G. M.: Intrinsic factors in the development of spinal deformities with paralysis. Paraplegia, *7:* 22, 1969

Burke, D. C.: Spinal cord trauma in children. Paraplegia, *9:* 1, 1971

Cattell, H. S., and Filtser, D. L.: Pseudo-subluxation and other normal variations in the cervical spine in children. J. Bone Joint Surg., *47A:* 1295, 1965

Fischer, L., Comtet, J. J., and Chappius, J. P.: Particularites radiologiques des fractures et luxations du rachis cervical chez l'enfant. Maroc Medical, *50:* 672, 1970

Gehrig, R., and Michaelis, L. S.: Statistics of acute paraplegia and tetraplegia on a national scale. Paraplegia, *6:* 93, 1968

Griffiths, S. C.: Fracture of odontoid process in children. J. Paediat. Surg., *7:* 680, 1972

Hunter, G. A.: Non-traumatic displacement of the atlanto-axial joint. J. Bone Joint Surg., *50B:* 44, 1968

Krenz, J., and Troup, J. D. G.: The structure of the pars interarticularis of the lower lumbar vertebrae. J. Bone Joint Surg., *55B:* 735, 1973

Kilfoyle, R. M., Foley, J. I., and Norton, P. L.: Spine and pelvic deformity in childhood and adolescent paraplegia. J. Bone Joint Surg., *47A:* 659, 1965

Melzak, J.: Paraplegia among children. Lancet, *2:* 45, 1969

Morgan, T. H., Wharton, G. W., and Austin, G. N.: The results of laminectomy in patients with incomplete spinal cord injuries. Paraplegia, *9:* 14, 1971

Nikitin, M. N.: Treatment of active rotational subluxation of the atlas. Orthopediya, Traumatologiya i Protezirovanie, *1:* 11, 1971

Stern, E. W., and Rand, R. W.: Birth injuries to the cord. Amer. J. Obstet. and Gynecol., *78:* 498, 1959

Tator, C. H.: Acute spinal cord injury: a review of recent studies of treatment and pathophysiology. Canad. Med. Ass. J., *107:* 143, 1972

Wiltse, L. L., and Widell, E. H.: Stress fracture—the basic lesion in isthmic spondylolisthesis. J. Bone Joint Surg., *55A:* 1306, 1973

Wortzman, G., and Dewar, F. P.: Rotary fixation of the atlanto-axial joint. Radiology, *90:* 479, 1968

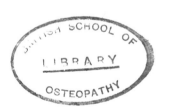

Appendix 1

Accident Prevention

The municipality opened a new adventure playground one weekend. Within a few hours, the orthopaedic resident had seen four fractures from the new giant rope swing. The resident called the police, who promptly closed the brand new playground. This caused much rumpus later, because the playground had been the apple of a politician's eye. But as a form of accident prevention, closing it was very effective.

Usually, it is difficult to do much by direct action. But if you discover a new hazard, you should write to your local Accident Prevention Society. This may be the Safety Committee of the hospital, the Standards Association, or the Safety League.

A friend, Dr. Alex Kates, cared for two children suffering crushing, degloving injuries of the foot. They were on escalators, wearing rubber boots, when the boots caught in the gap between the moving tread and the stationary side. He started a campaign that resulted in a better design for escalators.

A year after I reported a boy who nearly twisted off his arm in a high-speed laundry-dryer, the Canadian Standards Association has written a new standard that should prevent this type of injury.

At present I am hoping to institute some Safety standards for bicycle brakes. The traditional back-pedalling brake is being replaced by hand brakes in this region. When Scott borrowed his friend's bike he tried to stop on the hill, but back-pedalling did not help. He hit a truck, and damaged not only his femur, but also his femoral artery. If he had known where the hand brake was, he would have avoided permanent injury.

Power wringers remain a hazard that years of agitation have not changed. Last year, we treated 61 children with power-wringer injuries.

Practice preventive orthopaedics once in a while. Report the next hazard you meet that injures someone.

Appendix 2

Grief and Disaster

A doctor has to deal with grief every time a patient develops problems as a result of his care. Sometimes he may feel he has been negligent or made a wrong decision. At other times, a patient moves from one complication to another even more serious, in the course of the exemplary treatment of a trivial condition. The surgeon grieves for the patient, regrets the exhibition of his own stupidity, and perhaps has fears of litigation. These patients keep coming back, and the surgeon's grief can prevent any further useful intervention. The patient senses this change from optimism, bred of competence, to ineffectiveness. Complaints are stated more forcefully, in order to stir the doctor into activity again; but this only makes things worse. Indeed, the doctor's whole outlook on this particular problem may be permanently altered. For example, after missing one case of acute appendicitis he may feel compelled to remove the appendix from everyone with the vaguest suggestion of acute appendicitis, until he trusts his judgment once again. Many doctors show cyclical behavior in the treatment of disease.

At the moment, I can think of a number of patients I dread meeting because of the memories they bring back.

Why was I so stupid?

Why did I try to obtain a perfect rather than an adequate result, only to be left with a disaster?

Why did I treat this patient at all?

He had so many injuries, I thought that this one was the least of his problems.

I should have asked him back for a check radiograph and ignored that he lived a hundred miles away.

It didn't look 100 percent right, but I thought I would get away with it.

Grief is certainly a learning experience. But how do you live with this feeling? You can become a heavy drinker, become more secretive, become obsessional about every detail, seek a less demanding practice, have second opinions whenever you sniff danger, and create scenes every time one of your assistants makes an error.

My own practical solutions to the problem of professional grief are these: (1) Accept that persons in every occupation make errors, and we cannot expect to be immune. (2) Look at the patients of other surgeons. When I hear a paper at a meeting I am led to imagine that the author never makes a mistake. But statistics hide many faults, and quiet many a complaining tongue. Seeing somebody else's work, you will realize that you are not alone with disasters. There is nothing more comforting than listening to the justifiable complaints of a patient mismanaged by a senior man you admire. (3) Get on with treating your patient again. Forget the reason for the problem long enough to make a decision about the next step. For example, if a patient has a supracondylar fracture that goes on to malunion because you misinterpreted a radiograph, there is nothing to be gained by looking at it every month and hoping that it will go away. Instead, you should book the child for corrective osteotomy in 3 months' time.

Behind this feeling of grief, you will also have very real fears of litigation. A doctor needs courage to admit even a trivial error because of the risk of painful and expensive consequences. This seems unrealistic. Most industries and businesses have mechanisms for dealing with error. The whole system of guarantees on manufactured goods is designed to handle errors in an easy way, and more particularly to limit the liability of the company.

In Ontario, and in other places, legislation exists to provide modest recompense by simple means for the innocent victims of crime. It would seem timely to provide some comparable method of recompensing patients with iatrogenic problems by something less elaborate than suing the doctor or the hospital. For the patient without subsidized legal aid, the cost can be prohibitive. For the doctor, the commotion and opprobrium generated make litigation something to be avoided by all means. There is much to be said for making admission of error possible. The Workman's Compensation Board has done this for industrial accidents. Perhaps the Medical Protection Association and the Ministry of Health could do something in the same direction. Even the car insurance industry has accepted a 'no fault' plan because of the costs and difficulties of establishing liability. The main problem to be expected from such a plan is that it might soon be swamped with claims by patients who believe that every consequence of an illness is due to medical negligence. Until these legal innovations are made, the surgeon has to struggle with the sense of grief, and try to be honest.

Appendix 3

Writing a Medicolegal Report

You will probably write many reports. At first they will seem useful as a lucrative adjunct to your practice, but as time goes by you will meet many parents who can ill afford the cost of your report for an action that is unlikely to succeed. Reports are time-consuming to prepare, because very much more detail is required than you normally use for the purpose of making a diagnosis and recording and assessing treatment.

The quality of reports varies a great deal, yet lawyers very seldom send them back for improvement. Perhaps they don't read them. You can improve your reports by writing in a clear, unambiguous, accurate, and detailed fashion. Remember that you are writing as an unbiased expert, and you should not write an extravagant report for the plaintiff and a deprecating report for the defendant. "This dear little child was struck down by a speeding motorist;" "the unsupervised child of an unemployed workman ran out in front of a car without warning." Statements like these, in addition to putting you on one side or the other, have no place in a medical report. Your report should deal with the health of the child, not with hearsay evidence. Stick to facts.

Release form. Before sending any report, be sure that you have a release note from the lawyers, signed by the child's guardian.

The Report. Lay the report out clearly, using headings as a guide to the organization. Try to distinguish clearly between factual observations and opinion. Try to indicate which observations have been made by you personally and which have been made by others.

Identification. Identify the subject of the report by name, address, date of birth and the date of the accident.

History of accident. This history can be very brief, because you have only the secondhand impression of the events. It is the lawyer's job to investigate this, not yours. When you use other people's testimony, make this clear on the report by words such as: "His mother told me that. . . ."

Initial examination. The hospital record will describe the time, date, and mode of arrival; include this. If you examined the child, write: "When I examined him, I found. . . ." If you are using the notes of somebody else, put this down clearly: "On arrival at the hospital, he was examined by Dr. So-and-so, who noted. . . ."

Put down the positive findings or diagnoses first, with mention of investigations used to support them. Then describe negative findings, such as, "he was not unconscious." If other specialists have examined the child at this time, list their names, and note the diagnoses they reached.

Treatment and progress. Lawyers are not interested in minutiae. They want a broad picture from which to form an image of "pain and suffering." State the number of days traction was used, the number of days that intravenous fluid balance was maintained. Do not get involved with drug dosage or your own little dilemmas. You are not being sued.

Give the date that the cast was removed and the number of visits made and how long the child was on crutches.

Present state. If the lawyer wants a current examination list the complaints and physical findings. Many lawyers do not ask for a special examination for medicolegal purposes, particularly if it is a year or more after the accident. It is my custom to leave out the heading "Present State" in this situation and to replace it with a phrase such as, "I have not examined the child since the 21st October 1971 and if complaints are made regarding permanent disability, the child should be brought to see me for an up-to-date examination."

Summary and conclusions. Put down the diagnosis and list any current sequelae or complaints. Announce your prognosis, with the introduction: "In my opinion," for each particular complaint. When the child complains of symptoms outside of your particular specialty, you should not attempt to give a prognosis on these complaints; rather, refer the lawyer to the specialist who is familiar with the given body system.

Children rarely complain about the sequelae of injury. Parents are more concerned with the possibility of late effects. Unlike adults, who often seem to exaggerate the consequence of injury, children seldom do. Writing an opinion is very much easier. Special mention should be made about the possibility of a growth disturbance following injury. Few fractures affect growth, but lawyers have been trained to expect a definite statement. In Chapter 17, you will find advice on how to deal with leg-length discrepancy in report writing.

You should also mention the possibility of late osteo-arthritis, although very little data is available. Whatever you put in your report would be hard to refute. Try to state if late problems are (1) probable (indicate the percentage of probability) or (2) possible (probable and possible have two distinct meanings). Indicate the treatment that may be required for any late problems together with the morbidity rate of that procedure.

When you send the report, be sure to keep a copy of it; read it carefully before posting, and initial any alterations that you make. A covering letter, offering to clarify any points that are not clear, together with an account of the cost of the report, of the cost of past and possible future medical treatment, should be enclosed.

Finally, remember that often parents will be given the report to read by their lawyer, and that the only occupational hazard to life that an orthopaedic surgeon faces is murder by the patient who feels that he has been wronged in a compensation suit.

Appendix 4

The Role of Muscles in Fracture Patterns

Fractures happen so quickly that it is impossible to reconstruct the direction of forces responsible. A given type of injury is apparently capable of producing many different patterns of fracture. For example, a valgus force at the elbow may damage the radial neck, the medial epicondyle, or the medial condyle in children of a given age. But a judo expert would be able to ride such a force by yielding to it.

I think that many fractures associated with falls are produced by muscle holding the limb so rigidly that bone-breaking forces are generated. The evidence in favor of this hypothesis is as follows:

(1) Muscle contraction alone is strong enough to produce a fracture. Athletes avulse apophyses. Grenade throwers get spiral fractures of the humerus. Patients receiving E.C.T. and those with uncontrollable convulsions sustain many fractures.

(2) A limb with a rigidly immobilized joint, for example by arthrodesis, is more likely to fracture than a mobile limb. If muscles are holding a limb rigid during a fall less energy can be absorbed before injury.

(3) "He put his arm out to save himself." If he puts his arm out from the body as fast as the ground is coming up the velocity of impact is double what it would have been if he had done nothing. The risk of injury to the wrist has been increased while the risk of a head injury has been diminished. Certainly people do tense their muscles when they sense a fall (as been shown on E.M.G. by Carlsoo and Johansson and by Watt and Jones).

(4) Wrestlers and paratroopers can be trained to avoid injury when they fall. Cats do it instinctively. Wrestlers, who are thrown from one side of the ring to the other, "go with the fall," they do not resist it.

If it can be accepted that many fractures are the result of resisted falls, perhaps it could be accepted that the *site* of the fracture depends on which muscles are contracting. Tomkins has put forward the view that the radial head is dislocated in a Monteggia fracture by strong contraction of biceps when a hyperextension force is applied to the arm. In the autopsy room (when muscles are ineffective) hyperextension produces a supracondylar fracture.

It may well be that the level at which a forearm fractures is determined by the extent of muscle activity. If triceps alone is contracting, a high fracture may be anticipated; when pronator teres is contracting, a fracture just distal to its insertion may be expected; and if the wrist flexors are active, a wrist fracture should occur. Similar hypotheses can be invoked to resolve the mechanism whereby similar forces produce fractures at many different sites. Muscle contraction may concentrate the force of the injury at a particular site.

A greenstick fracture is the result of force too short-lived to produce a complete fracture, and not the result of force too weak to produce a complete fracture, because a bone with a greenstick fracture is weaker than an intact bone. A greenstick fracture avoids becoming a complete fracture, either because the child has come to rest on the ground or because the muscles relax in the nick of time.

In conclusion, muscle action may produce fractures and may determine the site of injury.

REFERENCES

Kelly, J. P.: Fractures complicating electro-convulsive therapy and chronic epilepsy. J. Bone Joint Surg., *36B:* 70, 1954

Tompkins, D.G.: The anterior Monteggia fracture. J. Bone Joint Surg., *53A:* 1109, 1971

Carlsöo, S., and Johansson, O.: Stabilization of and load on the elbow in some protective movements, an experimental study. Acta. Anat., *48:* 224, 1962

Watt, D., and Jones, G. M.: The functional role of the myostatic reflex in man. Proc. Canad. Fed. Biol. Soc., *9:* 13, 1966

Appendix 5

References

This is a short list of references. Tachdjian has recently published an excellent bibliography in "Pediatric Orthopedics" and there is little point in recording an exhaustive list again. I have recorded only the more recent references at the end of each chapter because these will lead back to the older ones.

GENERAL READING

Blount, W. P.: Fractures in Children. Baltimore, Williams & Wilkins, 1955

Charnley, J.: The Closed Treatment of Common Fractures. ed. 3. Edinburgh, E. & S. Livingstone, 1970

Cooper, R. G.: Fractures in Children: fundamentals of management. J. Iowa Med. Soc., *54:* 472, 1964

Judet, R., Judet, J., and Lagrange, J.: Les fractures des membres chez l'enfant. Paris, Libraire Maloine, 1958

Poland, J.: Traumatic Separation of the Epiphyses. London, Smith Elder, 1898. [This is a masterpiece and should be studied by anyone who thinks they have anything new to write.]

Pollen, A. G.: Fractures and Dislocations in Children. Edinburgh, Churchill Livingstone, 1973

Salter, R. B.: Textbook of Disorders and Injuries of the Musculoskeletal System. Baltimore, Williams & Wilkins, 1970

Sharrard, W. J. W.: Paediatric Orthopaedics and Fractures. Oxford, Blackwell, 1971.

Tachdjian, M. O.: Pediatric Orthopedics. Philadelphia, W. B. Saunders, 1972

Watson-Jones, R.: Fractures and Joint Injuries. Edinburgh, E. & S. Livingstone, 1962

Index

Numerals in italics indicate a figure; "t" following a page number indicates a table.

Abdomen, injury(ies) of, 69–72
  care of, nonoperative, 70
    operative, 70
  diagnosis of, 70
  incidence of, 69
  initial management of, 70
  penetrating, 72
  physical signs of, 67, 70
Accident(s), as cause of death, 66
  prevention of, 225
Adult(s), and child, anatomical differences of, 1
  biomechanical differences of, 1–5
  fracture of hip in, compared, 155–156
  physiological differences of, 5–6
  separations at ankle in, compared, 198, 198
Air splint, in osteogenesis imperfecta, 41, 43
Airway, maintenance of, in severe injuries, 66–67
  in unconscious patient, 82
  obstructed, and craniocerebral injury, 78
Amputation, fingertip, 61–62, 62
  in unsalvageable degloved extremity, 63
Analgesics, in initial care in severe injury, 67
Angiography, in craniocerebral injury, 80
Angulation, as problem in finger fractures, 141, 142
  as problem in fracture of tibia, 197
  correction of, in second-hand case, 45
  deformity, forearm, causes of, 140
  in fracture of femur, three-week-old case of, 179
  volar, and fractures of forearm, 126
Ankle, 198–209
  bone. See Talus
  epiphyseal separations at, in children and adults, compared, 198, 198
  fracture(s) of, adult, 208, 208
    at medial malleolus, 205–206, 203, 204, 205
    diagnosis of, 198–200, 199
    epiphyseal, at medial malleolus, 206, 206
    open, 209, 208
    patterns of, 200–206, 200

  rotated, 208, 207
  Tillaux, 204, 202
  triplane, 204–205, 203
  holding of, for application of below-knee cast, 208
  injuries of, miscellaneous, 206–209
    Type VI, 206, 206
  ligaments, 198, 198
Apophysis, displacement of, in pelvic fracture, 153–154
Arm(s). See also Limb(s)
  reconstruction of, following vascular damage, 34
Arteriography, cerebral, in craniocerebral injury, 80
  in ischemia, 31
Artery(ies), damage to, importance of early recognition of, case illustrating, 31–32, 30–31
  in proximal metaphyseal fracture of tibia, 189–191, 190
  See also Vascular damage
  lesions of, and compression, 30
    in continuity, 29–30
      treatment of, 32–33
    in discontinuity, 29
      treatment of, 33
    intimal, 29
    and spasm, 29–30
      treatment of, 32–33
  occlusion of, compensated, 28–29, 29
    complete, 28
    incomplete, 28, 29
    physical signs of, 28
  repair of, for complete ischemia, expectation of, 32
Arthrogram, as diagnostic aid, 19
Asphyxia, traumatic, 69
Atlantoaxial joint, rotatory fixation of, 221–222, 222

Backache, leg length discrepancy and, 178, 177
Bandage, figure-of-eight, in fracture of clavicle, 84, 85
Battered child, 36–39, 197, 206
  management of, 37–38
  recognition of, 36–37, 36, 37
Battering children, 38–39
Bayonet apposition, in femur, 169
Bennett's fracture dislocation of thumb, 144, 143

Bicipital tuberosity, position of, and rotation of radius, 126, 127
Bladder, injury to, 77
Bleeding. See Hemorrhage
Blood, loss, in severe injuries, treatment in, 67
  See also Hemorrhage
  supply, of epiphyses, 9
    in fracture of radial neck, 114
    of growth plate, 9, 8
    obstruction. See Ischemia
  transfusion, technique in, 67
Blood vessels, effects of fractures of forearm on, 127
  injuries of. See Vascular damage
Bone(s), bend of, 2, 3
  biomechanics of, 1
  cyst, simple, 39, 38
  disease, general, 41
  flake of, as complication of fracture of radial neck, 117, 119
  grafting, in fractures caused by bone cysts, 39, 39
  growth of, disturbed, reasons for, 8
  growth remodelling of, 5, 5
  lesions of, local, 39
    in supracondylar fracture of elbow, 101–102, 102, 103
  long, fractures of, head injuries with, 41, 44
  nonunion of, 6
  overgrowth of, 5
  porosity of, of adult and child, compared, 1, 1, 2
  progressive deformity of, 5
  weakness, general, 39–41
Bowel, injuries of, 72
Bowing, volar, and fractures of forearm, 126
Brain, burr hole exploration of, 81
  edema of, in head injuries, 81
  injury of, emergency measures in, 79
  See also Craniocerebral injury
Brain scanning, in craniocerebral injury, 80
Bronchopneumonia, in severe head injuries, 82
Brush burn, simple, 53
  with tissue loss, 53–54, 55, 56
Buckle fracture(s), 1–2, 2
  of femur, 179, 178
  of forearm, 134, 135
  of thumb, 141–143, 142

Bumper fracture, site of, age and, 155, *155*
Burn, brush, simple, 53
    with tissue loss, 53–54, *55, 56*
Butterfly fragment, following fracture of femur, 178, *178*

Callus, fracture, following perichondrial ring injury, 17
    hyperplastic, in osteogenesis imperfecta, *43*
    in paraplegia, 40, *41*
Cartilage, growth, as diagnostic trap, 19
    biomechanics of, 2–4
        injury through, in pelvic fracture, 153
Cast(s), application of, 23–25
        distraction of child during, 24
    below-knee, holding of ankle for, *208*
    bracing, in midshaft fracture of femur, 172
    in complete fractures of radius and ulna, 130, 131, *132, 133, 134*
    loose, recognition of, 27, *25*
    position of limb for, 24, *24*
    slippage in, in elbow injury, 93–94
    Statue of Liberty, 89, *88*
    stovepipe, *178*
    three-point molding of, 24–25, *24*
    in Type II shoulder injury, 89, *88*
    unsatisfactory, 23, *23*
Cerebral palsy, 40
Chest, flail, 69
    injury(ies) of, 68–69
        closed, 68
        penetrating, 69
    problems, in severe head injuries, 82
Child(ren), and adult, anatomical differences of, 1
        biomechanical differences of, 1–5
        fracture of hip in, compared, 155–156
        physiological differences of, 5–6
        separations at ankle in, compared, 198, *198*
    battered, 36–39, 197, 206
        management of, 37–38
        recognition of, 36–37, *36, 37*
    battering, 38–39
    distraction of, during application of cast, 24
    limping, 196
    newborn, fractures in, 42, *44*
    relationship with, during diagnosis, 18
    uncooperative, as warning, 26
Chloride, metabolism, disorders to, in severe head injuries, 82
Chondrolysis, in growth plate injuries, 16
Clavicle, injuries of, sites of, 84–86
    medial end of, separation of, 84–85
    outer end of, fracture of, 86, *86*
    shaft of, fractures of, 84, *84, 85*
Cleidocranial dysostosis, 85

Closed reduction, and cast, in supracondylar fracture of elbow, 97–98
    in complete fractures of radius and ulna, 130–131, *132, 133 134*
    complications after, in medial epicondylar fractures of elbow, 107
    follow-up of, in supracondylar fracture of elbow, 100
    in growth plate injuries, 15–16
    and percutaneous wire, in supracondylar fracture of elbow, 98, *96*
    technique of, in supracondylar fracture of elbow, 98–99, *97, 98, 99, 100, 101*
    with traction, in complete fractures of radius and ulna, 131–132
Coccyx, fractures of, 223
Complications, possible, recognition of, 26
Compression, and arterial lesions, 30
Concussion, 217
Condyle, medial, injury of, diagnosis of, 19, *20*
Consciousness, level of, recording of, in craniocerebral injury, 78, 79
Contracture, quadriceps, following fracture of femur, 178
    Volkmann's, 20, 28
        in supracondylar fracture of elbow, 101
Coracoid process, fracture of, 87, *87*
Coxa magna luxans, 162–164
Coxa vara, 156, 161, *160*
Craniocerebral injury, 78–83
    diagnosis of, 80
    examination in, 78–80
    positioning of patient in, 78, 81, *79*
    problems associated with, 81–82
    prognosis in, 82
        grave, signs of, 83
    signs of deterioration in, 80
    surgical intervention in, 81
    treatment of, 80–81
        summary of, 82–83
Cranium, examination of, in craniocerebral injury, 78–79
Crush-avulsion injuries, 53, *53*
Cubitus valgus, 128
Cyst, bone, simple, 39, *38*

Death, accidents as cause of, 66
Deformity, angular, forearm, causes of, 140
    bone, progressive, 5
    degree of, diagnosis of, 19–20, *21*
    flexion, in fracture of base of thumb, 141–143, *142*
    gunstock, in supracondylar fracture of elbow, 103, *104*
    Madelung's, 128, *130*
    mallet, in phalangeal fractures, 144, *144*
    progressive, 5
        following perichondrial ring injury, 17, *17*

rotational, in fracture of forearm, 124, *124*
        recognition of, 125–126, *126*
    valgus, in proximal metaphyseal fracture of tibia, 191–194, *190, 191*
        in supracondylar fracture of elbow, 103–104
    varus, in ablation of perichondrial ring, 206, *206*
        in fracture of tibia with intact fibula, 196, *192*
        in supracondylar fracture of elbow, 103–104, *104*
Degloving injury(ies), of extremity, unsalvageable, 63, *62*
    partial, 58–60, *60, 61*
    total, complex, 62–63, *62*
        simple, 60–62, *61, 62*
Dermatomes, *51*
Diabetes insipidus, in severe head injuries, 82
Diagnosis, relationship with parents and child during, 18
    traps to, 18–20
Diaphragm, rupture of, 68
Dislocation(s), of elbow, 108, *107*
    of elbow joint. See Elbow, joint, dislocation(s) of
    of fingers and thumb, 148, *148*
    fracture, Bennett's, of thumb, 144, *143*
        of radius and ulna, 136–140
    of hip, 166–167, *164, 165, 166, 167*
    of patella, 183–184, *183, 184*
    of shoulder, 87
    vertebral, cord injury with, 217–218, 217t
Displacement, degree of, diagnosis of, 19–20, *21*
Down's syndrome, dislocation of hip in, 166, *164*
Duodenum, injuries of, 72
Dysostosis, cleidocranial, 85
Dystrophy, muscular, 39–40, *41*

Edema, cerebral, in head injuries, 81
Elbow, 93–123
    dislocation of, 108, *107*
    fracture(s) of, diagnosis of, 93, *93, 94*
        lateral condylar, 109–111
            complications of, 109
            displaced, 109, 110, *109, 110*
                treatment of, results of, 110–111, *112*
                    technique in, 110, *111*
            late cases of, 111, *113*
            mechanism of, 109, *108*
            undisplaced, 109, *109*
                treatment of, 109–110
        lateral epicondylar, 109
        medial condylar, 112, *114*
        medial epicondylar, diagnostic traps in, 105–106, *105*
            treatment of, closed reduction in, complications after, 107

in displacement, 106, *106*
and dislocation, 107, *106*
minimal, 106
open reduction in, 107, *106*
problem after, 107
problems in, 107
with trapped fragment, 107
varieties of, 105, *105*
proximal radial, 112–118
reduction of, 93
complications in, 93–95
supracondylar, 95–105
angulated greenstick, 96, *95*
classical displaced, closed reduction in, and cast, 97–98
follow-up of, 100
and percutaneous wire, 98, *96*
technique of, 98–99, *97, 98, 99, 100, 101*
initial care in, 97
open reduction in, and internal fixation, 98
reduction in, problems with, 102–103
varus and valgus deformity following, 103–104, *104*
requiring reduction, problems associated with, 100–102, *102, 103*
traction in, 97, *95*
extension, experimental production of, 95–96, *94*
joint, dislocation(s) of, at articular surface of ulna, 120
medial epicondylar, 119
true, 120
with obvious fractures, 120
with occult fragments, 119–120
medial hinge of, and closed reduction of fracture, 98, *97, 98*
pulled, 122, *121*
pathology of, 122, *121*
treatment of, 122
Electrolyte balance, maintenance of, in severe injury, 81–82
Emergency room, initial care of severe injuries in, 66
Emphysema, subcutaneous, 69
Epicondyle, medial, separation of, diagnosis of, 19, *20*
Epiphysis(es), blood supply of, *9*
cartilaginous, 10
of clavicle, separation of, 84–85
comminuted fractures of, 7, *7*
fractures of, in child abuse, 36, *36, 37*
not involving growth plate, 7, *7*
ligamentous attachment of, avulsion at, 7, *7*
ossified, 10–11
osteochondral fragments of, 7, *7*
proximal, of shoulder, separation of, 87, *87*
separation of, from metaphysis, experiments in, 2–4, *4*
slipped, in hip fracture, 158

totally clad with cartilage, 9
unossified, separation of, 19
with soft-tissue attachments, 9
Escharectomy-fasciotomy, in wringer injury, 58, *58*
Examination, in craniocerebral injury, 78–80
immediate, in severe injuries, 66
Exostosis, traumatic, 17, *16*
Extremity(ies). *See* Limb(s)

Fasciotomy, and exploration, 32
subcutaneous, 33, *33*
Fasciotomy-fibulectomy, 33
Fat embolism, in fracture of femur, 177
pulmonary, in severe head injuries, 82
Fat fracture, 47–48, *48*
Fat pad sign, in elbow fracture, *95*
Femur, distal epiphysis of, separation of, 180, *178, 180*
fracture(s) of, intraarticular, 185, *185, 186*
management of, in restless child, 41
supracondylar, buckle, 179, *178*
displaced, 179–180
stress, 179, *179*
and tibia, fractured, in same leg, 197, *194–195, 196*
shaft of, 169–180
fracture(s) of, abducted, 173
abducted, 173
classical midshaft, 171–173, *169, 170*
in child 2 years and over, 172, *170–171, 172*
in child under 2 years, 172, *172*
classification of, 171–173, *169*
difficulties associated with, 170
examination in, 170–171
extended, 173, *173, 174*
problems in, early, 173–177
late, 178–179
with multiple injuries, 173–174, *175*
shortening of, management of, in second-hand case, 45
Fibroma, nonossifying, 39, *40*
Fibula, epiphysis of, displaced, 208, *207*
fracture of, in fracture of tibia, 196, *192, 193*
with intraarticular fragment, 206, *199*
injury of, Type I, 200, *1*
intact, in fracture of tibia, 195–196, *191*
loss of, 208, *207*
Finger(s), fracture(s) of, problems of, 141
metacarpophalangeal joint of, dislocations of, 148
phalanx(ges) of, fractures of. *See* Phalanx(ges), of finger(s)

Fingertip amputation, 61–62, *62*
Fixation, internal, of growth plate injuries, 11
in hip fracture, 156, 160–161, *156, 159, 161*
in supracondylar fracture of elbow, 98
in vascular damage, 33
intramedullary, in fracture of femur with multiple injuries, 174, *175*
Flail chest, 69
Flexion deformity, in fracture of base of thumb, 141–143, *142*
Fluid(s), balance, maintenance of, in severe head injury, 82
replacement of, in craniocerebral injury, 78
Fluorothane shakes, 41
Follow-up, importance of, 20–21, 26–27
Foot(Feet), 210–215
reconstruction of, following vascular damage, 34–35
Forearm, anatomy of, 124–128
bones of, remodelling and, 22–23, *5*
fractures of, follow-up care in, 140
mechanism of, 124
remodelling and, 126, *128, 129*
rotational deformity in, 124, *124*
recognition of, 125–126, *126*
radiographs of, 138, *137*
rotation, 124–125, *125*
Foreign body(ies), in knee, 188, *187*
removal of, 48
Fracture(s), buckle. *See* Buckle fracture(s)
bumper, site of, age and, 155, *155*
classification of, 1–2, *2*
complete, 5
displaced, supracondylar, of femur, 179–180
epiphyseal, 7, *7*
fat, 47–48, *48*
greenstick. *See* Greenstick fracture(s)
lucky, 44, *46*
multiple, in child abuse, 36, *37*
in newborn, 42, *44*
nonconforming, 19, *21*
pathological, 39–41
patterns, role of muscles in, 229
Robert Gillespie's, 197, *196*
slip of, recognition of, 27, *26*
stress, 42–43, *45*
of femur, 179, *179*
of metatarsal, 215, *215*
Tillaux, 204, *202*
torus. *See* Buckle fracture(s)
triplane, 204–205, *203*
uneducated beliefs concerning, 26
with vascular damage. *See* Vascular damage, fractures with
Fracture, dislocation(s), Bennett's, of thumb, 144, *143*
of radius and ulna, 136–140

Fragment(s), butterfly, following fracture of femur, 178, *178*
    detached, in fracture of tibial spine, 182–183, *182*
    intraarticular, in fracture of fibula, 206, *199*
    osteochondral, in dislocation of patella, 184, *183*
    of epiphysis, 7, *7*
Frostbite, 148–149, *148*

Galeazzi's fracture dislocation, 139–140, *140*
Gallows traction, in midshaft fracture of femur, 172, *172*
Genitourinary tract, injuries of, 74–77
    diagnosis of, 75
        presentation of, 75
        urologic evaluation in, techniques for, 75–76, *75*
    upper, injuries of, specific, 76, *75, 76t*
Gillespie's fracture, 197, *196*
Grafting, bone, in fractures caused by bone cysts, 39, *39*
Grafts, skin. *See* Skin, graft(s)
Greenstick fracture(s), 2, 229, *3, 4*
    of femur, *178*
    of radius, 128–129, *131*
    of tibia, 191–194, *189, 190, 191*
Grief, professional, solutions to problems of, 226
Growth, effects of fractures of forearm on, 128, *130*
    effects of frostbite on, 148–149, *148*
    effects of wringer injuries on, 149, *149*
Growth cartilage, as diagnostic trap, 19
    biomechanics of, 2–4
    injury through, in pelvic fracture, 153
Growth plate, anatomy of, 8–9, *8*
    biomechanics of, 2–4
    blood supply of, 9, *8*
    closure of, premature, as complication of fracture of hip, 158–159, *159*
        as complication of fracture of radial neck, 117, *120*
    disruption, management of, in second-hand case, 46
    fractures of epiphysis not involving, 7, *7*
    healing reactions of, 9–11, *10*
    injuries of, 7–16
        at medial malleolus, 205–206, *203, 204*
        care of, 14–16
        classification of, Poland, *11*
            Salter-Harris, 11–16, *10*
        consequences of, 7–8
        defining line of fracture in, 14–15
        immobilization in, 16
        internal fixation of, 11
        presenting late, 16
        reduction methods in, 15–16
        treatment of child and parents in, 15
        Type I, 11–12, *10, 11, 12*
        Type II, 12–13, *10, 13*
        Type III, 13, *10, 13*

Type IV, 13–14, *10, 14*
Type V, 14–15, *10, 15, 16*
    proximal tibial, injuries of, 189, *190*
    transverse section of, histology of, 9, *9*
Gunstock deformity, in supracondylar fracture of elbow, 103, *104*

Hand, 141–149
Head, examination of, in craniocerebral injury, 78–79
    injury(ies) of, 67
        severe. *See* Craniocerebral injury with long bone fractures, 41, *44*
Healing, speed of, 6
Heel bone, fractures of, 210–211, *213*
Hemarthrosis, traumatic, of knee, 181
Hematoma(s), 47
    extradural, in craniocerebral injury, 80
Hematuria, in genitourinary injuries, 75
Hemobilia, traumatic, 71
Hemophilia, 42
Hemorrhage, control of, in penetrating chest injuries, 69
    extradural, in craniocerebral injury, 80
    gastrointestinal, 72
    intraperitoneal, in rupture of liver, 70–71
        in rupture of spleen, 70
        in severe injuries, 68
        signs of, 70
    in pelvic fracture, 151–152
    retroperitoneal, in abdominal injuries, 71
        in pelvic fracture, 71–72, 151–152
    severe occult, evidence of, 75
    urethral, in genitourinary injuries, 75
Heparin, postoperative, in vascular damage, 33
Heterotopic ossification, as complication of fracture of radial neck, 117, *119*
Hip, 155–168
    dislocation of, 166, *164*
        complications of, 166–167, *166, 167*
        recurrent, 166
        trapped intraarticular fragment in, 166, *166, 167*
        treatment of, 166, *165*
        results of, 167
    fracture(s) of, adult and child, compared, 155–156
        basal, 158–161
        displaced, fixation of, 159
            treatment of, 161–162, *160, 161*
        fixation of, internal, 156, 160–161, *156, 159, 161*
        transcervical, 158–161
        undisplaced, fixation of, 159–160
            treatment of, 161, *160*
    osteoarthritis of, following fracture of femur, 178
    slipped epiphysis of, 158
    traumatic separation of, 158
    Type I injuries of, 158, *156, 157*
Hip spica, in midshaft fracture of femur, 172, 173

Humerus, fracture(s) of, and bone cysts, 39, *38*
    management of, in restless child, 41
    shaft of, fracture of, management of, 90–91, *90, 91, 92*
        special problems associated with, 91-92
Hyperbaric oxygen, in vascular damage, 33
Hyperpigmentation, skin graft, 65, *65*
Hypertrophic scars, 63, *63*

Immobilization, child and, 155–156
    in growth plate injuries, 16
Infant, limping, 196
Infection, growth plate injuries and, 16
Injury(ies), crush-avulsion, 53, *53*
    degloving. *See* Degloving injury(ies)
    multiple, with fracture of femur, 173–174, *175*
        and fracture of tibia in same leg, 197, *194–195, 196*
    severe, initial care of, 66–68
Internal fixation. *See* Fixation, internal
Interposition, as problem in finger fractures, 141
Intertrochanteric fractures, treatment of, 164-166, *162, 163*
Ischemia, after reduction, 28
    aftermath of, 33–34
    compartment, 28, *29*
    complete, expectations of arterial repair for, *32*
    in fracture of femur, 176–177
    muscle, 28, *29*
    prevention of, 30
    reconstruction of limb following, 34–35
    treatment of, 30–33
    Volkmann's, 28, *29*

Joint(s), atlantoaxial, rotatory fixation of, 221–222, *222*
    elbow. *See* Elbow, joint
    knee. *See* Knee joint
    metacarpophalangeal, dislocations of, 148, *148*
        fracture dislocation at, in wringer injury, 55, *56*
    metatarsophalangeal, dislocation of, skin graft contracture and, 64, *64*
    surface, irregularity, finger fractures and, 141, *142*
        management of, in second-hand case, 46
    tibiofibular, proximal, subluxation of, 188

Kidney(s), injury of, 67-68
    trauma to, surgical management of, 76
        indications for, 76, 77
        types of, *75*
            correlated with clinical and radiographic findings, 76t

Knee cap, dislocation of, 183–184, *183, 184*
  fractures of, 184–185, *184*
Knee joint, 181–188
  foreign bodies in, 188, *187*
  injuries of, capsular, 186
    ligamentous, 186
  locking of, apparent, 188
    benign, 188
  puncture wounds of, 188, *187*

Laceration(s). *See also* Wound(s)
  tidy, 48
    closure of, direct, 50–51, *49*
      skin graft, 51, *50, 51, 52*
    initial care of, 50
  untidy, 48
    closure of, 53
    initial care of, 52–53, *52*
Laminectomy, 223
Laparotomy, in duodenal and pancreatic injuries, 72
  in hepatic rupture, 71
  in penetrating abdominal injury, 72
Leg(s). *See also* Limb(s)
  length, as problem in fracture of femur, 178, *176*
    as problem in fracture of tibia, 197
  discrepancy, and backache, 178, *177*
  reconstruction of, following vascular damage, 34
Ligament(s), ankle, 198, *198*
  of knee, injuries of, 186
Limb(s), fractures of, in severe head injuries, 82
  lower, problems of, following spinal fracture, 221, *221*
  reconstruction of, in vascular damage, 34–35
  severed, 35, *34*
  unsalvageable degloved, 63, *62*
Limp, following fracture of femur, 172, 178
  following fracture of tibia, 196
Litigation, admission of error and, 226
Liver, rupture of, 70–71
Lumbar puncture, in craniocerebral injury, 80
Lung, contusion, 68
  fat embolism in, severe head injuries, 82
  laceration, in penetrating chest injuries, 69

Madelung's deformity, 128, *130*
Malarticulation, as problem in finger fractures, 141, *142*
Malleolus, medial, epiphyseal fractures of, 206, *206*
  fractures around, 205–206, *203, 204, 205*
  removal of, 17, *17*
Mallet deformity, in phalangeal fractures, 144, *144*

Malrotation, finger fractures and, 141, *141*
  following fracture of femur, 179
  radial, 126, *126*
  and rotation of forearm, 124, *125*
Malunion, in elbow injury, 94–95
  and rotation of forearm, 124, *125*
  in supracondylar fracture of elbow, 103–105, *103, 104*
Medicolegal report, writing of, 227–228
Meniscus, 186–187
  torn, treatment of, 188
Metacarpophalangeal joint, fracture dislocation at, in wringer injury, 55, *56*
Metacarpus, fifth, injuries of, 144
  shaft of, fractures of, 144
  thumb, injuries of, 141–144
Metaphysis, separation of epiphysis from, experiments in, 2–4, *4*
  upper, of shoulder, fractures of, 90
Metatarsal(s), fifth, base of, Robert Jones fracture of, 212–213, *214*
  fractures of, 212–215
    multiple, 215, *214*
    stress, 215, *215*
Metatarsophalangeal joint(s), dislocation of, skin graft contracture and, 64, *64*
Midtarsal injuries, 211–212, *214*
Monteggia's fracture dislocation, 121, 136–138, *137, 138*
  treatment of, 139, *139*
Muscular dystrophy, 39–40, *41*
Muscle(s), displacement, in pelvic fracture, 153–154
  gastrocnemius, in midshaft fracture of femur, 172, *169*
  ischemia, of, 28, *29*
  role of, in fracture patterns, 229
Myelography, 223

Necrosis, avascular, as complication of basal and transcervical hip fractures, 158–159, *158*
  as complication of fracture of radial neck, 117, *119*
  in dislocation of hip, 166, 167, *165 166*
  following internal fixation of hip fracture, 160, *159*
  in hip fracture, 155
  signs of, 162, *162*
Nerve(s), effects of fractures of forearm on, 127
  injury(ies) of, in medial epicondylar fracture of elbow, 107
  in pelvic fracture, 152
  in supracondylar fracture of elbow, 100–101
Nerve palsy(ies), in elbow injury, 93
  radial, in fracture of humeral shaft, 91–92
  in supracondylar fracture of elbow, 97, *95*
  in tibial fractures, 197

Nervous system, central, examination of, in craniocerebral injury, 79–80
Neuromuscular disorders, 39
Newborn, fracture in, 42, *44*
Nonunion, 6
  as complication of fracture of radial neck, 118
Note-keeping, in vascular damage, 33

Olecranon, fracture(s) of, 118, *121*
  and fracture of radial neck of elbow, 116–117, *116, 117*
Open reduction, in complete fractures of radius and ulna, 132–133, *135*
  in growth plate injuries, 15–16
  indications for, 25–26
  and internal fixation, in supracondylar fracture of elbow, 98
  problem of, in medial epicondylar fracture of elbow, 107
  technique of, in medial epicondylar fracture of elbow, 107, *106*
  in Type II shoulder injury, 89, *89*
Os calcis, fractures of, 210–211, *213*
Osteoarthritis, of hip, following fracture of femur, 178
Osteodystrophy, renal, 42, *44*
Osteogenesis imperfecta, 41
Osteomyelitis, healing, protection from fracture in, *41*
Osteopetrosis, 41
Osteotomy, supracondylar, in varus and valgus deformity, 103–104, *104*, 104t
Overdiagnosis, 19
Overgrowth of bone, 5
Overlap, 23
  in fracture of femur, 179
Oxygen, hyperbaric, in vascular damage, 33

Palsy(ies), cerebral, 40
  nerve, in elbow injury, 93
    in supracondylar fracture of elbow, 97, *95*
    in tibial fractures, 197
  radial nerve, in fracture of humeral shaft, 91–92
Pancreas, injuries of, 72
Paraplegia, 40–41, *41*
  causes of, 216
Parent(s), attitude of, in child abuse, 36–37
  informing of, 26, 27
  relationship with, during diagnosis, 18
Patella, dislocation of, 183–184, *183, 184*
  fractures of, 184–185, *184*
Patient(s), second-hand, diplomatic considerations in, 44–45
  technical considerations in, 45–46

Pelvis, 150–154
fracture(s) of, associated injuries in, 150
classification of, 150
hemorrhage in, 71–72, 151–152
initial management in, 150–154
patterns of, 152–153, *151, 152, 153 154*
treatment of, 154
Perichondrial ring, ablation of, 206, *206*
injuries of, 17, *16*
removal of, 17
Perineum, extravasation in, in genitourinary injuries, 75
Periosteum, biomechanics of, 4–5
separation of epiphysis and, 2–3
Phalanx(ges), of finger(s), distal end of, injuries of, bicondylar, 146–148, *147*
cartilaginous, 145–146, *147*
unicondylar, 146, *147*
proximal end of, injuries of, Type I, 144, *144*
Type II, 144–145, *145*
Type III, 145, *146*
shaft of, fractures of, 145
of toe(s), fractures of, 215, *16, 215*
Pinning, percutaneous, in supracondylar fracture of elbow, 98, *96*
Steinmann, in fractures of tibia and fibula, 196, *192–193*
supracondylar in, extended fracture of femur, 173, *174*
Pneumothorax, simple, 68
subcutaneous emphysema and, 69
tension, 67, 68
treatment of, 68–69
treatment of, in penetrating chest injury, 69
Poland classification of growth plate injuries, *11*
Poliomyelitis, 39
Positioning of patient, in craniocerebral injury, 78, 81, *79*
Pronation, radius in, 126, *127*
Public relations, in vascular damage, 33

Quadriceps contracture following fracture of femur, 178

Radiograph(s), of ankle, 198–200, *199*
in cervical spine injuries, 221
in closed reduction of supracondylar fracture of elbow, 99–100, *100, 101*
in complete fractures of radius and ulna, 130–131
in craniocerebral injury, 80
diagnostic, 18, *18*
scope of, ℸ9–20, *19, 20, 21*
in elbow injury, 93, *93*
of forearm, 138, *137*
in fracture of radial neck, 113–114
in fractures of forearm, 126, *126*
in knee joint injury, 181

in lateral condylar fracture of elbow, 109, 110–111, *93, 108, 112*
in midshaft fracture of femur, 172, *173*
oblique, in ankle injuries, 19, *19*
in pelvic fracture, 151, 152–153, *151*
in penetrating abdominal injury, 72
in rotatory fixation of atlantoaxial joint, 221–222, *222*
in severe injuries, 67
stress, in diagnosis, 19, *1*
in elbow injury, 93, *94*
in tibial growth plate injuries, 189, *190*
in Type II shoulder injury, 88
Radiohumeral dislocation, 121, *121*
Radius, anatomy of, 124–128
distal, epiphyseal separation of, Type I, 133–134
Type II, 134, *135*
fracture of, displaced, and displaced fracture of distal ulna, 136, *137*
fracture(s) of, 124–140
clinical examination in, 125, *126*
effects of, on growth, 128, *130*
on nerves and vessels, 127
follow-up care in, 140
and fracture of ulna, complete, 129–130
closed reduction in, techniques of, 130–132, *132, 133, 134*
open reduction in, technique of, 132–133, *135*
greenstick, angulated, 128–129, *131*
displaced, 128, *131*
mechanism of, 124
radiographic aids in, 126, *126*
remodelling and, 126, *128, 129*
rotational deformity in, 124, *124*
recognition of, 125–126, *126*
solitary, medially displaced, 136, *135*
overlapping, 134–135, *136*
fracture dislocations of, 136–140
head of, dislocation of, 120–121
long-standing, 121, *138*
solitary, 121, *138*
separation of, 138, *138*
malrotation of, 126, *126*
neck of, dislocation of, congenital, 138, *138*
fracture of, associated injuries in, 114
blood supply in, 114
concomitant injuries in, 116–117, *116, 117*
displacement in, 113–114
minimally displaced, treatment of, 115, *116*
moderately displaced, treatment of, 115–116
posteriorly displaced, 113, *115*
results of treatment of, 117–118
site of, 114, *115*
valgus, 112–113, *114*
Record-keeping, in vascular damage, 33
Rectum, examination of, in genitourinary injuries, 75

Reduction, closed. *See* Closed reduction
contraindications to, 22
open. *See* Open reduction
Remodelling, awaiting of, contraindications to, 22–23, *5*
indications for, 22
and fractures of forearm, 126, *128, 129*
growth, 5, *5*
principles of, 22
process of, 22
Report, medicolegal, writing of, 227–228
Resuscitation in severe injuries, 66–68
Rickets, 42, *45*
Rotation, deformity of, in fractures of forearm, 124, *124*
recognition of, 125–126, *126*
forearm, 124–125, *125*

Sacrum, fractures of, 223
Salter-Harris classification of growth plate injuries, 11–16, *10*
Scapula, fractures of, 87, *87*
Scars, donor site, as complication of skin grafting, 63–64, *64*
hypertrophic, 63, *63*
Scoliosis, following spinal fracture, 219, *220*
Second-hand cases, diplomatic considerations in, 44–45
technical considerations in, 45–46
Shock, and craniocerebral injury, 78
in fracture of femur, 174
initial care in, 67
Shortening, femoral, management of, in second-hand case, 45
Shoulder, dislocation of, 87
injury of, Type II, degrees of displacement in, 88–89
description of, 87–88, *88*
management of, 88–89
prognosis in, 89–90
upper metaphysis of, fractures of, 90
Skin, deficiency of, at laceration, test for, 50
degloved. *See* Degloving injury(ies)
flaps, avulsion of, complex, with exposure of vital structures, 58, *59*
simple, 58, *58, 59*
in brush burn with tissue loss, 54, *56*
pedicle, in complex total degloving, 62
tube, in complex total degloving, 62–63
graft(s), in brush burn with tissue loss, 53–54, *55, 56*
care of, 51
contraction of, 64–65, *64*
donor sites for, 63–64
full-thickness, 51
in fingertip amputation, 61–62, *62*
hyperpigmentation, 65, *65*
instruments for obtaining, 51, *51*
levels of cutting of, 51, *50*

split-thickness, 51
  in complex total degloving, 62
  in simple total degloving, 60, *61*
  technique for obtaining, 64
  techniques, 51, *51, 52*
margins, in laceration, closure of, 51, *49*
traction, fixed, in midshaft fracture of femur, 172, *172*
  in fracture of humeral shaft, 91, *91*
Skull, burr hole exploration through, 81
Sling, in Type II shoulder injury, 89
Smith-Petersen nail, in hip fracture, 156, *156*
Soft tissue(s), deficiency of, at laceration, test for, 50
injuries of, 47–65
  complications of, 63–65
  diagnosis of, 20, *22*
  in supracondylar fracture of elbow, 100–101
Spasm, and arterial lesions, 29–30
  treatment of, 32–33
Spina bifida, 40–41
Spinal cord, contusion of, 217
infarction of, 217
injury(ies) of, general features of, 216
  with vertebral fracture or dislocation, 217–218, 217t
  without fracture or open injury, 217
Spine, cervical, fractures of, treatment of, 223
injuries of, 218–219, *219*
  common, 221–222
  radiographs in, 221
  rare, 222–223
  lower, fractures of, 223
dens of, separation of, from neural arch, 216, *216*
fracture(s) of, lower limb problems associated with, 221, *221*
  spinal problems associated with, 219–220, *220*
  types of, 218–221
  urological problems associated with, 221
fusion of, following spinal fracture, 219–220, *220*
injury(ies) of, assessment of, 223
  classification of, 216–218, 217t
  curative measures in, 223
  diagnosis of, 80
  general features of, 216
  preventive measures in, 223
  rehabilitation following, 223
lumbar, injuries of, 219, 223, *222*
thoracic, injuries of, 218, 223, *218*
Spleen, rupture of, 70
Splenectomy, indications for, 70
Splint(s), air, in osteogenesis imperfecta, 41, *43*
as first aid in supracondylar fracture of elbow, 97
prior to diagnostic radiograph, 18

Spurs, bony, following fracture of femur, 178, *178*
Stiffness, following reduction of elbow fracture, 95, 103
Stockinette Velpeau, in fracture of humeral shaft, 90, *90*
Stress fracture(s), 42–43, *45*
of femur, 179, *179*
of metatarsal, 215, *215*
Stress radiographs. *See* Radiograph(s), stress
Subtrochanteric fracture, open, 173, *174*
with multiple injuries, 174, *175*
Supination, radius in, 126, *127*
Suture(s), interrupted, in skin closure, 51, *49*
polyglycolic acid, in subcutaneous closure, 50, *49*
subcuticular, in skin closure, 51, *49*
Synostosis, as complication of fracture of radial neck, 117, *118*

Talus, body of, fracture of, 210, *212*
lateral wall of, fracture of, 210, *213*
neck of, fracture of, 210, *210, 211*
Tattooing, traumatic, 53, *54*
Tendons, peroneus longus and brevis, rupture of, 54
Thoracobrachial box, in fracture of humeral shaft, 90–91, *91*
Thrombosis, 30, 33
Thumb, base of, impacted fracture of, 141–143, *142*
metacarpophalangeal joint of, dislocation of, 148, *148*
metacarpus of, injuries of, 141–144
Type II injuries of, 143–144, *143*
Type III injuries of, 144, *143*
Tibia, 189–197
distal, diaphysis of, Robert Gillespie's fracture of, 197, *196*
fracture(s) of, associated injuries in, 197
  complications of, 197
  diaphyseal, 194–195, *191*
  and femur, fractured, in same leg, 197, *194–195, 196*
  and fibula, fractured, 196, *192, 193*
  intact, 195–196, *191*
  intraarticular, 204–206
  metaphyseal, 197
  open, 196
  and pathological fractures, 197
  variations of, common, 195–196
  uncommon, 196–197
injury of, Type I, 204, *202*
  Type II, 200–204, *201*
proximal, fracture(s) of, metaphyseal, arterial hazard, 189–191, *189, 190*
  valgus greenstick, 191–194, *189, 190, 191*
injuries of, classification of, 189, *189*
  growth plate, 189, *190*

Tibial plateau, fracture(s) of, 185–186, *186*
Tibial spine, fracture(s) of, 181–183, *181, 182*
Tibial tubercle, avulsion of, 186
Tibiofibular joint, proximal, subluxation of, 188
Tightness, linear, as complication of soft-tissue injury, 63, *64*
Tillaux fracture, 204, *202*
Toe(s), phalanx(ges) of, fractures of, 215, *16, 215*
Torus fracture(s). *See* Buckle fracture(s)
Tracheastomy, indications for, 82
Traction, and closed reduction, in complete fractures of radius and ulna, 131–132
gallows, in midshaft fracture of femur, 172, *172*
skin, fixed, in midshaft fracture of femur, 172, *172*
  in fracture of humeral shaft, 91, *91*
  in supracondylar fracture of elbow, 97, 102–103, *95*
  in Type II shoulder injury, 89
ulnar pin, in fracture of humeral shaft, 91, *91*
Transfusion, blood, in severe injuries, 67
Traumatic tattooing, 53, *54*
Treatment, correct, traps between you and, 20–26
traps arising during, 26–27
Triffin pins, in hip fracture, 156, *156*
Triplane fracture, 204–205, *203*
Trochanter, fracture(s) of, 155, 164–166, *155, 162, 163*
Tuberosity, bicipital, position of, and rotation of radius, 126, *127*

Ulna, anatomy of, 124–128
bending of, in dislocation of radial head, 138, *138*
distal, fracture of, displaced, and displaced fracture of distal radius, 136, *137*
fracture(s) of, 124–140
  clinical examination in, 125, *126*
  effects of, on nerves and vessels, 127
  follow-up care in, 140
  and fracture of radius, complete, 129–130
    closed reduction in, techniques of, 130–132, *132, 133, 134*
    open reduction in, technique of, 132–133, *135*
  mechanism of, 124
  radiographic aids in, 126, *126*
  remodelling and, 126, *128*
  rotational deformity in, 124, *124*
  recognition of, 125–126, *126*
fracture dislocations of, 136–140
metaphysis of, fractures of, malalignment in, 124, *125*

Unconsciousness, problems associated with, 81–82
    in severe injuries, 67
Ureter, injury to, 77
Urethra, hemorrhage of, in genitourinary injuries, 75
    injury to, 77
Urethrogram, retrograde, in genitourinary injuries, 76, *75*
Urinary tract, of child, 74
    congenital anomalies of, and trauma, 74, *74*
Urogram, intravenous, in genitourinary injuries, 75–76
Urological investigation in severe injuries, 67–68
U-Slab, in fracture of humeral shaft, 90, *91*

Valgus deformity, in proximal metaphyseal fracture of tibia, 191–194, *190, 191*
    in supracondylar fracture of elbow, 103–104
Varus deformity, in ablation of perichondrial ring, 206, *206*

in fracture of tibia with intact fibula, 196, *192*
in supracondylar fracture of elbow, 103–104, *104*
Vascular damage, in elbow injury, 93
    fractures with, 28–35
        care of fracture in, 33
        management of, 30–34
        physical signs of, 28
        reconstruction of limb in, 34–35
        sites of, 29, *29*
    in penetrating chest injuries, 69
    in supracondylar fracture of elbow, 101
    in tibial fractures, 189–191, 197, *190*
Vein(s), damage to. *See* Vascular damage
    subclavian, compression of, in fracture of clavicle, 84
Vena cava, inferior, laceration of, treatment of, 71
Vertebra(ae), C1, lateral mass of, Jefferson's fracture of, 222
    subluxation or dislocation of, on C2, 222
    C2, fractures of, 223
    fracture(s) of, 221–223

or dislocation of, cord injury with, 217–218, 217t
Vital signs, charting of, in craniocerebral injury, 82
Volkmann's contracture, 20, 28
    in supracondylar fracture of elbow, 101
Volkmann's ischemia, 28, *29*

Waddell's triad of injuries, 41, *44*
Water deprivation, in severe head injuries, 82
Wet-lung, traumatic, 68
Whiplash injuries, 222
Wound(s). *See also* Laceration(s)
    abraded, 53–54
    puncture, of knee, 188, *187*
Wringer injuries, 54–58, *56, 57, 58*
Wringer injuries, growth arrest and, 149, *149*
Wrist, fracture(s) of, 141
    of, reduction in, 22
Z-plasty(ies), for skin closure in tidy laceration, 50
    for wound revision in hypertrophic scarring, 63, *63*